Novak's
Gynecology
Self-Assessment and Review

Second Edition

Novak's
Gynecology
Self-Assessment and Review

Second Edition

Editor

Jonathan S. Berek, MD, MMSc

Professor and Chair, College of Applied Anatomy
Executive Vice Chair, Department of Obstetrics and Gynecology
Chief of Gynecology, Division of Gynecologic Oncology
David Geffen School of Medicine at U.C.L.A.
Los Angeles, California

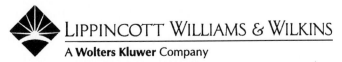

LIPPINCOTT WILLIAMS & WILKINS
A **Wolters Kluwer** Company

Philadelphia • Baltimore • New York • London
Buenos Aires • Hong Kong • Sydney • Tokyo

Acquisitions Editor: Lisa McAllister
Developmental Editor: Raymond E. Reter
Production Editor: Frank Aversa
Manufacturing Manager: Colin J. Warnock
Cover Designer: Christine Jenny
Compositor: TechBooks
Printer: Quebecor-World Dubuque

© **2003 by LIPPINCOTT WILLIAMS & WILKINS**
530 Walnut Street
Philadelphia, PA 19106 USA
LWW.com

Printed in the USA

Library of Congress Cataloging-in-Publication Data

Novak's gynecology self-assessment and review / [edited by] Jonathan S. Berek.—2nd ed.
    p. ; cm.
    Companion v. to: Novak's gynecology. 13th ed. 2002.
    Includes bibliographical references.
    ISBN 0-7817-3756-7
      1. Gynecology—Examinations, questions, etc. 2. Gynecology—Outlines, syllabi, etc.
    I. Title: Gynecology self-assessment and review. II. Berek, Jonathan S. III. Novak's
    gynecology.
      [DNLM: 1. Genital Diseases, Female–Examination Questions. 2. Gynecology—
    methods—Examination Questions. 3. Pregnancy
    Complications—Examination Questions. WP 100 N9351 2002 Suppl. 2003]
    RG111 .N68 2003
    618.1′0076—dc21
                                          2002069381

10 9 8 7 6 5 4 3 2 1

To my wife, Deborah,
whose love, patience, and support made this endeavor possible.

Preface

Novak's Gynecology has established a proud tradition, and I am pleased to offer this *Self-Assessment and Review* for the substantially updated thirteenth edition. The purpose of this book is to facilitate a careful review of the comprehensive information presented in the textbook.

The format is identical to the textbook, and several figures and tables are reproduced to assist the reader in a more detailed analysis of its key points. Each of the study guide's chapters presents questions derived from the subject matter in the corresponding chapter in the textbook, along with brief explanations of their answers and references to the source material in *Novak's Gynecology, 13th edition.*

My hope is that this companion study guide will enhance the usefulness of *Novak's Gynecology, 13th edition,* and encourage a better understanding and application of its principles.

Jonathan S. Berek, MD

Contributing Authors

Angeles Alvarez, MD

Associate Professor
Department of Obstetrics and Gynecology
Duke University Medical Center
Durham, North Carolina

Lawrence S. Amesse, MD, PhD

Assistant Professor
Department of Obstetrics and Gynecology
Wright State University
Associate Program Director
Miami Valley Hospital
Dayton, Ohio

Jean R. Anderson, MD

Associate Professor
Department of Gynecology and Obstetrics
The Johns Hopkins Medical Institutions
Baltimore, Maryland

Vicki V. Baker, MD

Professor
Department of Obstetrics and Gynecology
Division of Gynecologic Oncology
Wayne State University
Detroit, Michigan

David Allen Baram, MD

Clinical Assistant Professor
Department of Obstetrics and Gynecology
University of Minnesota School of Medicine
Minneapolis, Minnesota
Attending Physician
Regions Hospital
St. Paul, Minnesota

Jonathan S. Berek, MD, MMSc

Professor and Chair, College of Applied Anatomy
Executive Vice Chair, Department of Obstetrics and
    Gynecology
Chief of Gynecology and Division of Gynecologic
    Oncology
David Geffen School of Medicine at UCLA
Los Angeles, California

Ross S. Berkowitz, MD

William H. Baker Professor of Gynecology
Department of Obstetrics and Gynecology
Harvard Medical School
Director, Gynecology and Gynecologic Oncology
Brigham and Women's Hospital
Dana Farber Cancer Institute
Boston, Massachusetts

Andrew I. Brill, MD

Professor
Chief of General Obstetrics and Gynecology
Department of Obstetrics and Gyncology
University of Illinois at Chicago
Chicago, Illinois

Robert E. Bristow, MD

Assistant Professor
Department of Gynecology and Obstetrics
The Johns Hopkins Medical Institutions
Baltimore, Maryland

Joanna M. Cain, MD

Professor and Chair
Department of Obstetrics and Gynecology
Oregon Health and Science University
Portland, Oregon

Bum Chae Choi, MD

Center for Recurrent Miscarriage and Infertility
Creation and Love Women's Hospital
Gwangju, Korea

Daniel L. Clarke-Pearson, MD

James M. Ingram Professor and Director of Gynecologic
    Oncology
Department of Obstetrics and Gynecology
Duke University Medical Center
Durham, North Carolina

Daniel W. Cramer, MD, ScD

Professor
Department of Obstetrics and Gynecology
Harvard Medical School
Gynecologist
Brigham and Women's Hospital
Boston, Massachusetts

Dayton W. Daberkow, II, MD

Associate Professor of Medicine
Internal Medicine Residency Program Director
Louisiana State University Health Science Center
New Orleans, Louisiana

Thomas M. D'Hooghe, MD, PhD

Professor, Faculty of Medicine
Leuven University
Coordinator, Fertility Center
Leuven University
University Hospital Gasthuisberg
Leuven, Belgium

John C. Elkas, MD

Assistant Professor
Department of Obstetrics and Gynecology
Uniformed Services University of the Health Sciences
Bethesda, Maryland
Attending Physician
Department of Obstetrics and Gynecology
Walter Reed Army Medical Center
Washington, DC

Joseph C. Gambone, DO, MPH

Associate Professor
Department of Obstetrics and Gynecology
David Geffen School of Medicine at UCLA
Los Angeles, California

Rene Genadry, MD

Associate Professor
Department of Gynecology and Obstetrics
The Johns Hopkins Medical Institutions
Baltimore, Maryland

Armando E. Giuliano, MD

Chief of Surgical Oncology
John Wayne Cancer Institute
Clinical Professor, Department of Surgery
David Geffen School of Medicine at UCLA
Los Angeles, California
Director, Joyce Eisenberg Keefer Breast Center
Saint John's Hospital and Health Center
Santa Monica, California

Paul A. Gluck, MD

Associate Clinical Professor
Department of Obstetrics and Gynecology
University of Miami School of Medicine;
Attending Physician
Department of Obstetrics and Gynecology
Baptist Hospital of Miami
Miami, Florida

Donald Peter Goldstein, MD

Professor
Department of Obstetrics, Gynecology, and Reproductive
   Biology
Harvard Medical School
Senior Gynecologist
Department of Obstetrics and Gynecology
Brigham and Women's Hospital
Boston, Massachusetts

Baiba J. Grube, MD

Assistant Director, Joyce Eisenberg Keefer Breast Cancer
Department of Surgical Oncology
John Wayne Cancer Institute
Saint John's Health Center
Santa Monica, California

Laura J. Havrilesky, MD

Fellow, Department of Obstetrics, Gynecology, and
   Gynecologic Oncology
Duke University Medical Center
Durham, North Carolina

Avner Hershlag, MD

Associate Professor
Department of Obstetrics and Gynecology
New York University School of Medicine
New York, New York
Medical Director
Department of Obstetrics and Gynecology
North Shore University Hospital
Manhasset, New York

Joseph A. Hill, MD

Reproductive Endocrinologist
Fertility Center of New England
Reading, Massachusetts

Paula J. Adams Hillard, MD

Professor
Departments of Obstetrics and Gynecology,
   and Pediatrics
University of Cincinnati
Chief
Department of Gynecology
Cincinnati Children's Hospital
Cincinnati, Ohio

Christine H. Holschneider, MD

Clinical Instructor
Department of Obstetrics and Gynecology
David Geffen School of Medicine at UCLA
Los Angeles, California

William W. Hurd, MD

Nicolas J. Thompson Professor and Chairman
Department of Obstetrics and Gynecology
Wright State University School of Medicine
Dayton, Ohio

Julie A. Jolin, MD

Resident
Department of Gynecology and Obstetrics
The Johns Hopkins Medical Institutions
Baltimore, Maryland

Thomas C. Krivak, MD

Fellow, Gynecologic Oncology
Walter Reed Army Medical Center
Washington, DC

Johnathan Lancaster, MD

Associate, Department of Obstetrics and Gynecology
Duke University Medical Center
Durham, North Carolina

John R. Lurain, MD

John and Ruth Brewer Professor of Gynecology
   and Cancer Research
Head, Section of Gynecologic Oncology
Northwestern University Medical School
Chief, Gynecologic Oncology
Department of Obstetrics and Gynecology
Northwestern Memorial Hospital/Prentice Women's
   Hospital
Chicago, Illinois

Otoniel Martínez-Maza, PhD

Professor
Departments of Obstetrics and Gynecology, and
   Microbiology, Immunology, and Molecular Genetics
David Geffen School of Medicine at UCLA
Los Angeles, California

John W. McBroom, MD

Fellow, Gynecologic Oncology
Walter Reed Army Medical Center
Washington, DC

Howard D. McClamrock, MD

Associate Professor and Director
Department of Obstetrics, Gynecology, and Reproductive
   Sciences
Division of Reproductive Endocrinology and Infertility
University of Maryland
Baltimore, Maryland

Shawn A. Menefee, MD

Assistant Clinical Professor
Department of Reproductive Medicine
University of California, San Diego
Co-director, Section of Female Pelvic Medicine and
   Reconstructive Surgery
Department of Obstetrics and Gynecology
Kaiser Permanente
San Diego, California

Malcolm Gordon Munro, MD, FACOG, FRCS(C)

Professor
Department of Obstetrics and Gynecology
David Geffen School of Medicine at UCLA
Los Angeles, California

Thomas E. Nolan, MD, MBA

Professor
Departments of Obstetrics, Gynecology, and Medicine
Louisiana State University
Hospital Center Director
Department of Women's and Newborn Services
Medical Center of Louisiana
New Orleans, Louisiana

Dean T. Nora, MD

Fellow, Senior Surgical Oncology
John Wayne Cancer Institute
Santa Monica, California

David L. Olive, MD

Professor
Department of Obstetrics and Gynecology
Chief
Department of Reproductive Endocrinology and Infertility
University of Wisconsin–Madison School of Medicine
Madison, Wisconsin

Steven F. Palter, MD

Medical and Scientific Director
Reproductive Medicine and Surgery Center
Plainview, New York
Clinical Assistant Professor
Division of Reproductive Endocrinology and Infertility
Yale University School of Medicine
New Haven, Connecticut

C. Matthew Peterson, MD

Associate Professor
Division of Reproductive Endocrinology
Department of Obstetrics and Gynecology
University of Utah Medical Center
Director of Reproductive Endocrinology
LDS Hospital
Salt Lake City, Utah

John F. Randolph, Jr., MD

Associate Professor
Department of Obstetrics and Gynecology
University of Michigan
Ann Arbor, Michigan

Andrea J. Rapkin, MD

Professor
Department of Obstetrics and Gynecology
David Geffen School of Medicine at UCLA
Los Angeles, California

Robert W. Rebar, MD

Associate Executive Director
American Society for Reproductive Medicine
Birmingham, Alabama

Robert C. Reiter, MD

Vice President
Quality and Clinical Performance Improvement
ProMedica Health System
Toledo, Ohio

Wendy J. Schillings, MD

Clinical Associate Professor
Department of Obstetrics and Gynecology
Penn State College of Medicine
Hershey, Pennsylvania
Reproductive Endocrinology and Infertility Specialist
Department of Obstetrics and Gynecology
Lehigh Valley Health Network
Allentown, Pennsylvania

Daniel Joseph Schust, MD

Assistant Professor
Department of Obstetrics, Gynecology, and Reproductive
  Biology
Harvard Medical School
Associate Obstetrician and Gynecologist
Brigham and Women's Hospital
Boston, Massachusetts

David E. Soper, MD

Professor and Vice Chairman
Department of Obstetrics and Gynecology
Medical University of South Carolina
Charleston, South Carolina

Nada L. Stotland, MD, MPH

Professor
Department of Psychiatry and Obstetrics
  and Gynecology
Rush Medical College
Chicago, Illinois

Thomas G. Stovall, MD

Professor
Department of Obstetrics and Gynecology
University of Tennessee, Memphis
Memphis, Tennessee

Phillip G. Stubblefield, MD

Professor and Chairman
Department of Obstetrics and Gynecology
Boston University School of Medicine
Boston Medical Center
Boston, Massachusetts

L. Lewis Wall, MD, DPhil

Associate Professor
Section of Female Pelvic Medicine and Reconstructive
  Surgery
Department of Obstetrics and Gynecology
Washington University School of Medicine
St. Louis, Missouri

Mylene W. Yao, MD

Assistant Professor
Department of Obstetrics and Gynecology
Columbia University College of Physicians
  and Surgeons
New York, New York

Contents

Acknowledgments

I am grateful for the support I received from the publisher, especially Lisa McAllister, Raymond Reter, and Frank Aversa; from my excellent editorial assistant, Rebecca Rinehart; from my superb illustrator, Tim Hengst; from my hardworking manuscript processor, Sergio Huidor; and from my colleagues who contributed their time and effort to assist in the completion of this study guide.

PRINCIPLES
OF PRACTICE

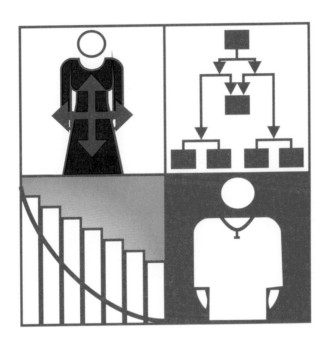

1

Initial Assessment and Communication

Paula A. Hillard
Jonathan S. Berek

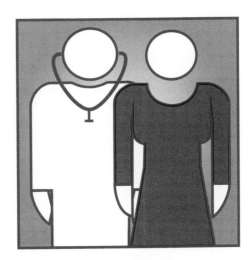

Learning Objectives

1. Be aware of the importance of communication in physician/patient interactions.

2. Recognize the value of open-ended questions in interviewing.

3. Be aware of the extent to which the patient's psychological reaction to her illness affects her responses.

4. Be able to describe and document the female genital examination for the medical record.

5. Be able to recognize and choose an appropriately sized vaginal speculum for individual patients.

Questions

1. A 30-year-old married woman comes to the office with the stated symptom of a vaginal discharge. During the interview, she appears anxious. She describes a yellow, malodorous discharge. Each of the following techniques would be helpful in determining the cause of her distress **except**

   A. Asking her what she fears may be the cause of her symptoms
   B. Allowing her to describe her symptoms without interruption
   C. Direct questioning about the possibility of sexually transmitted diseases
   D. Confronting her with suspicions about her sexual practices
   E. Asking her about associated psychological symptoms

2. Of the following techniques for communication with a patient, the physician should

   A. Listen more and talk less
   B. Interrupt the patient when she comes to the essential point in her history
   C. Provide a lecture to the patient on her disease
   D. Avoid open-ended questions

3. Of the following, which portion of the physical examination should be performed last:

   A. Uterine palpation
   B. Vulvar inspection
   C. Rectal examination
   D. Cervical inspection
   E. Abdominal palpation

4. A 42-year-old woman presents to the office with pelvic and abdominal pain, bloating, painful but regular menses, and weight loss. Each of the following is indicated during the physical examination **except**

   A. Pap smear
   B. Bimanual examination
   C. Rectovaginal examination
   D. Examination of stool for occult blood
   E. Endometrial biopsy

5. A 16-year-old girl presents to the emergency department with severe abdominal and pelvic pain. Her last menstrual period was 6 weeks ago, and a urine pregnancy test is positive. She states that she has been sexually active and that condoms were used inconsistently. She states that she has never had a pelvic examination. The most appropriate vaginal speculum for this patient would be

   A. Grave's extralong
   B. Grave's regular
   C. Pederson extralong
   D. Pederson regular
   E. Pediatric short speculum

Answers

1. **D**

   The art and techniques of obtaining a medical history vary with the patient, the type of problem with which she presents, and the physician's style. Techniques not conducive to appropriate communication between the physician and the patient, and which are generally best avoided, include behavior that is confrontational, combative, condescending, overbearing, or judgmental. Open-ended questions that allow the patient

to talk about her chief complaint are appropriate. After allowing her to describe the symptoms most bothersome to her, additional information can be obtained by direct questioning. This allows the clinician to formulate hypotheses that can be tested using additional questioning to formulate a differential diagnosis. A review of symptoms also may be helpful if the diagnosis does not seem obvious. The clinician should be aware of the influence of the patient's emotional state on her reaction to disease. Psychological factors or a psychiatric diagnosis may be complicating the presentation of illness. In addition, the patient may well have a different understanding, interpretation, or concern about her symptoms. It is often helpful to elicit that information.
Reference: Pages 4–6

2. A

In general, the physician needs to be a good listener. The physician needs to give the patient maximum opportunity to speak freely, avoiding interruptions, lectures, and soliloquies. It is advisable to ask open-ended questions to encourage maximum responses. The following are techniques to help achieve rapport with patients:

- Use positive language (e.g., agreement, approval, and humor).
- Build a partnership (e.g., acknowledge understanding, ask for opinions, paraphrase and interpret the patient's words).
- Ask rephrased questions.
- Give complete responses to the patient's questions.

Some general guidelines that help to improve communication follow:

- Listen more and talk less.
- Encourage the pursuit of topics introduced by and important to the patient.
- Minimize controlling speech habits such as interrupting, issuing commands, and lecturing.
- Seek out questions and provide full and understandable answers.
- Become aware of discomfort in an interview, recognize when it originates in an attempt by the physician to take control, and redirect that attempt.
- Assure patients that they have the opportunity to fully discuss their problem.
- Recognize when patients may be seeking empathy and validation of their feelings rather than a solution. Sometimes all that is necessary is to be a compassionate human being.

An interview that permits maximum transmission of information to the physician is best achieved by the following approach:

- Begin with an "open-ended" question.
- As the patient begins to speak, pay attention not only to her answers but also to her emotions and general body language.
- Extend a second question or comment, encouraging the patient to talk.
- Allow the patient to respond without interrupting, perhaps by using silence, nods, or small facilitative comments to encourage the patient to talk while the physician is listening.
- Summarize and express empathy and understanding at the completion of the interview.

Attentiveness, rapport, and collaboration characterize good medical interviewing techniques. Open-ended questions are generally desirable, particularly when coupled with good listening skills.
Reference: Pages 6–10

3. C

Typically, the abdominal examination should be done prior to the pelvic examination. The rectal examination should be performed after the direct examination and should be performed in premenopausal women as needed to assist the examiner in the assessment of the pelvic structures; when there is a suspicion of colorectal pathology (e.g., when

appendicitis has been excluded, or the patient complains of passing blood per rectum); and routinely in postmenopausal women.
Reference: Pages 12–17

4. E

The patient described could have a number of gynecologic problems, including ovarian or cervical cancer. The possibility of rectal disease or a gastrointestinal malignancy should also be kept in mind. The examination is designed to evaluate these possible causes of her symptoms. Screening for cervical cancer with a Pap smear and for colon cancer using a test for occult blood in the stool are both appropriate tests. A rectovaginal examination or a rectal exam alone is indicated given these symptoms. An endometrial biopsy is not indicated, given that the patient describes only dysmenorrhea, without menstrual abnormalities.
Reference: Pages 13–18

5. D (see Fig. 1.2)

The choice of an appropriate vaginal speculum can make the difference between an examination that is painful for the patient and thus relatively unrevealing, and an exam that is uncomfortable, yet tolerable, which allows valuable information to be gained. In general, the smallest speculum necessary to produce adequate visualization should be used. The speculum should be warmed (on a heating pad or with warm water) prior to insertion. The most appropriate speculum for *most* individuals during a routine examination is the Pederson speculum. Sexually active adult women may require a Grave's speculum if the vagina is particularly redundant or cervical procedures are indicated. A long speculum is rarely required, but may be indicated if the woman's buttocks preclude sufficient depth of insertion. The first pelvic examination for an adolescent is typically an anxiety-provoking experience. Most young women, even those who have not been sexually active, can tolerate an examination with the Pederson speculum. Some young women who are virginal may require a Huffman speculum (also called the narrow or virginal speculum) if the hymenal ring is tight. The so-called "pediatric" speculum, a short speculum, is almost never indicated in prepubertal girls for an examination in the office, but may occasionally be required for an examination under anesthesia. Its short length is inadequate to allow visualization of the cervix in menarchal women, and thus should not be used.
Reference: Pages 16–17

Figure 1.2 Vaginal specula. Grave's extralong (**1**), Grave's regular (**2**), Pederson extralong (**3**), Pederson regular (**4**), Huffman "virginal" (**5**), pediatric regular (**6**), and pediatric narrow (**7**).

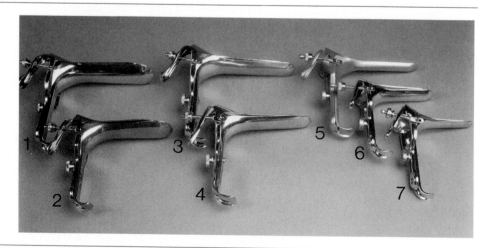

2 Principles of Patient Care

Joanna M. Cain

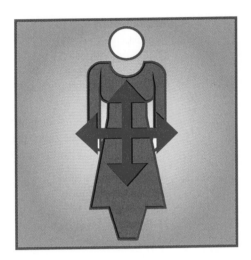

Learning Objectives

1. Know the concepts for use of ethical principles to assist in decision-making.

2. Understand the purpose of confidentiality and informed consent.

3. Be able to identify and deal with conflicts of interest.

4. Understand the concept of just allocation in the provision of health care.

Questions

1. A patient presents to her physician's office for human immunodeficiency virus (HIV) testing, but is concerned that the information resulting from the test could be damaging to her career if released. The ethical principle that supports confidentiality in this example is

   A. Autonomy
   B. Justice
   C. Double-effect
   D. Nonmaleficence
   E. Beneficence

2. An interactive discussion in which one participant has greater knowledge about medical information and the other participant has greater knowledge about that individual's value system and circumstances affected by the information is termed

   A. Informed consent
   B. Patient autonomy
   C. Paternalism
   D. Information allocation

3. A patient with severe pelvic pain presents to your office after seven prior surgeries in the previous 2 years. You assess her situation, review her records, examine her, and conclude that her best option is to begin medical therapy and that surgery has no role in her future care. She refuses and demands surgery immediately. Your ethical obligation is to

   A. Operate on the patient
   B. Insist upon medical therapy
   C. Offer medical therapy, but refuse to operate
   D. Have the situation arbitrated by a third party

4. The effect of therapy on the patient's experience of living, based on her perspective, is called

   A. Experiential care
   B. Quality of life (QOL)
   C. Patient-based outcome assessment
   D. Intervention efficacy

5. A local physician owns partial interest in an in-house magnetic resonance imaging (MRI) scanner. He sees a patient with multiple leiomyomata desiring conservative surgery. He believes that to perform optimal surgery, MRI assessment of the exact size and location of the tumors is required prior to the procedure. There is no state law that addresses the appropriate actions of the physician in this setting. His most appropriate course of action to avoid conflict of interest is

   A. Avoid the MRI and proceed directly to surgery.
   B. Perform the MRI at the local scanner, but inform the patient of the partial interest.
   C. Perform an alternative imaging study, such as ultrasound.
   D. Send the patient to an MRI scanner in another location.

6. The fair and equitable distribution of the burdens and benefits of health care delivery is termed

   A. Justice
   B. Nonmaleficence
   C. Fiduciary interest
   D. Beneficence

Answers

The practice of gynecology, as true for all aspects of medicine, is based on ethical principles that guide patient care. These principles and concepts create a framework for ethical decision making that applies to all aspects of practice:

- Autonomy: A person's right to self-rule, to establish personal norms of conduct, and to choose a course of action based on a set of personal values and principles derived from them.
- Beneficence: The obligation to promote the well-being of others, to achieve a goal of medicine.
- Confidentiality: A person's right to decide how and to whom personal medical information will be communicated.
- Covenant: A binding agreement between two or more parties for the performance of some action.
- Fiduciary Relationship: A relationship founded on faith and trust.
- Informed Consent: The patient's acceptance of a medical intervention after adequate disclosure of the nature of the procedure, its risks and benefits, and alternatives.
- Justice: The right of individuals to claim what is due them based on certain personal properties or characteristics.
- Nonmaleficence: The obligation to avoid harm while offering interventions.

1. D

Confidentiality is an expression of the trust or covenantal relationship between physician and patient. The patient seeking assistance from a health professional has the right to be assured that the information exchanged during the interaction is private. This assures that no harm occurs while a beneficence test is being performed. The right to privacy prohibits a physician from revealing information regarding the patient unless the patient waives that privilege. The only exceptions to this principle are when this right impinges on the legal and ethical rights of institutions and society at large, or if so declared by legislation.
Reference: Page 22

2. A

Informed consent is a process that involves an exchange of information directed toward reaching mutual understanding and informed decision making. Ideally, informed consent should be the practical manifestation of respect for patient preferences (autonomy). In essence, informed consent is a conversation between physician and patient that teaches the patient about the medical condition, explores her values, and informs her about the reasonable medical alternatives.
Reference: Page 23

3. C

Autonomy, the patient's right to choose to receive or refuse medical care, is an important ethical principle. However, it is **not** respect for a patient's wishes regardless of good medical judgment. The physician's ethical obligation is to seek the best for the patient's care (beneficence) and avoid harm (nonmaleficence) of surgery, even if that is what the patient wants. Physicians are not obligated to offer treatment they believe to be of no benefit to the patient. The patient does, however, have the right to refuse treatment if it does not conform with her values. Thus, the patient can refuse medical therapy, but she has no right to demand any treatment she wishes.
Reference: Pages 24–25

4. B

QOL is a much-used but often-unclear term. Basically, it refers to assessing the results of treatment intervention from the patient's perspective, not that of the physician, family members, or other interested parties. It is perilous and wholly speculative to assume that physicians know what QOL represents for a particular patient. Often, the patient may bring a host of modifying feelings, attitudes, and desires to any decision-making or evaluative process—factors known or understood only by the patient herself.

Controversy exists regarding whether currently available QOL measurement systems will provide information to help patients make decisions. Informing patients of others' experiences with alternative treatments may help in their decision making, but this is never a substitute for individual patient decision making.
Reference: Pages 25–26

5. B

The reality of care in the 2000's is that health care givers must make many decisions under the pressure of multiple conflicts of interest. Physicians are continually caught between self-interest and professional integrity. Focusing clearly on meeting the patient's best interest and responsibly rejecting choices that compromise the patient's needs are ethical requirements. Frequently, state law will address physician behavior in these situations. However, in the absence of such directive, it is still ethically necessary for financial conflicts of interest to be revealed to patients.
Reference: Pages 26–27

6. A

Justice is the right of individuals to claim what is due them based on certain personal properties or characteristics. However, distributing benefits in an equitable manner is a matter of great debate. There are various methods of proposed distribution:

- Equal shares (everyone has the same number of health care dollars per year).
- Need (only those people who need health care get the dollars).
- Queuing (the first in line for a transplant gets it).
- Merit (those with more serious illnesses receive special benefits).
- Contribution (those who have paid more into their health care fund get more health care).

Each may be just in some situations, but each will affect an individual patient in a different way. The principle of justice applies when a resource is desired or beneficial and to some extent scarce. With scarce resources, the overall benefits for all patients are considered in conjunction with the individual benefits for one patient. These decisions are frequently among the most difficult in health care delivery.
Reference: Pages 28–29

3

Quality Assessment and Improvement

Joseph C. Gambone
Robert C. Reiter
Paul A. Gluck

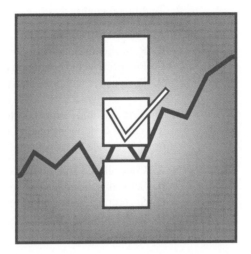

Learning Objectives

1. Understand the concepts of quality assurance, quality management, and patient safety.

2. Be able to enumerate the principles of quality assessment for health care.

3. Understand the principles of outcomes assessment, including quality-of-life measurement.

4. Be aware of the mechanisms for quality improvement and patient safety.

Questions

1. The annual United States health care expenditure of more than 14% of gross domestic product (GDP) is:

   A. About the same as other industrialized countries
   B. Less than other countries because of decreased access to care in the United States
   C. Higher than most but with much better outcomes
   D. Higher than any other country with lower overall outcomes

2. Traditional quality assurance (QA) compared to quality improvement (QI) is:

   A. Prospective and periodic rather than retrospective and continuous
   B. Retrospective and periodic rather than prospective and continuous
   C. Prospective and continuous rather than retrospective and periodic
   D. Prospective and preventative rather than retrospective and self-imposed

3. The first essential element or step to establish a QI process in any organization, whether it is called continuous quality improvement (CQI), total quality management (TQM), or performance improvement (PI) is:

   A. Controlling variation by using scientific methods
   B. Selecting strong leaders and putting them totally in charge
   C. Spending a great deal of money
   D. Understanding the customer(s) and incorporating this knowledge into the system

4. The terms efficacy, effectiveness, and efficiency are similar but differ importantly in the following way:

   A. Working under ideal conditions versus working under ordinary practice conditions versus representing the best value
   B. Working under ordinary practice conditions versus the best value versus working under ideal conditions
   C. The best value versus working under ideal conditions versus working under ordinary practice conditions
   D. Best practice versus best outcomes versus best value

5. Optimally effective health care is most closely related to

   A. Effectiveness
   B. Value
   C. Efficiency
   D. Efficacy

6. Improvement in health-related quality of life is primarily determined by

   A. The process of care, or how the care is delivered
   B. The structure of care, or the quality of the people and equipment
   C. The outcomes of care, or how the patient actually is helped
   D. All of the above

7. Variation or differences in the way that medical or surgical care is delivered:

   A. Should be totally eliminated
   B. Is always appropriate and represents the "art of medicine"
   C. Should be controlled in a way that allows for desirable variation due to patient differences
   D. Is due to financial considerations

8. Studying the variation in resources used (procedures and tests) in women's health care can help improve health care services by:

   A. Identifying overutilization and waste
   B. Identifying underutilization and lack of access to care
   C. Identifying uncertainty and the need for outcomes research
   D. All of the above

9. The PDCA cycle is a quality improvement tool that is used to test small-scale change. The acronym stands for

   A. Plan, Do, Control, and Advance
   B. Process, Do, Check, and Adjust
   C. Plan, Do, Check, and Act
   D. Process, Direct, Control, and Adjust

10. The basic "essential" element(s) of adequate informed consent are

    A. Risks and benefits
    B. Risks and alternatives
    C. Rationale, risks, benefits, and alternatives
    D. A thorough discussion of risks and complications

11. Effective patient safety initiatives are

    A. Designed to eliminate substandard providers.
    B. Multidisciplinary, nonpunitive, and focused on individual providers.
    C. Multidisciplinary, punitive, and focused on bad processes.
    D. Multidisciplinary, nonpunitive, and focused on system deficiencies.

Answers

1. **D**

   Overall health care spending in the United States has exceeded 14% of GDP since the early 1990's. This percent of gross domestic spending has been rising since health care spending statistics were first calculated in the early 1960's, when only 6% of gross domestic product was spent for health care goods and services. Figure 3.1 shows the dramatic drop in out-of-pocket expenditures as compared to those monies that are spent by governments, including federal, state, and local, and by insurance companies. No other country in the world spends as much of their GDP on health care. Despite this, the United States has overall health outcomes, such as longevity and perinatal and neonatal mortality rates, that are less than other industrialized countries including the United Kingdom, Japan, and Canada where health care spending is significantly less.
   Reference: Pages 33–34

2. **B**

   The traditional methods for assessing and improving quality in health services has tended to be self-imposed and retrospective and takes the form of peer review. Studies indicate that this methodology is not very effective at bringing about improvements in the way that health care is delivered. Health services investigators believe that this retrospective and periodic method of review, with its emphasis on finding "bad apples," is less effective than a process that is designed to be prospective and continuous. This methodology emphasizes that periodic review leads to only periodic improvement, and in order for systems such as health care services to continually improve, the process for quality review must be continuous. Figure 3.2 illustrates how QA or quality assurance is designed to deal with the small percentage of substandard care which is represented on the left side of the figure. Sanctions are used to attempt to eliminate this kind of care. CQI, on the other hand, attempts to shift the level of care to the right by examining in a

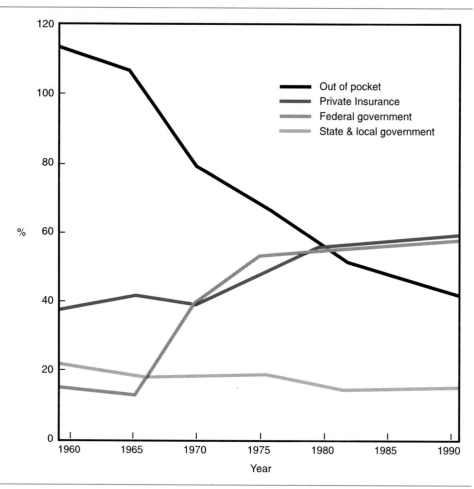

Figure 3.1 Sources of spending in U.S. health care, 1960–1990. Note that third-party payment had steadily replaced direct payment during this interval. (From U.S. Congressional Budget Office, 1992).

non-punitive fashion the processes of care. Traditional QA is retrospective and periodic rather than prospective and continuous.
Reference: Pages 34–36

3. D

Proponents of modern quality management recognize that in order to improve the quality of goods and services, the providers of these products must have a thorough understanding of who their customers are and how these customers view the goods or services in terms of quality and value. The presence of strong leadership and controlling variation using scientific methods, however, are important as a first step.
Reference: Pages 34–36

4. A

Knowing how well health care interventions really work is an essential element for quality assessment and quality improvement. Unfortunately, measurements of the success of health care interventions have tended to be based upon more theoretical or "off-line" measurements of true effectiveness. The Institute of Medicine (IOM), along with a number of other organizations and agencies, has defined theoretical effectiveness, or efficacy of a health care intervention, as how it works under ideal conditions that usually exist in traditional clinical trials. Effectiveness, on the other hand, indicates the measurement of how interventions work under ordinary every day clinical practice. A third term, efficiency, is similar to both efficacy and effectiveness; however, efficiency indicates the

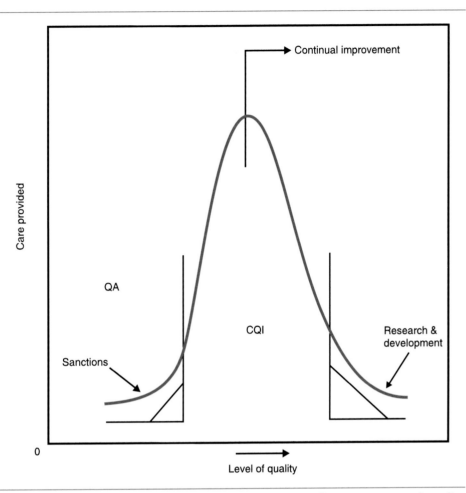

Figure 3.2   The hypothetical relationship between quality assurance and quality improvement.

measurement of effectiveness with the least waste in terms of cost and complications. In other words, efficiency indicates the best value in a given health care intervention.
Reference: Page 36

5. B

Donabedian has differentiated between optimally effective additions to health care and maximally effective additions to that care. Figure 3.3 identifies a "Point A" where the additional benefits for a health care intervention begin to level off or even decrease at a time when costs continue to increase at a greater rate. In the bottom panel, considering costs along with benefits results in a curve that begins to decrease further to "Point B." Point B identifies maximal benefits, but does not consider the proportionately higher addition of costs and, therefore, does not identify the optimally effective level or the level of greatest value.
Reference: Pages 36–37

6. C

The consumers of health care services—patients and potential patients—are increasingly more concerned about health-related quality of life and how it is affected or improved by health care services. Donabedian's model for assessing the quality of health care involves evaluating the structure of care (i.e., the resources, equipment, and people who provide the care), the process of care (i.e., the method by which a health care procedure or treatment is carried out), and, finally, the outcomes of care, which include both short-term adverse events such as complications and side effects as well as the

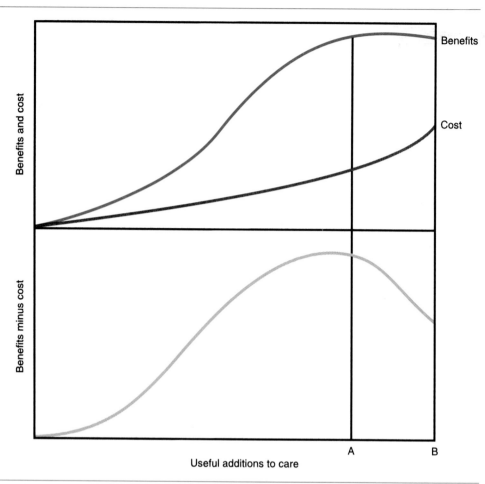

Figure 3.3   The "optimal" versus the "maximal" benefits and costs of medical treatments. *On the top panel,* the benefits to health and the costs of care are plotted. *On the bottom panel,* the cost is subtracted from the benefits, illustrating that after a certain point, additions of care may detract from the benefits. (From **Donabedian A.** The quality of care: how can it be assessed. *JAMA* 1988;260:1743, with permission.)

longer term outcomes of health and functional status and health-related quality of life. Improvement, therefore, in health-related quality of life and functional status is most related to outcomes of care or how a patient is actually helped by a procedure or treatment.
Reference: Pages 37–38

7. **C**

Variation is present in every aspect of life, including health care processes. Also, variation may be either desirable or undesirable. Examples of undesirable variation in health care would be allowing for individual provider preferences for medication, suture materials, catheters, and other equipment without scientifically based reasons for these expensive variations; or allowing for significant variation in the technique or the equipment used during a procedure, resulting in more time and expense, without evidence of improved patient outcomes. It is important to reduce undesirable variation in order to increase efficiency, while at the same time preserving desirable or intended variation that is needed to account for legitimate patient differences and preferences and to allow for innovation in health care technology.
Reference: Pages 40–42

8. **D**

The scientific study of variation in utilization rates allows clinicians to identify both over- and underutilization of health care services including health care procedures such as hysterectomy and cesarean delivery. Variation in utilization of health care services can be categorized as follows:

- Necessary and intended variation due to well-recognized patient differences such as severity of illness, comorbidity, and legitimate patient preferences.
- Acceptable but reducible variation because of uncertainty and lack of accurate information about outcomes.
- Unacceptable variation because of nonclinical factors such as habitual differences in practice style that are not grounded in knowledge or reason.

The identification of variation can identify over- and underutilization of health care services.

Reference: Pages 40–42

9. C

One model for scientifically testing changes in health care improvement, also used in other industries, is the PDCA cycle, which stands for Plan, Do, Check, and Act. "Do" means to implement the plan or process and collect the data. "Check" means to check the data to determine if the change to the process represents an improvement; and "Act" means to incorporate the change into the process if it is found to be an improvement. Another cycle with a different change is initiated if an improvement was not measured in the first cycle.

Reference: Pages 42–43

10. C

The process of informed consent evolved in the United States largely because of medical-legal liability that arose secondary to failure to properly inform patients before treatment, in particular, surgical procedures. Recent research has indicated that even the four basic or essential elements for adequate informed consent are not always covered during the informed consent process. Results from the study illustrated that rationale was covered only 43% of the time, a discussion of the benefits only 34% of the time, a discussion of the risks only 14% of the time, and alternatives, 12% of the time. Because clinical outcomes have been shown to improve with more participation of the patient in both decision-making and the delivery of care, researchers are now suggesting a process of informed collaborative choice. One model to accomplish this is the PREPARED checklist.

Procedure:	The course of action being considered
Reason:	The indication or rationale
Expectation:	The chances of benefit and failure
Preferences:	Patient-centered priorities (utilities) affecting choice
Alternatives:	Other reasonable options
Risks:	The potential for harm from procedures
Expenses:	All direct and indirect costs
Decision:	Fully informed collaborative choice

This sequenced checklist has been shown to improve health care decision-making by increasing patient satisfaction and self-efficacy and, therefore, facilitating more appropriate patient choice.

Reference: Pages 42–43

11. D

The most effective patient safety programs are modeled after aviation safety initiatives, which have been highly effective over the years. Individuals are encouraged to report system errors and problems with solutions for any problem emphasizing corrections to the process by understanding how "teams" of individuals can improve performance.

Reference: Pages 44–46

4

Epidemiology for the Gynecologist

Daniel W. Cramer

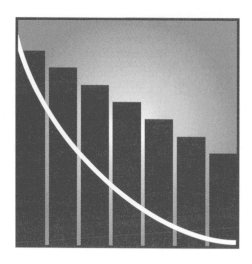

Learning Objectives

1. Be able to distinguish a descriptive study, a nonexperimental study, and an experimental analytic study.

2. Know the difference between incidence and prevalence.

3. Know the difference between a case-control and a cohort study.

4. Be able to define the measures of validity for a screening test including sensitivity and specificity.

5. Know what information is conveyed by a "*P* value" and a "confidence interval" and the principal types of statistical biases that may affect analytic studies.

6. Gain an appreciation of key exposures that can affect women's health.

7. Gain an appreciation of the principal cancers and other causes of death that occur in women of various age groups.

8. Gain an appreciation of the frequency of key benign gynecologic conditions such as endometriosis, fibroids, ovarian cysts, and pelvic inflammatory disease (PID).

Questions

1. An important association established through case reports, without etiologic studies like case-control or cohort ever being performed, includes

   A. Thalidomide and limb reduction birth defects
   B. The Dalkon shield intrauterine device (IUD) and septic abortion
   C. Sequential oral contraceptives and endometrial cancer in young women
   D. All of the above

2. An example of an incidence rate would be:

   A. The percentage of occult breast cancers found at autopsy
   B. The percentage of women still alive in 5 years after a diagnosis of ovarian cancer
   C. The number of women who develop endometrial cancer during a 1-year period divided by the estimated total population of women
   D. All of the above

3. A cohort study is distinguished from a case-control study in all of the following ways **except:**

   A. It can yield attributable risk
   B. Is less susceptible to selection bias
   C. Is always prospective
   D. Is usually more costly and difficult to conduct

4. A case-control study

   A. Begins with cases who have had a particular exposure and controls who have not
   B. Yields a term called the *exposure odds ratio* that is equivalent to attributable risk
   C. Is best for examining a relatively rare exposure and relatively common disease
   D. May be affected by recall bias

5. What is the purpose of randomization in a clinical trial?

   A. To minimize bias in selecting the overall target population
   B. To ensure an equal distribution of known and unknown confounders between treatment groups
   C. To ensure blindness in observing outcomes between treatment groups
   D. All of the above

6. The sensitivity of a diagnostic test is defined as:

   A. The number with a true-positive screening result out of all those who have the disease
   B. The number with a true-negative screening result out of all those who do not have the disease
   C. The number of true-positive results out of all those screened with positive results
   D. The number of true-negative results out of all those screened with negative results

7. A tendency for cases included in a particular study to have a different profile of exposures than the entire pool of potential cases would be an example of what type of bias:

   A. Information bias
   B. Selection bias
   C. Confounding
   D. Misclassification

8. If a relative risk of 1.5 is found in a study investigating a particular exposure and a particular disease is found, this means

   A. For every 100 women exposed, there were 1.5 additional diseased cases.
   B. The diseased women were 50% more likely to have the exposure than nondiseased women
   C. Exposed women were 50% more likely to develop disease than nonexposed women
   D. The association is significant

9. As applied to epidemiologic studies such as case-control, multivariate analysis is used

   A. To be certain the study is free of bias
   B. To minimize the effect of recall bias
   C. To control for known potential confounders
   D. All of the above

10. The process of pooling data from a number of separate studies addressing the same association in order to calculate a common measure of an association is called

   A. Conducting a metaanalysis
   B. Calculating a confidence interval
   C. Assessing biologic credibility
   D. Performing a stratified analysis

11. All of the following are appreciated risks (or benefits) of oral contraceptive use **except:**

   A. A decreased risk of ovarian cancer
   B. An increased risk for myocardial infarction in older users who smoked
   C. A decreased risk for benign breast disease
   D. An increased risk for pituitary adenomas

12. Which of the following statement about mortality in U.S. women is incorrect?

   A. Heart disease is the leading cause of death overall.
   B. Accidents are the leading cause of death in women aged 1 through 14 years.
   C. Cancer is the leading cause of death in women aged 20 to 39 years.
   D. Cancer is the leading cause of death in women aged 40 to 59 years.

13. The most common cause of hospitalization for women aged 15 to 44 years in the United States is

   A. Fibroids
   B. Endometriosis
   C. PID
   D. Cervical neoplasia

14. Which of the following statements about cancer in women in the United States is incorrect?

   A. The leading cause of cancer death is breast cancer.
   B. Endometrial cancer has a higher incidence than ovarian cancer.
   C. Ovarian cancer accounts for more deaths than endometrial cancer.
   D. Colon cancer is the third leading cause of cancer deaths.

Answers

1. D

Clinicians can make important public health contributions even if they may not be able to conduct expensive and complicated epidemiologic studies. All of these

associations were established through well-described case reports prepared by observant clinicians.
Reference: Page 50

2. C

The term *incidence* refers to the rate of occurrence of new cases of diseases or conditions over a specific time interval. The others would be examples of prevalence or simple frequency.
Reference: Page 51

3. C

A retrospective cohort study is possible when individuals who did or did not have a particular exposure are identified from medical record many years back and those (or other) records are traced to see who had a particular outcome.
Reference: Pages 51–54

4. D

A potential bias in most case-control studies is that the cases are more likely to recall or admit to a particular exposure than controls. Independent assessment of the exposure would be the ideal way to handle this potential bias but is often not possible.
Reference: Pages 51–54

5. B

The purpose of randomization is to ensure an equal distribution of known and unknown confounders between treatment groups. Randomization does not insure that the investigator has selected an appropriate study group or that there will be no bias in observing results (unless the trial is also double-blinded).
Reference: Pages 54–56

6. A

Sensitivity is the number with a true-positive screening result out of all those who have the disease. The remaining proportions (in order) define specificity, predictive value of a positive test, and predictive value of a negative test.
Reference: Page 55

7. B

A selection bias may occur when cases (or controls) selected for study differs substantially from the larger population of potential cases or control. A possible example may include the tendency for women with leg pains who are using oral contraceptives to be more likely to receive a diagnosis of a deep vein thrombosis than women with comparable symptoms who are not using oral contraceptives.
Reference: Page 56

8. C

Relative risk is defined as the risk for disease in exposed relative to risk for disease in nonexposed.
Reference: Page 53

9. C

A confounder is a variable like age or socioeconomic status that is associated with both the exposure and the illness. Multivariate analysis is a technique that "adjusts" for a number of potential confounders. It would not ensure that the study is free of all biases, especially selection or recall bias.
Reference: Page 56

10. A

Metaanalysis is the process of combining results from several independent studies examining the same exposure (or treatment) and same outcome in order to achieve

greater statistical power in examining an association. A metaanalysis is conducted by assembling measures of an association from different studies, like relative risks, weighting each by the variance of the measure, and taking an overall average.
Reference: Pages 56–57

11. D

There is good evidence to suggest all of these risks and benefits related to the use of oral contraceptives except pituitary adenomas.
Reference: Page 57

12. C

Accidents, suicides, and homicides account for almost twice as many deaths as cancer does in the 20 to 39 age group. Gynecologists should assess use of seat belts and risk for domestic violence in this age group.
Reference: Page 59

13. C

Based on data collected by the National Hospital Discharge Survey for 1988 to 1990 and by the Division of Reproductive Health of the Centers for Disease Control and Prevention, PID is the most frequent discharge diagnosis, with nearly 300,000 women hospitalized annually.
Reference: Page 62

14. A

Lung cancer is now the leading cause of cancer death in women, thus, emphasizing the importance that gynecologists encourage smoking cessation in women.
Reference: Pages 59–60

BASIC SCIENCE

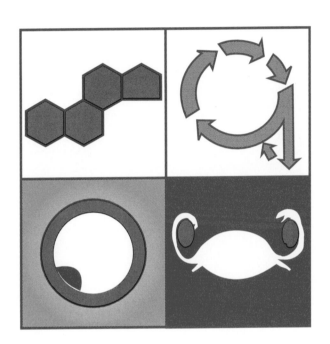

5 Anatomy and Embryology

Jean R. Anderson
Rene Genadry

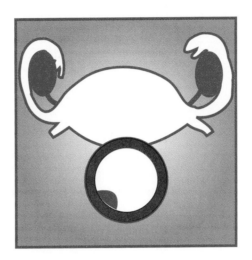

Learning Objectives

1. Be able to identify the bony structures, muscles, blood vessels, lymphatics, nerves and viscera of the pelvis.

2. Understand the special characteristics of the pelvic vascular system:

   A. Anatomic variation in branching patterns
   B. Extensive collateral connections
   C. Expansive capabilities

3. Understand the embryologic development of the pelvic viscera.

4. Know the anatomy of the anterior abdominal wall.

5. Understand the development of the urinary tract.

6. Know the anatomy of the perineum and pelvic floor.

7. Be able to identify the retroperitoneal spaces.

8. Know the complete course of the ureter, including its relationship to other important anatomic structures.

Questions

1. The ischial spine is an anatomic landmark for which of the following?

    A. Pudendal nerve block
    B. Sacrospinous ligament vaginal suspension
    C. Determination of level of fetal descent
    D. All of the above

2. A 60-year-old woman with a lateral paravaginal defect undergoes abdominal repair. During the course of the procedure, there is sudden profuse bleeding from the operative field. Which of the following vessels is most likely to have been injured?

    A. Inferior gluteal artery
    B. Obturator artery
    C. Internal pudendal artery
    D. Vaginal artery
    E. Uterine artery

3. Major components for support of the pelvic floor include which of the following?

    A. Pelvic diaphragm
    B. Endopelvic fascia
    C. Urogenital diaphragm
    D. Perineal body
    E. Parietal component of transversalis fascia
    F. All of the above

4. Which of the following statements about the pelvic vasculature is not true?

    A. The pelvic vessels play an important role in pelvic support.
    B. Branches of the internal iliac arteries can always be identified by the order in which they divide from the parent vessel.
    C. The pelvic vasculature has the ability to significantly expand volume and flow during pregnancy.
    D. There is continued pelvic perfusion after ligation of both internal iliac (hypogastric) arteries because of the extensive collateral blood supply.

5. During placement of a lateral laparascopic port, the surgeon visualizes the medial umbilical fold. What vascular structure lies approximately 1.5 cm medially that is vulnerable to injury with trocar insertion?

    A. Inferior epigastric artery
    B. Obturator artery
    C. Uterine artery
    D. Superior epigastric artery
    E. None of the above

6. A 25-year-old nulliparous woman with intractable pain in the lower midabdomen. Laparoscopic evaluation demonstrates severe endometriosis. Transection of the presacral nerve is advised; during the course of the operation, there is profuse bleeding from the operative field. The most likely vessel injured is the

    A. Inferior mesenteric artery
    B. Iliolumbar artery
    C. Lateral sacral artery
    D. Middle sacral artery
    E. Obturator artery

7. A 72-year-old woman is found to have invasive vulvar carcinoma. Inguinal lymph node dissection reveals two positive nodes. If there has been further lymphatic dissemination of tumor, which lymph node group would next be involved?

    A. Paraaortic
    B. Obturator
    C. External iliac
    D. Parauterine
    E. Internal iliac

8. A 30-year-old woman complains of numbness in her upper lateral thigh region after undergoing prolonged pelvic surgery. The most likely cause of her symptoms is injury to the

    A. Lateral femoral cutaneous nerve
    B. Obturator nerve
    C. Femoral nerve
    D. Ilioinguinal nerve
    E. Genitofemoral nerve

9. During embryonic life, the absence of antimülerian hormone results in

    A. Regression of the paramesonephric duct system
    B. Differentiation of the medullary region of the gonad into Sertoli cells
    C. Development of the mesonephric duct system
    D. Development of the paramesonephric duct system
    E. Descent of the ovaries

10. In the female embryo, the structure destined to become the clitoris is known as

    A. Genital tubercle
    B. Urogenital fold
    C. Labioscrotal swelling
    D. Urogenital sinus
    E. Cloaca

11. A dilatation and curettage is performed on a 46-year-old woman with abnormal uterine bleeding. Laparoscopy is performed because of persistent bleeding and suspected perforation. Perforation is noted in the anterior mid uterine corpus and is managed conservatively. The most likely uterine position predisposing to perforation in this location is

    A. Midposition
    B. Anteflexed
    C. Retroflexed
    D. Anteverted

12. A 32-year-old woman is undergoing oophorectomy because of a large, right-sided complex ovarian mass, believed to be an endometrioma. The ureter is found to be densely adherent to the mass. In preparing to dissect the ureter from the mass, the surgeon identifies the ureter proximal to the ovary. Which of the following best describes the position of the ureter as it enters the pelvis?

    A. Crosses the common iliac vessels at their bifurcation, just medial to the ovarian vessels
    B. Crosses the hypogastric (internal iliac) artery just proximal to the bifurcation of the obturator artery
    C. Crosses the common iliac vessels at their bifurcation, lateral to the ovarian vessels

D. Crosses the hypogastric artery at the level of the bifurcation of the posterior division

E. Crosses the hypogastric artery medial to the bifurcation of the uterine artery

Answers

1. D

The ischial spine is the point of fixation for the sacrospinous ligament. The pudendal nerve and internal pudendal vessels lie posterior to the sacrospinous ligament at its attachment at the ischial spine. The sacrospinous ligament is often used for vaginal suspension and the ischial spine is the landmark used in the performance of this procedure. Because of the proximity of the pudendal nerve, palpation of the ischial spine is also used to place pudendal nerve blocks. Palpation of the ischial spine is used during labor to assess progression of fetal descent.
Reference: Page 71

2. B

During dissection of the paravesical space to reach the lateral vaginal attachments to the arcus tendineus, the obturator vessels are vulnerable to injury as they course along the lateral pelvic sidewall to exit the pelvis through the obturator foramen. The inferior gluteal and internal pudendal arteries are vulnerable to injury during sacrospinous vaginal suspension.
Reference: Pages 77–82

3. F

For its support, the pelvic floor relies on the complementary role of the pelvic diaphragm and its fascia resting on the perineal fibromuscular complex, composed of the urogenital diaphragm anteriorly and the perineal body joined to the anococcygeal raphe by the external anal sphincter posteriorly. The fascia of the pelvic diaphragm is a continuation of the transversalis fascia and includes a parietal component and a visceral component (the endopelvic fascia); together these invest the pelvic organs and form ligaments and septa, which reinforce and help fixate the pelvic floor.
Reference: Pages 72–73

4. B

There is significant anatomic variation between individuals in the branching pattern of the internal iliac vessels. There is no constant order in which branches divide from the parent vessel and some branches may arise as common trunks or may spring from other branches rather than from the internal iliac. Occasionally a branch may arise from another vessel entirely. This variation may also be found in the branches of other major vessels. The pelvic surgeon must be prepared for deviations from "textbook" vascular patterns.
Reference: Pages 77–82

5. E

The inferior epigastric artery is vulnerable to injury with placement of lateral laparascopic ports. It lies approximately 1.5 cm lateral to the medial umbilical fold, which marks the site of the obliterated umbilical artery.
Reference: Page 82

6. D

The presacral nerve (superior hypogastric plexus) lies beneath the peritoneum in front of the terminal aorta, the fifth lumbar vertebra, and the sacral promontory medial to the ureters. Embedded in loose areolar tissue, the plexus overlies the middle sacral vessels, which are vulnerable to injury during transection of the two or three incompletely fused trunks, which usually make up the presacral nerve.
Reference: Pages 88–89

7. C

Lymphatic drainage of the vulva is to the superficial and deep inguinal nodes, which then drain to the external iliac chain of lymph nodes.
Reference: Pages 85–86

8. A

The lateral femoral cutaneous nerve derived from L-2–L-3 spinal segments provide sensory innervation to the lateral thigh to the level of the knee and injury to this nerve is the most likely cause of the patient's symptoms. The obturator nerve provides sensory innervation to the medial thigh and leg, the hip and knee joints. The femoral nerve provides sensory innervation to the anterior and medial thigh, the medial leg and foot, and hip and knee joint with motor innervation to the iliacus and anterior thigh muscles. The ilioinguinal nerve supplies sensory innervation to the upper medial thigh, mons and labia majora, while the genitofemoral nerve provides sensation to the anterior vulva with its genital branch and sensation to the middle/upper anterior thigh with its femoral branch.
Reference: Pages 87–88

9. D

In the absence of antimülerian hormone, the paramesonephric or mülerian duct system is able to develop into the female internal genital organs, whereas the presence of this hormone allows the mesonephric system to develop into male internal genital structures, with regression of the paramesonephric system. Testis-determining factor (TDY) is elaborated by the male gonad and results in degeneration of the gonadal cortex and differentiation of the medullary region of the gonad into Sertoli cells. Ovarian descent into the pelvis is under control of a ligamentous cord called the gubernaculum.
Reference: Pages 91–92

10. A

The genital tubercle in the female embryo becomes the clitoris. The urogenital folds become the labia minora and the labioscrotal swellings the labia majora. The cloaca is the early common opening of the genital, urinary, and gastrointestinal systems to the fetal exterior. It is partitioned by the mesenchymal urorectal septum into an anterior urogenital sinus and a posterior rectum.
Reference: Pages 93–95

11. C

The most common uterine position is mid-to-anterior in orientation. When the uterine corpus is at a posterior angle to the long axis of the cervix, particularly if deeply retroflexed, perforation more commonly occurs. This can be prevented by careful examination prior to insertion of instruments, traction on the cervix to reduce the degree of flexion, and careful introduction of dilators and curettes.
Reference: Page 100

12. A

The ovarian vessels cross over the ureter as it approaches the pelvic brim and lie in proximity just lateral to the ureter as it crosses over the common iliac vessels at their bifurcation to enter the pelvis.
Reference: Pages 79, 102–107

6

Molecular Biology and Genetics

Vicki V. Baker
Otoniel Martínez-Maza
Jonathan S. Berek

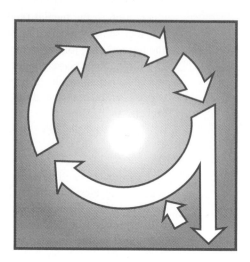

Learning Objectives

1. Be able to identify the phases of the normal cell cycle.

2. Be able to identify factors that regulate the normal cell cycle.

3. Understand the process of apoptosis.

4. Be able to identify the components of the immune system.

5. Be aware of the factors that trigger neoplasia.

Questions

1. Which of the following statements about the normal cell cycle is incorrect?

    A. Red blood cells, uterine muscle cells, and nerve cells are terminally differentiated cells and, therefore, cannot reenter the cell cycle.
    B. The G_2 phase of the cell cycle is the most variable phase.
    C. The DNA content of the cell is copied during the S phase of the cell cycle.
    D. During mitosis, the DNA content is equally distributed to each of the daughter cells to yield diploid genetic material.
    E. Proteins are synthesized during the G_2 phase of the cell cycle.

2. Which of the following effects is caused by the tumor suppressor gene *p53*?

    A. Cell cycle arrest at the G_2/M boundary
    B. Inhibition of microtubuli formation during mitosis
    C. Prevention of apoptosis
    D. Increased amount of cells in the G_2 phase
    E. Arrest of cells at the G_1/S boundary

3. Which of the following statements about apoptosis is incorrect?

    A. Apoptosis is a process that occurs in normal tissue to maintain a balance between cell proliferation and cell death.
    B. Apoptosis is an energy-dependent process.
    C. Apoptosis can hardly be distinguished from cell necrosis.
    D. Apoptotic cells exhibit cellular condensation and fragmentation of the nucleus.
    E. Apoptosis is an important factor in the growth of neoplasm.

4. Which of the following statements about oncogenes is correct?

    A. Examples of oncogenes are *erb*-b2, c-*myc*, and k-*ras*.
    B. *Erb*-b2 plays a role as oncogenic protein in ovarian cancer.
    C. Normal cells do not express oncogenes.
    D. Expression of oncogenes might be induced by environmental factors.
    E. The protooncogene *fms* encodes a receptor for colony stimulating factor.

5. Which of the following statements about transforming growth factor-β (TGF-β) is correct?

    A. TGF-β is exclusively produced by the embryo and theca cells.
    B. TGF-β has a mainly stimulating effect on the immune system.
    C. TGF-β activates intracytoplasmatic serine kinases.
    D. TGF-β does not play a role in gynecologic malignancies.
    E. None of the above statements is correct.

6. Which of the following statements about the effect of growth factors on intracellular signaling is incorrect?

    A. The interaction between growth factors and their receptors can result in activation of intracytoplasmatic kinases.
    B. Proteins encoded by protooncogenes do not participate in intracellular signal transduction.
    C. G proteins are guanyl nucleotide-binding proteins.
    D. G proteins display GTPase activity.
    E. Adenylate cyclase molecules can be activated by G proteins.

7. Which of the following DNA alterations play a role in gynecologic cancer?

   A. Amplification
   B. Point mutations
   C. Deletions
   D. Rearrangements
   E. All of the above

8. Which of the following gene therapy modalities has shown to be most effective in preclinical as well as clinical studies?

   A. Replacement of mutated *p53* tumor suppressor genes with wild-type *p53* gene
   B. Inhibition of oncogenes and protooncogenes
   C. Cytokine gene-modified tumor cell vaccines
   D. Suicide gene therapy
   E. None of the above

9. Which of the following tumor-associated antigens is specific for the associated gynecologic malignancy?

   A. Squamous cell carcinoma (SCC) antigen for cervical cancer
   B. Cancer antigen 125 (CA125) for ovarian cancer
   C. Carcinoembryonic antigen (CEA) for endometrial cancer
   D. β-Human chorionic gonadotropin (β-hCG) for ovarian germ cell tumor
   E. None of the above

10. Which of the following classes of cluster determinants (CD) are present in all mature T cells?

    A. CD3
    B. CD4
    C. CD8
    D. CD20
    E. CD56

11. Which of the following statements about differences between T and B cells is incorrect?

    A. T cells are part of the cellular immune response, B cells produce a humoral immune response.
    B. B cells are able to produce antibodies specific for a certain antigen.
    C. B-cell and T-cell receptors interact with the antigen in similar ways.
    D. Both B and T cells can go into clonal expansion upon recognition of an antigen.
    E. Both T cells and B cells have been isolated from gynecologic malignancies.

12. Which one of the following cell types is considered the most important and effective in mediating lysis of tumor cells?

    A. CD4$^+$ helper cells
    B. CD8$^+$ killer cells
    C. Macrophages
    D. Natural killer (NK) cells
    E. B cells

13. Which of the following cell types is able to generate a memory response?

    A. NK cells
    B. T cells
    C. Macrophages
    D. Eosinophils
    E. Monocytes

14. Which of the following cytokines is produced in a predominantly T_H1-like T-cell response?

    A. Interleukin (IL)-2
    B. IL-4
    C. IL-5
    D. IL-10
    E. Granulocyte-macrophage colony-stimulating factor (GM-CSF)

15. Which of the following cytokines is primarily involved in generation of inflammatory responses?

    A. IL-1
    B. IL-2
    C. IL-6
    D. IL-10
    E. IL-12

16. Which of the following cytokines is similar to GM-CSF in its biologic activities?

    A. IL-2
    B. IL-3
    C. IL-6
    D. IL-12
    E. Interferon-γ

17. Which of the following cytokines have been found in large amounts in ascites from patients with ovarian cancer?

    A. IL-2
    B. IL-8
    C. IL-10
    D. IL-15
    E. Interferon-α

18. Which of the following is a potentially lethal side effect of IL-2 therapy?

    A. Anaphylaxis
    B. Neutropenia
    C. Dehydration
    D. Vascular leak syndrome
    E. T-cell lymphoma

19. Which of the following is the single most important risk factor for the development of cancer?

    A. Smoking
    B. Radiation
    C. Advanced age
    D. Exposure to environmental carcinogens
    E. Genetic disposition

Answers

1. B (see Fig. 6.2)
The highest degree of variation is found in the G_1 phase of the cell cycle. Depending on the cell type, the G_1 phase can range from 8 hours to more than 100 hours. These variations account for different generation times exhibited by various cell types. This

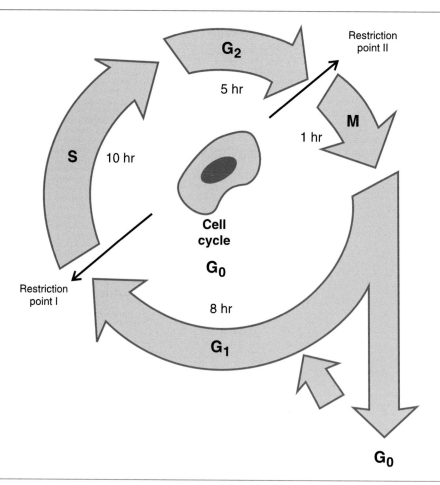

Figure 6.2   The cell cycle.

is an important biological phenomenon, because a number of antineoplastic drugs are active in the G_1 or G_1/S transition point of the cell cycle. This phase is characterized by diverse biosynthetic activity. Enzymes and regulatory proteins necessary for DNA synthesis are being produced to prepare the cell for the mitosis.

Terminally differentiated cells, such as red blood cells, uterine smooth muscle cells, and nerve cells, cannot reenter the cell cycle and must be generated from stem cells. They differ from cells in the quiescent G_0 phase. Cells in G_0 can be stimulated to enter the cell cycle following exposure to specific stimuli. The stimuli can include steroid hormones, irradiation, cytotoxic drugs, or trauma. Rapidly proliferating cells are in general more susceptible to the effect of antineoplastic drugs. These cells are mainly found in the gastrointestinal tract or the skin.

During the S phase, the DNA content of the cell is copied. After initiation of DNA synthesis, the replication of DNA proceeds as an "all-or-none" phenomenon. Cells that contain more than diploid genetic material, such as polyploid cancer cells for example, might produce either more or less than twice the amount of DNA during the S phase.

During the G_2 phase of the cell cycle, proteins are synthesized (e.g., proteins with structural and enzymatic properties). Errors of replication, which occur during DNA replication, are repaired in this phase. Failure to detect and correct genetic errors might allow genetically aberrant cells to continue through the cell cycle. These cells may ultimately avoid cell cycle control and display malignant transformation.
Reference: Pages 123–125

2. E

The *p53* tumor suppressor gene elicits its main function via cell cycle control by arresting cells in the G_1/S check boundary. Errors of replication not repaired in the G_2 phase or resulting from mitosis, are repaired in the G_1 phase. The tumor suppressor gene *p53* encodes for protein with diverse transcriptional activity. The induced mechanisms ultimately lead to growth arrest in the G_1/S transition point, allowing time for the cell to repair DNA damage. If DNA repair is successful, the cell will continue to cycle and undergo DNA replication during the S phase. If DNA repair fails, however, *p53* is able to induce apoptosis or cell suicide via a number of different pathways. A cell with extensive DNA damage would subsequently disintegrate and die. Cells with normal or nonmutated p53 protein, therefore, possess a strong control mechanism for preventing genetically aberrant cells from continuous proliferation.

The gene *p53* is still the most important tumor suppressor gene in gynecologic malignancies. Overall, approximately 30% of ovarian cancers have been found to display aberrant *p53* expression. The importance of mutations in the *p53* gene lies in the inability of the cell to arrest in the G_1/S transition point. The cell, therefore, has less time to repair DNA defects. Furthermore, the apoptosis-inducing effect of the wild-type p53 protein is missing in cells that have mutated *p53* gene sequences. The resulting mutated or truncated proteins fail to induce the transcriptional mechanisms that induce cell suicide or apoptosis. Knowledge of this mechanism had lead to the development of novel therapeutic approaches in cancer gene therapy. The introduction of the wild-type *p53* gene into cells with mutated *p53* has been shown to restore the growth arrest and apoptosis in a variety of different cancer cell lines.
Reference: Page 126

3. C

Apoptosis can be distinguished from necrosis by a number of features. In apoptosis, the cell condenses with fragmentation of the nucleus. This is an energy-dependent process, which is regulated by the expression of specific genes. In contrast, cell necrosis is an energy-independent process. In necrosis, cells undergo spontaneous lysis.

Apoptosis is required to maintain a balance between proliferation and cell death in normal tissue. This mechanism, for example, accounts for the development of intestinal mucosa or palatal fusion. It is regulated by complex interactions between certain genes such as *Bcl2*, *c-myc*, and *p53*.

Apoptosis is also an important factor in the genesis of neoplasms. Cancer cells fail to show an adequate rate of apoptosis as found in normal tissue. Genes involved in the regulation of apoptotic pathways are frequently mutated in cancer cells. Lack of functional apoptotic pathways contribute to increased and uncontrolled proliferation of cells. The development of novel therapies for cancer uses replacement of genes in cancer cells to restore the apoptotic machinery.
Reference: Pages 127–128

4. C (see Table 6.1)

Many oncogenes are expressed at low levels in normal cells and are required for cellular functions such as cell division. Although more than 100 oncogenes have been identified, only a small minority seem to participate in the development of most oncogene-associated tumors. Oncogenes exist within a cell in a latent state as a protooncogene and must be activated endogenously by genetic rearrangement or exogenously by environmental factors to produce the oncogenic effect.

A variety of different oncogenes has been associated with ovarian cancer, including *erb*-b2, c-*myc*, *jun*, or k-*ras*. The oncogene *erb*-b2 is a 185-kd oncogenic protein that directly correlates with prognosis. A protein present in normal adult tissue, *erb*-b2 is overexpressed in cancer tissue.

Table 6.1. Protooncogenes

Protooncogenes	Gene Product/Function
Growth factors	
fgf-5	Fibroblast growth factor
sis	Platelet-derived growth factor beta
hst, int-2	
Transmembrane receptors	
erb-B	Epidermal growth factor (EGF) receptor
HER-2/neu	EGF-related receptor
fms	Colony-stimulating factor (CSF) receptor
kit	Stem cell receptor
trk	Nerve growth factor receptor
Inner-membrane receptor	
bcl-2	
Ha-ras, N-ras, N-ras	
fgr, lck, src, yes	
Cytoplasmic messengers	
crk	
cot, plm-1, mos, raf/mil	
Nuclear DNA binding proteins	
erb-B1	
jun, ets-1, ets-2, fos, gil 1, rel, ski, vav	
lyl-1, maf, myb, myc, L-myc, N-myc, evi-1	

Protooncogenes encode growth factors as well as membrane and cytoplasmatic receptors. These proteins transmit signals from an extracellular ligand to the nucleus and activate DNA expression. In general, protooncogenes stimulate cellular proliferation. Examples of protooncogenes include *fms*, which encodes the transmembrane receptor for the colony-stimulating factor; *erb*-b2, which encodes the receptor for epidermal growth factor; and *sis*, which encodes the receptor for TGF-β. Oncogenes are a target for molecular therapies, because inhibition of oncogene overexpression has been shown to cause cell growth arrest in various cancer cell lines.
Reference: Pages 127–128

5. C (see Table 6.3)

TGF-β belongs to a family of proteins with a variety of effects on different cell systems. It mainly elicits inhibitory effects on the immune system. TGF-β inhibits stimulation and proliferation of T cells and, therefore inhibits important immune responses against tumor cells. TGF-β is produced by a variety of cells. It is important in embryonic development and induces production of the müullerian inhibiting substance (MIS). It exerts its effect via a complex of type-I and type-II receptors on the cell surface. Upon binding to the receptor complex, intracytoplasmatic serine kinases are activated. This activation induces a pathway, which ultimately leads to the induction of transcriptional activity. Most cells are growth inhibited by TGF-β; other cell lines, however, show growth activation with TGF-β.

TGF-β seems to play an important role in gynecologic malignancies. In ovarian cancer, TGF-β has been overexpressed. TGF-β was also a major immunosuppressive factor in ascites from patients with ovarian cancer. Ascites from ovarian cancer patients are able to inhibit the generation of lymphokine-activated killer cells mainly due to the presence of high amounts of TGF-β.
Reference: Pages 129–131

Table 6.3. Growth Factors that Play Important Roles in Female Reproductive Physiology

Growth Factor	Sources	Targets	Actions
Platelet-derived growth factor (PDGF)	Placenta, platelets, preimplantation embryo, endothelial cells	Endothelial cells Trophoblasts	Mitogen
Epidermal growth factor (EGF)	Submaxillary gland, theca cells	Granulosa cells Endometrium, cervix	Mitogen
Transforming growth factor–alpha (TGF-alpha)	Embryo, placenta, theca cell, ovarian stromal cell	Placenta Granulosa cells	Mitogen
Transforming growth factor–beta (TGF-beta)	Embryo, theca cells	Endometrium Granulosa cells Theca cells	Mitogen
Insulin-like growth factor 1 (IGF-1)	Granulosa cells	Theca cells Granulosa cells	Mediates growth hormone activity
Insulin-like growth factor 2 (IGF-2)	Theca cells	Theca cells	Insulin-like effects
Fibroblast growth factor (FGF)	Granulosa cells	Granulosa cells	Angiogenic activity Mitogen

6. B

Protooncogenes and G proteins participate in intracellular signal transduction. Growth factors elicit an effect on cells mainly by controlling cyclic adenosine monophosphate (AMP) levels via activating or inhibiting adenylate cyclase. In mammalian cells, different proteins couple the activated receptor to cyclase. Transmembrane receptors interact with a ligand at the cytoplasmic or membrane portion of the receptor. The receptor is subsequently activated and may dimerize with homologous or heterologous receptors. The cytoplasmatic portion of the activated receptor displays kinase activity, which induces a number of downstream effects on different intracytoplasmatic and intranuclear proteins. The receptor–growth factor complex activates G proteins, which undergo structural changes upon binding to guanosine triphosphate (GTP). Carrying the GTP, it now activates the adenylate cyclase molecule. The activated G protein keeps the cyclase active as long as the GTP is intact. Hydrolysis of the GTP to guanosine diphosphate (GDP) by the G protein terminates the action of the cyclase. These are important pathways for the understanding of receptor-induced cellular changes in normal and neoplastic cells.
Reference: Pages 131–132

7. E

Normal cells and tumor cells are dividing cells, constantly producing genetic material during the cell cycle. DNA synthesis may yield various errors in the replicated DNA, altering the structure and function of the cells. A number of these aberrations have been identified in premalignant, malignant, and benign neoplasms. Amplification, point mutations, deletions, and rearrangements are all mechanisms that lead to genetic errors. Amplification is an increase in the copy number of a gene and can enhance gene expression by increasing the amount of template DNA available for transcription. Protooncogene amplification is a common event in gynecologic malignancies. An example of oncogene amplification is *erb*-b2, which is found in 30% of all ovarian malignancies.

Point mutations can lead to altered code sequences and, subsequently, to gene products with modified activity. The *p53* tumor suppressor gene has a number of common genetic mutations termed "hot spots." Loss of p53 activity through genetic mutation increases the likelihood of uninhibited cell proliferation.

Deletions and rearrangements yield altered proteins that may, for example, encode mutant receptors such as the epidermal growth factor receptor, which is constitutively activated and transmits signals to the cytoplasm for cellular proliferation in the absence of ligand.
Reference: Pages 133–135

8. E

A number of preclinical studies in different animal models and ongoing clinical trials are currently investigating the therapeutic effect of genetic modification of cancer cells in gynecologic malignancies. Different approaches are currently being used. However, none of these approaches has been found to be effective in patients to date.

Advances in our understanding of the biology of tumors and novel techniques in molecular biology have led to a variety of therapeutic approaches that target different tumor characteristic phenomena. Genes for the expression of cytokines have been transferred into tumor cells. The resulting tumor cells co-present tumor-associated antigen on the cell surface and produce cytokines necessary to stimulate immune-effector cells. The close vicinity of tumor-associated antigen and immunostimulatory cytokine effectively stimulate a strong antitumor response in animals.

Inhibition of oncogene expression in cancer cells can result in reversal of the malignant phenotype. For example, the oncogene *erb*-b2 has been blocked in ovarian cancer cells yielding tumor cells with abrogated tumorigenicity in mice. Mutated or missing p53 protein can be replaced in cancer cells by insertion of the wild-type *p53* gene. The genetically modified cells are growth-arrested due to the cell cycle inhibitory effect of p53. Furthermore, these cells have a higher degree of apoptosis when transfected with the wild-type *p53* gene. In suicide cancer gene therapy, cancer cells are transfected with genes that encode an enzyme capable of converting a normal nontoxic substance into a toxic metabolite. Upon presentation of the appropriate substrate, the toxic metabolic is produced in transgene expressing tumor cells and induces cell death.
Reference: Pages 132–135

9. E

Although a variety of tumor-associated antigens such as SCC, CA125, and CEA have been described in gynecologic malignancy, unfortunately, none of these tumor markers are specific for a particular type of cancer. Tumor-associated antigens have been identified using monoclonal antibody techniques. They are useful markers in following the progression of the disease and the success of treatment. The combination of different tumor markers, for example CA125 and OVX1 in ovarian cancer, may improve the specificity and sensitivity of screening tests.

Monoclonal antibodies react with tumor-associated antigens and can be conjugated to toxins like recin, radioisotopes, or chemotherapeutic agents. These conjugated antibodies can be directed toward human ovarian carcinoma antigens to induce tumor cell killing. However, although the antitumor effects observed in animal studies have been very promising, conjugated monoclonal antibodies have not shown significant effects in patients with gynecologic malignancies. Recently, antigen-specific T cells have been used to identify novel antigens.
Reference: Pages 135–137

10. A

T cells can be distinguished from other lymphocytes by their cell surface phenotype. They express complexes of proteins on the cell surface that are responsible for various

functions in the different subsets of T cells. All mature T cells express the cluster determinant CD3. In addition to CD3, T cells classified as helper T cells express CD4 and killer T cells express CD8. CD20 molecules are found on B cells. The CD56 molecule is unique to NK cells. Immunofluorescence is used to identify cluster determinants on T cells and subsequently identification of different subsets.
Reference: Pages 136–137

11. C

T cells can respond to antigens only when the processed antigens are presented in association with Major histocompatibility complex (MHC) molecules on antigen-presenting cells. The CD4 helper T cell population recognizes antigens in association with MHC class II molecules. The CD8$^+$ T-cell killer cell population recognizes antigens in association with MHC class I molecules. B cells express antibodies on their cell surface that function as receptors for antigens. These antibody receptors do not need additional molecules for effective antigen recognition and binding.

T cells belong to the cellular immune system, whereas B cells produce antibodies and are responsible for the humoral immune response. Both B and T cells are able to effectively process antigens and clonally expand. As much as B cells produce specific antibodies against antigens, T cells specific for a certain antigen can expand in a clonal fashion. Both B and T cells have been isolated from gynecologic malignancies. Tumor infiltrating T cells can be isolated from tumors and stimulated to expand *in vitro* by IL-2. These lymphokine-activated tumor-infiltrating lymphocytes are the basis of cellular immunotherapy.
Reference: Pages 136–137

12. D

Cytotoxic killer T cells (or CD8$^+$ T cells) are considered to be the most effective mediators of tumor cell lysis. Killer T cells can recognize antigens associated with MHC class I molecules. Through antigen-specific T-cell receptors, a series of events involving cytokine production by CD4 helper T cells induces activation of cytotoxic T cells, which are able to lyse tumor cells directly.

Macrophages are professional antigen-presenting cells for CD4$^+$ helper T cells. Macrophages and B cells express MHC class II molecules. These cells are able to phagocytose antigen and subsequently present intracellularly processed antigen to CD4$^+$ helper T cells. Helper T cells possess T-cell receptors for the specific antigen and can produce a variety of cytokines.

One of the most important cytokines generated by CD4$^+$ T cells is IL-2, which is able to stimulate killer T cells. The killer T cells ultimately integrate signals from specific antigens and unspecific stimulation by different cytokines, mainly IL-2. NK cells have an innate immune response. They can generate nonspecific killing of tumor cells and virus-infected cells without stimulation by specific antigens.
Reference: Pages 136–137

13. B

T cells can generate a memory response. After first encounter with an antigen, specific T-cells clones are generated. These T-cell clones can be induced by a secondary presentation of the antigen to the T cells. A rapid clonal expansion upon secondary antigen recognition increases the velocity and magnitude of the immune response against the previously recognized antigen. This memory response is crucial, for instance, for the effect of immunization against viruses.

NK cell activity presents an innate form of immunity that is unspecific and unable to generate a memory response. Monocytes and their tissue form (macrophages) are

unspecific cytotoxic cells and are unable to mount a memory response. B cells can effectively generate immune responses particularly important in vaccination.
Reference: Pages 137–138

14. A

IL-2 is a T-cell–produced cytokine, part of the so-called type I T-helper cell–related immune response (T_H1). T_H1 and T_H2 are T-helper cell subpopulations, characterized by the nature of the induced immune response. Although originally described in mice, a similar dichotomy exists in humans. T_H1-type immune responses are characterized by the production of IL-2 and interferon-γ; T_H2-like responses produce IL-4, IL-5, IL-6, IL-10, and GM-CSF. In general, T_H1-type responses generate cellular immune responses compared to T_H2-type responses, which induce the production of antibodies by B cells. In ovarian cancer and other malignancies, a predominantly T_H2-like response has been found that contributes to the failure of the immune system to respond adequately to the tumor disease. Immunotherapy attempts to stimulate T_H1-type responses in order to generate the more effective cytotoxic T-cell population against the tumor.
Reference: Pages 139–140

15. A (see Table 6.4)

IL-1 is involved in fever and inflammatory responses. Its pleiotropic effects include the stimulation of T cells and B cells to produce cytokines. Two forms of IL-1 have been described with similar biologic activity, namely IL-1a and IL-1b. The primary sources of IL-1 are macrophages, some B cells, epithelial cells, brain cells, and the cells lining the synovial spaces. IL-1 is important in the pathomechanism of infertility and may be inhibiting nidation of the fertilized egg.
Reference: Pages 139–140

16. B

IL-3 is a cytokine that enhances the early differentiation of hematopoietic cells. It has stimulatory effects on hematopoietic stem cells. Similar to granulocyte macrophage colony stimulating factor, it enhances the activation and proliferation of macrophages and granulocytes. It is used *in vitro* as growth factor for hematopoietic cells. Similar effects can be generated with granulocyte macrophage colony stimulating factor, which is currently used in preventing and treating neutropenia in patients undergoing chemotherapy.
Reference: Page 140

17. C

High concentrations of IL-10 have been found in ascites from patients with ovarian cancer. Other cytokines such as IL-6, TNF-α, granulocyte colony-stimulating factor, and GM-CSF are also significantly increased in ascites from patients with ovarian cancer when compared to peritoneal fluid in patients without cancer.

IL-10 is a potentially immunosuppressive cytokine. Since high concentrations of IL-10 are found in the ascites of ovarian cancer patients, IL-10 might significantly contribute to the lack of effective immune responses against the tumor. IL-6 inhibits T_H2-type immune responses and potentially inhibits the generation and activation of cytotoxic T-cell responses. Furthermore, it is an autocrine and paracrine growth factor for certain ovarian cancer cell lines.
Reference: Pages 140–141

18. D

Vascular leak syndrome is a potentially lethal side effect of high-dose IL-2 therapy. IL-2 has been used in a variety of studies with different tumors including ovarian cancer for antitumor therapy. High doses of intravenously or intraperitoneally injected IL-2 might generate potent antitumor responses by stimulating cellular immune responses.

Table 6.4. Sources, Target Cells, and Biological Activities of Cytokines Involved in Immune Responses

Cytokine	Cellular Source	Target Cells	Biologic Effects
IL-1	Monocytes and macrophages Tumor cells	T cells, B cells Neurons Endothelial cells	Costimulator Pyrogen
IL-2	T cells (T_H1)	T cells B cells NK cells	Growth Activation and antibody production Activation and growth
IL-3	T cells	Immature hemopoietic stem cells	Growth and differentiation
IL-4	T cells (T_H2)	B cells T cells	Activation and growth; isotype switch to IgE; increased MHC II expression Growth
IL-6	Monocytes and macrophages T cells, B cells Ovarian cancer cells Other tumors	B cells T cells Hepatocytes Stem cells Tumor cells	Differentiation, antibody production Costimulator Induction of acute-phase response Growth and differentiation Autocrine/paracrine growth and viability-enhancing factor
IL-10	T cells (T_H2) Monocytes and macrophages 	T cells (T_H1) Monocytes and macrophages B cells	Inhibition of cytokine synthesis Inhibition of Ag presentation and cytokine production Activation
IL-12	Monocytes	NK cells, T cells (T_H1)	Induction
IFN-γ	T cells (T_H1) NK cells	Monocytes/macrophages NK cells, T cells, B cells	Activation Activation Enhances responses
TNF-α	Monocytes and macrophages T cells	Monocytes/macrophages T cells, B cells Neurons (hypothalamus) Endothelial cells Muscle and fat cells	Monokine production Costimulator Pyrogen Activation, inflammation Catabolism/cachexia

IL-1, interleukin-1; T_H1, type 1 T helper lymphocyte; NK cells, natural killer cells; T_H2, type 2 T helper lymphocyte; IgE, immunoglobulin E; MHCII, major histocompatibility complex class II; Ag, antigen; IFN, interferon; TNF, tumor necrosis factor.
From **Berek JS, Martinez-Maza O.** Immunology and immunotherapy. In: **Lawton FG, Neijt JP, Swenerton KD.** *Epithelial cancer of the ovary.* London: BMJ, 1995:224, with permission.

A number of side effects have been associated with IL-2 therapy. Vascular leak syndrome has been described in a number of patients. Disruption of endothelial membranes and subsequent leakage of fluids into the extravasal space may lead to brain and lung edema or lethal fluid and electrolyte imbalances. Vascular leak syndrome has been associated with high mortality.

Other side effects of IL-2 therapy, such as allergic reactions or hematopoietic side effects, are less likely to have lethal consequences. The administration of IL-2 and the associated side effects of high doses of IL-2 may be preventable by generating genetically modified tumor cells. The IL-2 gene can be transferred into tumor cells that function as a constant producer for IL-2 *in vivo.* However, because IL-2 is expressed

constitutively, low levels can be maintained with subsequently diminished side effects. This concept is currently under investigation. The clinical application of recombinant IL-2 in patients with ovarian cancer has not shown any significant antitumor effects. A number of studies in the last 10 years have revealed an overall response rate of 20% in patients with ovarian cancer. Malignancies such as melanoma or renal cell carcinoma have been found to be more responsive to this form of immunotherapy.
Reference: Pages 141–142

19. C

Advanced age is the single most important risk factor for the development of cancer. A possible explanation for the increase in risk of cancer with age might be the accumulation of critical genetic mutations over time with cumulation of exogenous, DNA-damaging factors.

Specific mutations have been found in cigarette smokers with a high frequency of G-T transversions in the sequence of the *p53* tumor suppressor gene. Radiation exposure should be considered an environmental carcinogen since diagnostic studies are not associated with an increased risk of cancer due to the quite low doses of radiation. More recently, immune function particularly in human immunodeficiency virus (HIV)—infected patients with the obvious increase of Kaposi's sarcoma, B-cell lymphoma, and cervical cancer have become important risk factors. High-fat diets correlate with the development of certain cancers (e.g., colon cancer). In contrast, vitamin C–rich foods and green leafy vegetables seem to decrease the incidence of lung cancer. More advanced studies are needed to evaluate the importance of these factors.
Reference: Pages 142–144

7

Reproductive Physiology

Steven F. Palter
David L. Olive

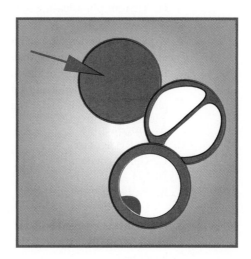

Learning Objectives

1. Understand the anatomy of the hypothalamic-pituitary-ovarian axis.

2. Be aware of the structure and function of reproductive hormones.

3. Understand menstrual cycle physiology, including endometrial changes and follicular development.

Questions

1. Major secretory products of the hypothalamus include all of the following except:

   A. Gonadotropin-releasing hormone (GnRH)
   B. Adrenocorticotrophic hormone
   C. Growth hormone-releasing hormone
   D. Thyrotropin-releasing hormone

2. A patient is undergoing induction of ovulation with exogenous gonadotropins. Her ultrasound examination reveals four follicles, 13-, 12-, 10-, and 9-mm mean diameters. In previous attempts to induce ovulation, she has spontaneously ovulated early due to a premature luteinizing hormone (LH) surge. To prevent the occurrence of this phenomenon in this cycle, you administer

   A. Progesterone
   B. GnRH agonist
   C. GnRH antagonist
   D. LH
   E. Prolactin

3. A chemist is charged with creating a drug that binds to the GnRH receptor but is not easily or rapidly degraded. She decides to modify the basic GnRH decapeptide at which locations?

   A. Amino terminus
   B. Amino acid 3 (Trp)
   C. Amino acid 6 (Glu)
   D. Carboxy terminus

4. A lesion in the pituitary stalk is likely to produce an increase in which pituitary hormone?

   A. Follicle-stimulating hormone (FSH)
   B. Growth hormone
   C. Prolactin
   D. Thyrotropin hormone

5. An assay is devised to measure LH concentrations in the blood. The method used is an immunoassay that recognizes the alpha subunit of the LH molecule. In clinical trials, there is a major discordance between this test and all commercially available tests. The reason for this apparent lack of accuracy is

   A. The alpha subunits of FSH, LH, and thyrotropin are identical and thus cross-react with the assay
   B. Only assays of beta subunits will detect available hormones
   C. All existing tests are inaccurate
   D. Successful assays are limited to recognizing carbohydrate moieties on the pituitary hormone molecules

6. Hormonal characteristics of the follicular phase of the menstrual cycle include:

   A. Frequent GnRH pulses, low progesterone, increasing estrogen
   B. Infrequent GnRH pulses, low progesterone, increasing estrogen
   C. Frequent GnRH pulses, high progesterone, decreasing estrogen
   D. Infrequent GnRH pulses, high progesterone, decreasing estrogen

7. A woman with severe hypogonadotropic hypogonadism (undetectable levels of FSH and LH) wishes to undergo ovulation induction. You induce ovulation with recombinant FSH only. As follicles grow, the serum estrogen concentration will

A. Rise normally
B. Rise initially, then stabilize
C. Fail to rise normally
D. Fail to rise initially, then rise rapidly
E. Rise faster than normal

8. Hormones that act to inhibit FSH release in the follicular phase include:

A. Estrogen
B. Inhibin-B
C. Estrogen and inhibin-B
D. None of the above

9. A reproductive age woman is being treated by another physician for a non-gynecologic problem with an angiotensin inhibitor, specifically targeted to inhibit vascular endothelial growth factor (VEGF). The likely effect upon her menstrual cycle is

A. Lower estrogen and progesterone serum concentrations in the luteal phase
B. Higher estrogen and progesterone serum concentration in the luteal phase
C. Lower estrogen serum concentrations in the follicular phase
D. Higher estrogen serum concentrations in the follicular phase
E. No effect upon estrogen and progesterone serum concentrations

Answers

1. B

The major secretory products of the hypothalamus are the pituitary-releasing factors (see Fig. 7.3).

- GnRH, which controls the secretion of LH and FSH.
- Corticotropin-releasing hormone (CRH), which controls the release of corticotropin.
- Growth hormone-releasing hormone (GHRH), which regulates the release of growth hormone (GH).
- Thyrotropin-releasing hormone (TRH), which regulates the secretion of thyrotropin.

Reference: Pages 150–153

2. C

GnRH antagonists produce a competitive blockade of GnRH receptors, preventing stimulation by endogenous GnRH and causing an immediate fall in gonadotropin and sex-steroid secretion. GnRH agonists, on the other hand, initially stimulate gonadotropin release before down-regulation. Progesterone in high doses may inhibit GnRH secretion from the hypothalamus, but it also promotes gonadotropin release initially. Exogenous LH and prolactin should play no role in control of premature LH surge.
Reference: Pages 152–155

3. C

As a peptide hormone, GnRH is degraded by enzymatic cleavage of bonds between its amino acids. Pharmacologic alterations of GnRH have led to the creation of agonists and antagonists. The primary sites of enzymatic cleavage are between amino acids 5 and 6, 6 and 7, and 9 and 10. Substitution of the amino acid glycine at the 6 position with large, bulky amino acid analogues makes degradation more difficult and creates a form of GnRH with a relatively long half-life. Substitution at the carboxy terminus produces a form of GnRH with increased receptor affinity. These two locations are thus the most commonly modified when producing such analogues. GnRH analogues are now widely

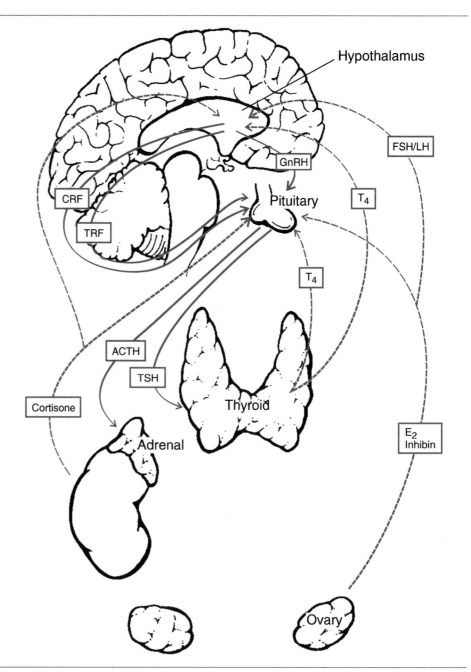

Figure 7.3 **The hypothalamic secretory products function as pituitary releasing factors that control the endocrine function of the ovaries, the thyroid, and the adrenal glands.**

used to treat disorders dependent on ovarian hormones, such as precocious puberty, ovarian hyperandrogenism, leiomyomas, endometriosis, and hormonally dependent cancers (see Fig. 7.4)
Reference: Pages 152–153

Figure 7.4 **Gonadotropin-releasing hormone (*GnRH*) is a decapeptide.**

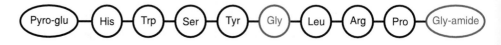

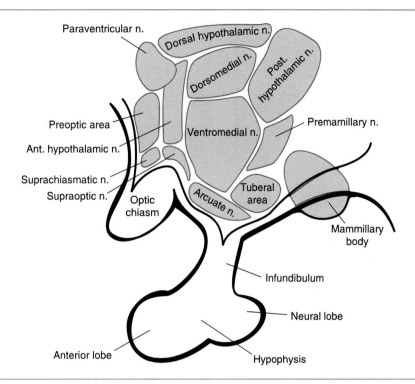

Figure 7.2   The neuronal cell bodies of the hypothalamus.

4. C

Prolactin production is under tonic inhibitory control by the hypothalamic secretion of dopamine. Therefore, interruption of dopamine transport down the infundibular stalk to the pituitary gland (see Fig. 7.2) will result in increased synthesis of prolactin. In this respect, prolactin is unique in comparison to all other pituitary hormones: it is predominantly under tonic inhibition, and release of control produces an increase in secretion.

Reference: Pages 151, 156

5. A

Structurally, there is great similarity between FSH and LH. They are both glycoproteins that share identical alpha subunits and differ only in the structure of their beta subunits, which confer receptor specificity. Thyrotropin and human chorionic gonadotropin (hCG) also share identical alpha subunits with the gonadotropins (see Fig. 7.6).

Reference: Pages 155–156

Figure 7.6   The structural similarity between follicle-stimulating hormone (FSH), luteinizing hormone (LH), and thyrotropin (TSH). The α subunits are identical and the β subunits differ.

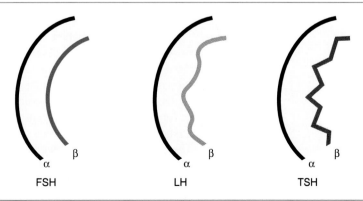

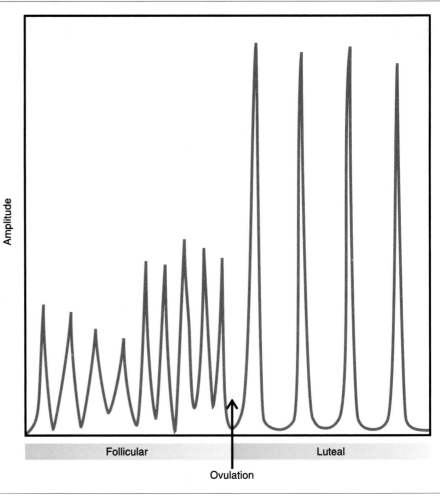

Figure 7.5   The pulsatile secretion of gonadotropin-releasing hormone in the follicular and luteal phases of the cycle.

6. A

Pulsatile secretion of GnRH in the follicular phase is frequent and of high amplitude (see Fig. 7.5). Progesterone is low throughout the follicular phase, but begins to climb just before ovulation and reaches a sustained peak throughout the luteal phase. Estrogen is low at the beginning of the follicular phase, but as follicular development proceeds the serum estrogen level rises (see Fig. 7.9).

Reference: Pages 154–155, 160

7. C

The fundamental tenet of follicular development is the two-cell, two-gonadotropin theory. This theory states that there is a subdivision and compartmentalization of steroid hormone synthesis activity in the developing follicle. In general, most aromatase activity for estrogen production is in the granulosa cells. Aromatase activity is enhanced by FSH stimulation of specific receptors on these cells. However, granulosa cells lack several enzymes that occur earlier in the steroidogenesis pathway and require androgens as a substrate for aromatization. Androgens, in turn, are synthesized primarily in response to stimulation by LH, and the theca cells possess most of the LH receptors at this stage. Therefore, a synergistic relationship must exist: LH stimulates the theca cells to produce androgens, which are transferred to the granulosa cells for FSH-stimulated aromatization into estrogens (see Fig. 7.12). In this patient, a lack of LH will result in

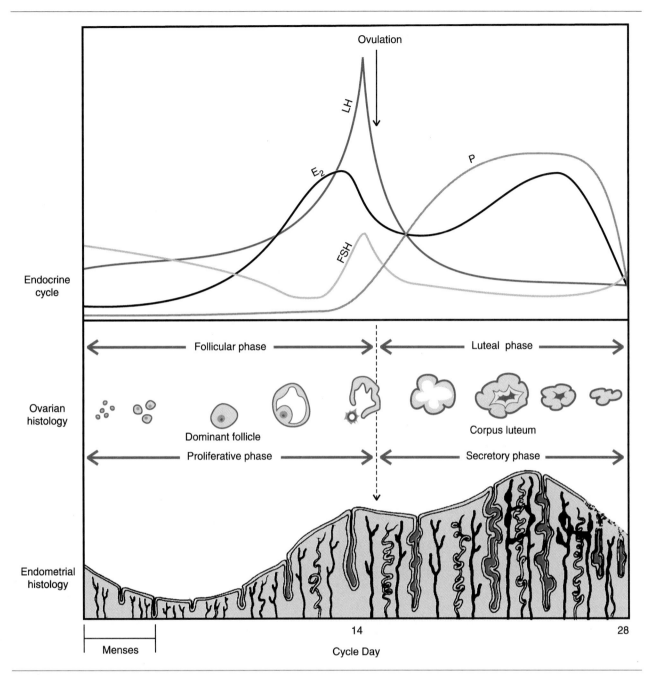

Figure 7.9   The menstrual cycle. The top panel shows the cyclic changes of follicle-stimulating hormone (*FSH*), luteinizing hormone (*LH*), estradiol (*E2*), and progesterone (*P*) relative to the time of ovulation. The bottom panel correlates the ovarian cycle in the follicular and luteal phases and the endometrial cycle in the proliferative and secretory phases.

little androgen substrate available to granulosa cells. Thus, estrogen levels will be low despite follicular growth.
Reference: Pages 165–167

8. C
Rising estrogen levels have a negative feedback effect on FSH secretion. Inhibin-B acts similarly: It is secreted primarily in the follicular phase and acts to inhibit FSH

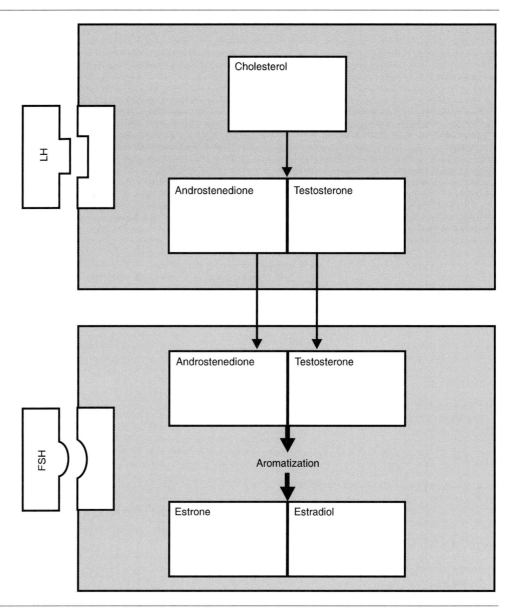

Figure 7.12 **The two-cell, two-gonadotropin theory of follicular development in which there is compartmentalization of steroid hormone synthesis in the developing follicle.**

synthesis and release. Together, these hormones cause a steady decline in the FSH concentration throughout the follicular phase.
Reference: Pages 165–167

9. A

Unlike in the developing follicle, the basement membrane of the corpus luteum degenerates to allow proliferating blood vessels to invade the granulosa–luteal cells in response to secretion of angiogenic factors such as vascular endothelial growth factor (VEGF). This angiogenic response allows large amounts of luteal hormones to enter the systemic circulation. In this patient, the angiogenic effect is inhibited and vessels will fail to adequately invade the corpus luteum, reducing the amount of estrogen and progesterone reaching the peripheral circulation.
Reference: Page 167

PREVENTIVE AND PRIMARY CARE

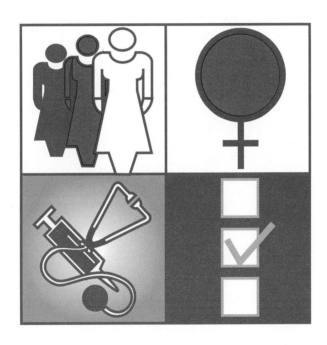

8

Preventive Health Care and Screening

Paula A. Hillard

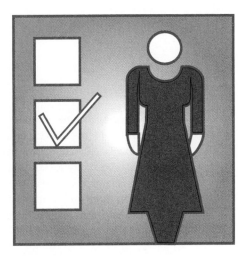

Learning Objectives

1. Be familiar with the major causes of morbidity and mortality by different age groups in order to provide a targeted approach to assessing patients' risks.

2. Be familiar with the quality of evidence ratings promoted by the Canadian and U.S. Task Forces on Preventive Health Services.

3. Be aware that the current health risks to adolescents are predominantly behavioral and be able to provide primary preventive services to adolescents based on the Guidelines for Adolescent Preventive Services (GAPS).

4. Be familiar with current recommendations for immunizations by age group and risk status.

5. Be able to calculate a patient's body mass index (BMI) and to counsel about daily food choices based on the Food Guide Pyramid.

Questions

1. Women taking oral contraceptives (OC) and antibiotics concurrently have been reported to have had pregnancies by anecdotal report only. Individuals taking antibiotics during OC have been advised to use a backup method during the course of antibiotic therapy, because of this risk of OC failure. The U.S. Preventive Services Task Force Quality of Evidence rating for this conclusion would be which of the following:

   A. I
   B. II-1
   C. II-2
   D. II-3
   E. III

2. A 17-year-old woman comes for an annual gynecologic examination. She reports no current symptoms or complaints, and is currently taking combination oral contraceptives. She states that she has had no major medical problems. A sexual history reveals that she is currently sexually active with one partner. Her partner usually uses condoms. She first had intercourse at age 14, and estimates that she has had six lifetime partners, including three within the last 6 months. She is uncertain of her past immunization history, but states that she has not seen her primary physician for over 4 years. Which of the following is indicated?

   A. Hepatitis B vaccine series
   B. Hepatitis A vaccine
   C. Tetanus-diphtheria (Td) vaccine
   D. Measles, mumps, rubella (MMR) trivalent vaccine
   E. Varicella zoster vaccine

3. A 51-year-old woman is seen for an annual gynecologic visit. She has no current symptoms and is having regular menses. She has no major illnesses, and her family history is negative for cardiovascular disease and malignancy. A screening mammogram is recommended. She asks how strong this recommendation is. According to the U.S. Preventive Services Task Force, the strength of this recommendation is based on good evidence. Thus, the strength of the recommendation would be:

   A. A
   B. B
   C. C
   D. D
   E. E

4. A 21-year-old woman comes to the office for a sports physical examination. She is a distance runner. She states that she has not had a menstrual period in 6 months. She weighs 104 lb (50 kg) and is 5 ft 6 in. (1.7 M) tall. Her BMI is

   A. 15
   B. 17
   C. 19
   D. 21
   E. 23

5. To identify a problem drinker, which of the following questionnaires can be used?

   A. T-ACE questionnaire
   B. COMCAT questionnaire
   C. BDI questionnaire

6. A 43-year-old woman asks what her target heart rate should be when she is in good condition from exercising. You tell her:

A. 120
B. 126
C. 133
D. 141

Answers

1. E

The U.S. Preventive Services Task Force has adopted a description of the quality of evidence from clinical studies from the Canadian Task Force on the Periodic Health Examination, 1979. This rating system describes three different levels of evidence (see Table 8.9).

As the data for this recommendation is based only on anecdotal, descriptive studies and several expert committee opinions, it is classified as Level III.
Reference: Pages 176, 181, 188–189

2. A

Recommendations for immunization have been established by a number of national organizations. The American Academy of Pediatrics has recommended immunizations for childhood and adolescence. The American College of Obstetricians and Gynecologists (ACOG) has also published recommendations for immunizations as part of the Guidelines for Primary and Preventive Care. In addition, the Centers for Disease Control (CDC) have suggested guidelines for the hepatitis B vaccine, . The consultants of *The Medical Letter* have made recommendations about two other vaccines: hepatitis A vaccine and varicella zoster vaccine. A group of expert consultants convened as a group by the American Medical Association has issued a set of guidelines for health care of adolescents entitled the *Guidelines for Adolescent Preventive Services* (GAPS) (see Table 8.11).

This patient's sexual behavior clearly places her in a high-risk category for risk of hepatitis B, and thus, according to the ACOG Guidelines, would dictate that hepatitis B vaccine series be given during adolescence. CDC guidelines recommend hepatitis B vaccination at a preadolescent visit at the ages of 11 to 12 years. These guidelines (**http://www.cdc.gov/nip**) emphasize the need for "catch-up" vaccinations for adolescents who missed either the neonatal vaccination or the preadolescent vaccination.

Table 8.9. Quality of Evidence—U.S. Preventive Services Task Force

I.	Evidence obtained from at least one properly designed randomized, controlled trial.
II-1.	Evidence obtained from well-designed controlled trials without randomization.
II-2.	Evidence obtained from well-designed cohort or case-control analytic studies, preferably from more than one center or research group.
II-3.	Evidence obtained from multiple time series with or without the intervention. Dramatic results in uncontrolled experiments (such as the results of the introduction of penicillin treatment in the 1940s) could also be regarded as this type of evidence.
III.	Opinions of respected authorities, based on clinical experience, descriptive studies, or reports of expert committees.

From **Canadian Task Force on the Periodic Health Examination.** The periodic health examination. *CMAJ* 1979;121:1193–254, with permission.

Table 8.11. Guidelines for Adolescent Preventive Services

1. From ages 11 to 21 years, all adolescents should have an annual routine health visit.

2. Preventive services should be age and developmentally appropriate, and they should be sensitive to individual and sociocultural differences.

3. Physicians should establish office policies regarding confidential care for adolescents and how parents will be involved in that care. These policies should be made clear to adolescent and the parents.

4. Parents or other adult caregivers of adolescents should receive health guidance at least once during early adolescence, once during middle adolescence and, preferably, once during late adolescence.

5. All adolescents should receive health guidance annually to promote a better understanding of their physical growth, psychosocial and psychosexual development, and the importance of becoming actively involved in decisions regarding their health care.

6. All adolescents should receive health guidance annually to promote the reduction of injuries.

7. All adolescents should receive health guidance annually about dietary habits, including the benefits of a healthy diet, ways to achieve a healthy diet, and safe weight management.

8. All adolescents should receive health guidance annually about the benefits of exercise and should be encouraged to engage in safe exercise on a regular basis.

9. All adolescents should receive health guidance annually regarding responsible sexual behaviors, including abstinence. Latex condoms to prevent sexually transmitted diseases (STDs) (including human immunodeficiency virus [HIV] infection) and appropriate methods of birth control should be made available with instructions on how to use them effectively.

10. All adolescents should receive health guidance annually to promote avoidance of the use of tobacco, alcohol, abusable substances, and anabolic steroids.

11. All adolescents should be screened annually for hypertension according to the protocol developed by the National Heart, Lung, and Blood Institute Second Task Force on Blood Pressure Control in Children (18).

12. Selected adolescents should be screened to determine their risk of developing hyperlipidemia and adult coronary heart disease following the protocol by the Expert Panel on Blood Cholesterol Levels in Children and Adolescents (19).

13. All adolescents should be screened annually for eating disorders and obesity by determining weight and stature and asking about body image and dieting patterns.

14. All adolescents should be asked annually about their use of tobacco products, including cigarettes and smokeless tobacco.

15. All adolescents should be asked annually about their use of alcohol and other abusable substances and about their use of over-the-counter or prescription drugs for nonmedical purposes, including anabolic steroids.

16. All adolescents should be asked annually about involvement in sexual behaviors that may result in unintended pregnancies and STDs, including HIV infection.

17. Sexually active adolescents should be screened for STDs.

18. Adolescents at risk for HIV infection should be offered confidential HIV screening with the enzyme-linked immunosorbent assay and confirmatory testing.

19. Female adolescents who are sexually active or any female 18 years of age or older should be screened annually for cervical cancer by use of a Papanicolaou (Pap) test.

20. All adolescents should be asked annually about behaviors or emotions that indicate recurrent or severe depression or risk of suicide.

21. All adolescents should be asked annually about a history of emotional, physical, and sexual abuse.

22. All adolescents should be asked annually about learning or school problems.

Table 8.11.—continued

23. Adolescents should receive a tuberculin skin test if they have been exposed to active tuberculosis, have lived in a homeless shelter, have been incarcerated, have lived in or come from an area with a high prevalence of tuberculosis, or currently work in a health care setting.

24. All adolescents should receive prophylactic immunizations according to the guidelines established by the federally convened Advisory Committee on Immunization Practices: a bivalent tetanus-diphtheria vaccine 10 years after their previous diphtheria vaccination (usually 5 to 66 years old). All adolescents should receive a second trivalent measles-mumps-rubella vaccination, unless there is documentation of two vaccinations earlier during childhood. A measles-mumps-rubella vaccination should not be given to adolescents who are pregnant—susceptible adolescents who engage in high-risk behaviors should be vaccinated against hepatitis B virus. This includes adolescents who have had more than one sexual partner during the previous 6 months, have exchanged sex for drugs or money, are males who have engaged in sex with other males, or have used intravenous drugs. Widespread use of the hepatitis B vaccine is encouraged because risk factors are often not easily identifiable among adolescents.

From **Elster AB, Kuznets NJ.** *AMA Guidelines for adolescent preventive services (GAPS): recommendations and rationale.* Baltimore: Williams & Wilkins, 1994:1–191.

The current recommendations for tetanus include the recommendation for a repeat of the bivalent Td (diphtheria/tetanus) vaccine 10 years after the previous vaccination. The previous immunization usually occurred at ages 5 to 6; the booster should be given at ages 15 to 16. Since pertussis is relatively benign in adolescents, reimmunization with pertussis vaccine is unnecessary.

The MMR vaccinations should be given if an adolescent (a) has not had measles, mumps, or rubella infections documented by a physician; (b) lacks laboratory evidence of immunity; or (c) has not had two doses of MMR. Preferably, the second MMR should be given during early puberty, prior to the time when an adolescent is at risk for pregnancy. Adolescents who are sexually active should be cautioned not to become pregnant for 3 months following the MMR vaccination, although this remains a theoretical precaution.

A live attenuated varicella vaccine was approved in mid-1995. Chickenpox occurs mainly in children younger than 8 years; by the age of 12, less than 10% are still susceptible. Adults account for only 2% of cases of chickenpox, although they account for 50% of the deaths. *The Medical Letter* recommends vaccination for everyone older than 1 year who is in good health and has no history of clinical varicella. It should not be given to pregnant women. It is not clear how long immunity lasts or whether a booster will be necessary in adulthood.

A vaccine to prevent hepatitis A is also now available in the United States. Many adults in the United States are immune to hepatitis A. Antibody testing costs less than the two doses, which are recommended for travelers to endemic areas and members of other high-risk groups including homosexual men and intravenous drug abusers. Thus it is *not* recommended for most adolescents.
Reference: Pages 186–190

3. A

The U.S. Preventive Services Task Force has rated the strength of clinical recommendations; see the scale in Table 8.10. Because mammography has been shown to be effective in reducing the mortality from breast cancer by randomized clinical trials, the strength of recommendation is A.
Reference: Page 189

Table 8.10. The Task Force Graded the *Strength of Recommendations* for or Against Preventive Interventions as Follows

Strength of Recommendations

A: There is good evidence to support the recommendation that the condition be specifically considered in a periodic health examination.

B: There is fair evidence to support the recommendation that the condition be specifically considered in a periodic health examination.

C: There is insufficient evidence to recommend for or against the inclusion of the condition in a periodic health examination, but recommendations may be made on other grounds.

D: There is fair evidence to support the recommendation that the condition be excluded from consideration in a periodic health examination.

E: There is good evidence to support the recommendation that the condition be excluded from consideration in a periodic health examination.

U.S. Preventive Services Task Force. *Guide to Clinical Preventive Services,* 2nd ed. Baltimore: Williams & Wilkins, 1996.

---

4. B

The BMI is calculated by dividing the weight in kilograms by the height in meters squared. This calculated value gives a good assessment of nutritional status. Tables facilitate these calculations and the conversions from pounds to kilograms and inches to meters. In addition, tables also indicate the percentiles of weight. Patients who are 20% above or below the normal range (BMI of approximately 22) should be assessed for systemic disease or eating disorder. This patient's BMI of 17 suggests that further questioning about bulimic behaviors, distorted body image, and excessive dieting or exercise is indicated. In women with anorexia nervosa, hypoestrogenism with attendant risk for osteoporosis is a concern. Menstrual disturbances are also common in these young women, and amenorrhea is one of the diagnostic criteria for anorexia nervosa. Psychiatric evaluation and treatment are indicated; hospitalization may be necessary in severe cases.
Reference: Pages 191–193

5. A (see Table 8.12)

Alcoholic beverages should be limited to less than 1 oz of absolute alcohol per day (equivalent to two cans of beer, two glasses of wine, or two average cocktails). A simple device called the T-ACE questionnaire can be used to elicit information about alcohol

---

Table 8.12. T-ACE Questionnaire

Do you have a drinking problem?

Experts in treating alcohol abuse use the T-ACE questions below to help them find out whether a person has a drinking problem. These questions can also apply to other drugs.

T How many drinks does it take to make you feel high (Tolerance)?

A Have people Annoyed you by criticizing your drinking?

C Have you ever felt you ought to Cut down on your drinking?

E Have you ever had a drink first thing in the morning to steady your nerves or get rid of a hangover (Eye opener)?

If your answer to the tolerance questions is more than two drinks, give yourself a score of 2. If you answer yes to any of the other questions, give yourself a score of 1 each. If your total score is 2 or more, you may have a drinking problem.

From **Sokol RJ, Martier SS, Ager JW.** The T-ACE questions: practical prenatal detection of risk-drinking. *Am J Obstet Gynecol* 1989;160:865.

use and identify problem drinkers. Women should be questioned in a nonjudgmental fashion about their alcohol use and directed to counseling services as required.
Reference: Page 193

6. **C**
Cardiovascular fitness can be evaluated by measurement of heart rate during exercise. As conditioning improves, the heart rate stabilizes at a fixed level. The heart rate at which conditioning will develop is called the target heart rate (THR). The formula for calculating the target heart rate is 220 minus the patient's age times 0.75. In the above example, the THR would be $(220 - 43) \times 0.75 = 133$.
Reference: Pages 193–194

9 Primary Medical Care

Dayton Daberkow II
Thomas Nolan

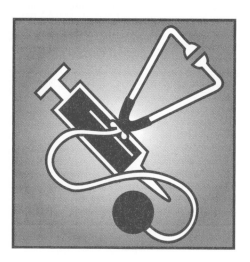

Learning Objectives

1. Be able to describe common respiratory diseases of women, their diagnoses, and their treatment.

2. Understand the role of hypertension in health and disease.

3. Know how to diagnose and treat hyperlipidemia.

4. Know the classification, diagnosis, and treatment of diabetes mellitus.

5. Understand the scope of thyroid disease in the female.

Questions

1. A 38-year-old woman presents to your office with a productive cough for 8 days. She has had a fever and has been unable to work because of fatigue. She takes no medicines, has no medical problems, and does not smoke. A chest x-ray reveals a right middle lobe infiltrate. Her vital signs are as follows: heart rate, 82 beats per minute; blood pressure, 130/88 mm Hg; temperature, 39°C; and respiratory rate, 12 per minute. You recommend which of the following?

   A. Admit to the hospital and start intravenous antibiotics.
   B. Begin a *macrolide* and have patient return in 2 days if not better.
   C. Begin *penicillin* and have patient return in 2 days if not better.
   D. Begin *amoxicillin* and have patient return in 2 days if not better.

2. A 33-year-old female teacher presents for her annual health maintenance examination and states she has "sinus problems" and desires antibiotics. She has had a runny nose for 3 days, no purulent discharge, no tooth pain and her physical exam is significant for a clear discharge seen on her nasal turbinates. You recommend the following:

   A. If she is currently on oral contraceptives, then *tetracycline* 250 mg four times daily is an excellent choice.
   B. Her infection is probably viral, reassure her and prescribe decongestants and have her return in 2 to 3 days if she is not better.
   C. You have found that *ampicillin* 250 mg four times daily works well and warn her about yeast infections.
   D. Order sinus films, which show normal findings. Reassure her and prescribe heat and decongestants.

3. A 45-year-old obese woman (5 ft 4 in., 290 lb) presents with blood pressures of 140/100 mm Hg and 146/98 mm Hg in the past 3 months. Her physical examination is unremarkable and she does not smoke or have a family history of coronary artery disease. You then do the following:

   A. Perform a basic laboratory work up (complete blood count [CBC]; urinalysis; electrocardiogram [ECG]; sodium, creatinine, and fasting glucose levels; and lipid profile) and prescribe weight loss and exercise therapy for 6 months.
   B. Perform a basic laboratory work up (CBC; urinalysis; ECG; sodium, creatinine, and fasting glucose levels; and lipid profile) and begin a diuretic.
   C. Perform a basic laboratory work up (CBC; urinalysis; ECG; sodium, creatinine, and fasting glucose levels; and lipid profile), and begin an angiotensin converting enzyme (ACE) inhibitor.
   D. Counsel her on the health consequences of her obesity and begin a thiazide diuretic.

4. Certain hypertensive agents in nonpregnant individuals are more useful in specific conditions. Which of the following has not been proven to have a beneficial effect?

   A. ACE inhibitors in diabetics.
   B. β-Blockers with coexisting coronary artery disease.
   C. Calcium channel blockers with heart failure.
   D. β-Blockers with migraine headaches.

5. A 58-year-old woman on hormone replacement therapy who is a nonsmoker presents with a family history of premature cardiovascular deaths. Recently, she had her lipid profile done, which revealed

   Total cholesterol: 270 mg/L
   Triglycerides: 110 mg/L

Low-density lipoprotein (LDL) cholesterol 210 mg/L
High-density lipoprotein (HDL) cholesterol 45 mg/L

She has been on a low cholesterol diet (step 2) for 6 months. Her workup for secondary dyslipidemia is unrevealing and her liver function tests are normal. You recommend

A. She has several risk factors and that she should start on a "statin" drug (lovastatin, pravastatin, or simvastatin).

B. She should be tried on a step 2 diet (<7% saturated fats as a percentage of total calories and <200 mg cholesterol daily) for an additional 2 to 3 months and have her lipid profile repeated.

C. She should attempt to get her LDL-cholesterol lowered by exercise and moderate alcohol consumption.

D. She should be started on nicotinic acid at a dosage of 500 mg four times daily.

6. A 31-year-old woman presents with a family history of coronary artery disease. Her grandmother and grandfather both died in their late 70s with myocardial infarctions. Both her parents are in their 50s with no problems. She does not smoke or drink alcohol. Her lipid profile is as follows:

Total cholesterol:	230 mg/dL
Triglycerides:	115 mg/dL
LDL:	130 mg/dL
HDL:	50 mg/dL

You recommend

A. She should be started on drug therapy immediately.

B. She needs to start drug therapy in addition to lifestyle changes.

C. She is at no higher risk of coronary heart disease and should have her cholesterol checked every 3 to 5 years and maintain a healthy lifestyle.

D. She is at higher risk for coronary heart disease because of her family history. Therefore, because her LDL is elevated she should start taking a "statin" drug.

7. The diagnosis of diabetes mellitus can be determined by the following:

A. A random blood glucose level of 180 mg/dL in an individual with signs and symptoms of diabetes mellitus.

B. A single fasting blood glucose of more than 140 mg/dL on two separate occasions.

C. A single fasting blood glucose of more than 136 mg/dL on two separate occasions.

D. A single fasting blood glucose of more than 126 mg/dL on two separate occasions.

8. What are the recommended clinical practice guidelines for nonpregnant adults with diabetes mellitus?

A. Hemaglobin 1Ac yearly

B. Yearly urinalysis for microalbuminuria

C. Dilated retinal eye examination every 4 months

D. Comprehensive foot examination every 2 years

9. A 32-year-old woman sees you for a check-up. She was diagnosed with hypothyroidism in her early 20s and has been on replacement therapy (0.15 mg of *levothyroxine* daily) since then. She has had no complaints but asks you during your assessment whether she is getting adequate therapy. You then

A. Tell her that the dose she is taking is probably adequate (1.6 μg/kg), especially because she feels well.

B. Draw thyrotropin and T$_4$ levels, which reveal a thyrotropin of 10 μU/mL (0.4–6 μU/mL [normal ranges]) and T$_4$ of 0.2 ng/dL (0.7–1.8 ng/dL). Reassure her these results are normal.

C. Draw thyrotropin and T$_4$ levels, which reveal a thyrotropin of 10 μU/mL (0.4–6 μU/mL) and T$_4$ of 0.2 ng/dL (0.7–1.8 ng/dL). Increase her dose to 0.175 mg daily and check her levels in a week.

D. Draw thyrotropin and T$_4$ levels, which reveal a thyrotropin of 10 μU/mL (0.4–6 μU/mL) and T$_4$ of 0.2 ng/dL (0.7–1.8 ng/dL). Increase her dose to 0.2 mg daily and check her levels in 6 weeks.

E. Draw thyrotropin and T$_4$ levels, which reveal a thyrotropin of less than 1.0 μU/mL (0.4–6 μU/ml) and a T$_4$ level of 13 ng/dL (0.7–1.8 ng/dL). Reassure her that these results are normal.

Answers

1. B

Pneumonia in patients who are 60 years or younger without coexisting conditions like heart disease, lung disease, liver disease, renal failure, or other comorbid medical illnesses and who do not appear toxic may be treated with a *macrolide* or *doxycycline* as an outpatient with close follow-up.
Reference: Pages 200–201

2. B

The five clinical findings of maxillary toothache, poor response to nasal decongestants, abnormal transillumination, and a colored discharge by history or physical examination are the most useful in the diagnosis of acute sinusitis. When none of these findings is present, the diagnosis is highly unlikely and antibiotic therapy is not warranted. Systemic decongestants help to shrink the obstructive ostia, promote sinus drainage and ventilation, and possibly prevent the development of an acute maxillary bacterial sinusitis. Initial episodes of sinusitis do not require imaging studies and therapy is usually empiric. When persistent sinus infections occur, studies and referral are indicated.
Reference: Pages 197–199

3. A

Diagnosis and management of hypertension are based on the classification of blood pressure readings (Table 9.5) and the risk-group stratification (Table 9.6). Certain laboratory tests and procedures are recommended in the initial evaluation of uncomplicated hypertension (Table 9.4). For patients with stage 1 hypertension and in risk

Table 9.5. Blood Pressure Classification (Adults 18 years and Older)

Category	Systolic BP (mm Hg)	Diastolic BP (mm Hg)
Optimal	<120	<80
Normal	<130	<85
High normal	130–139	85–89
Hypertension	—	—
Stage 1	140–159	90–99
Stage 2	160–179	100–109
Stage 3	≥180	≥110

BP, blood pressure.
Adapted from *The Sixth Report of the Joint National Committee on Prevention, Detection, Evaluation, and Treatment of High Blood Pressure (JNC VI).* Bethesda, MD: National Institutes of Health, National Heart, Lung, and Blood Institute; 1997; NIH publication 99-4080.

Table 9.6. JNC Blood Pressure Risk Group Stratification

Risk Group A: No major risk factors and no target-organ damage or clinical cardiovascular disease.

Risk Group B: At least one major risk factor, not including diabetes; no target-organ damage or clinical cardiovascular disease.

Risk Group C: Any target-organ damage, clinical cardiovascular disease, or diabetes, with or without other risk factors.

JNC, Joint National Commission.
Adapted from The Sixth Report of the Joint National Committee on Prevention, Detection, Evaluation, and Treatment of High Blood Pressure (JNC VI). Bethesda, MD: National Institutes of Health, National Heart, Lung, and Blood Institute; 1997; NIH publication 99-4080.

Table 9.4. Laboratory Tests and Procedures Recommended in the Evaluation of Uncomplicated Hypertension[a]

Urinalysis

Complete blood count

Potassium, sodium, creatinine

Fasting glucose

Total cholesterol, high-density lipoprotein cholesterol

12-lead electrocardiogram

[a]If any of the above are abnormal, consultation or referral to an internist is indicated.
Adapted from The Sixth Report of the Joint National Committee on Prevention, Detection, Evaluation, and Treatment of High Blood Pressure (JNC VI). Bethesda, MD: National Institutes of Health, National Heart, Lung, and Blood Institute; 1997; NIH publication 99-4080.

Figure 9.2 Algorithm for the treatment of uncomplicated hypertension. (From The Sixth Report of the Joint National Committee on Prevention, Detection, Evaluation, and Treatment of High Blood Pressure (JNC VI). Bethesda, MD.: National Institutes of Health, National Heart, Lung, and Blood Institute; 1997. NIH publication 99-4080. See Table 9.6 for definitions of risk groups A, B, and C.)

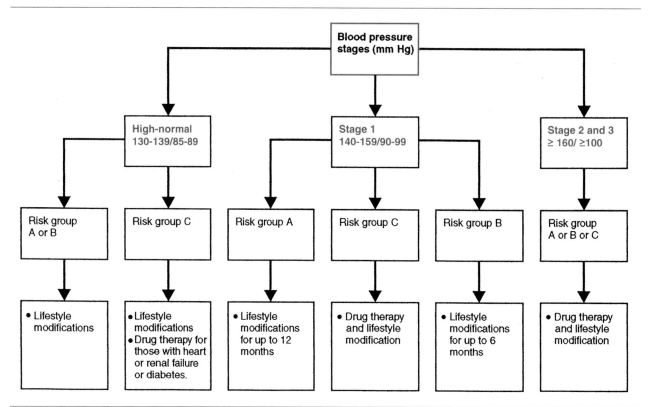

group B (at least one major risk factor not including diabetes and have no target-organ damage or clinical cardiovascular disease) lifestyle modifications should be attempted for up to 6 months before initiating drug therapy.
Reference: Figure 9.2; Pages 203–206

4. **C**

Calcium channel blockers are not recommended for use in patients with heart failure from left ventricular failure. Certain drugs in this class can worsen the systolic dysfunction. Angiotensin converting enzyme inhibitors have fewer adverse effects on glucose homeostasis and are the preferred drug in patients with diabetic nephropathy. β-Blockers without intrinsic sympathomimetic activity have been shown to reduce the risk for subsequent myocardial infarctions or sudden cardiac death in patients with coronary artery disease. In addition, β-blockers can decrease the frequency of recurrent migraine headaches.
Reference: Pages 207–210

5. **A**

Patients with two or more risk factors should aim for LDL cholesterol below 130 mg/dL. If the LDL remains greater or equal to 130 mg/dL after 3 months of therapeutic lifestyle changes, drug therapy should be initiated. While *nicotinic acid* will help lower the LDL, the side effects and frequency of dosing preclude it from being a first-line drug for this patient.
Reference: Figure 9.4; Pages 211–217

Figure 9.4   Treatment decisions based on the low-density lipoprotein cholesterol. (Adapted from the Second Report of the National Cholesterol Education Program (NCEP) Expert Panel on the Detection, Evaluation, and Treatment of High Blood Cholesterol in Adults. *JAMA* 1993; 269:3015–3023.)

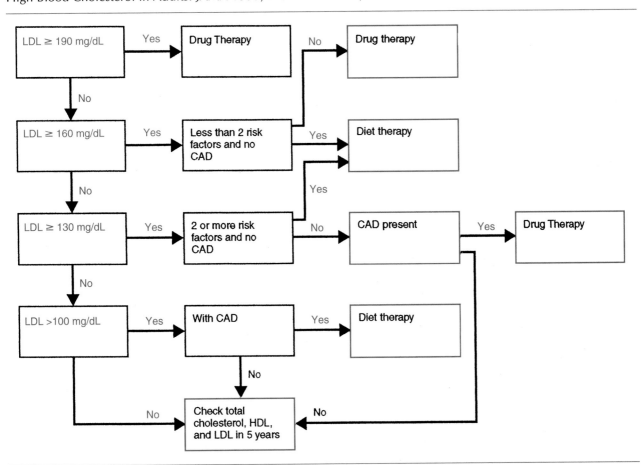

6. C

In young adults with zero to one risk factors and an LDL cholesterol below 160 mg/dL, a lipid profile may be repeated in 5 years. There is no indication to start drug therapy although therapeutic lifestyle changes may be encouraged. A grandmother and grandfather with a history of coronary heart disease are not considered risk factors because they are not first-degree relatives.
Reference: Pages 214–218

7. D

There are three methods available to diagnose diabetes mellitus in nonpregnant adults. A single fasting blood glucose greater or equal to 126 mg/dL on two separate occasions or a random blood glucose greater or equal to 200 mg/dL in someone with symptoms of diabetes (polydipsia, polyuria, polyphagia, or weight loss). A 2-hour oral glucose tolerance test may also be used but is more cumbersome to perform.
Reference: Pages 218–222

8. B

The recommended clinical practice guidelines for nonpregnant adults with diabetes mellitus are yearly urine analysis for microalbuminuria, Hg1Ac every 3 months if

---

Table 9.10. Physician Guidelines in the Therapy of Diabetes Mellitus

- Establish diagnosis and classify type of diabetes mellitus (DM).

- The oral glucose tolerance test (OGTT) is not recommended for routine clinical use because of its higher cost, time requirement, and limited reproducibility.

- Initiate diabetes education classes to learn blood glucose monitoring and diabetic medications, to learn signs and symptoms and complications, and to learn how to manage sick days.

- Place patient on ADA diet with appropriate caloric, sodium, and lipid restrictions.

- Establish cardiac risk factors, evaluate for baseline kidney function (serum creatinine, urine for microalbuminuria).

- If neuropathy is present, refer to a neurologist.

- Establish extent of funduscopic lesion (refer to ophthalmologist as needed).

- Check feet and toenails at each visit.

- Patient to use finger-stick blood glucose for daily diabetic control.

- Follow chronic glycemic control by HbA_{1c} every 2 to 3 months in the office.

- Initial general health evaluation should consist of a complete history and physical examination and the following laboratory tests: CBC with differential, chemistry profile, fasting lipid profile, urinalysis, thyroid function tests, urine for microalbuminuria and ECG (baseline at age 40 or older, repeat yearly).

- Oral hypoglycemic agents (OHA) like the sulfonylureas may be considered if fasting blood glucose does not decline or increase, if the patient has had diabetes for less than 10 years, does not have severe hepatic or renal disease, and is not pregnant or allergic to sulfa drugs.

- While on oral hypoglycemic agents, check the HbA_{1c} every 3 months.

- If the HbA_{1c} is <7% or the postprandial glucose is <200 mg/dl, omit the oral hypoglycemic agents, place on diet therapy alone, and follow every 3 months.

- If the fasting serum glucose is >200 mg/dl consistently or the HbA_{1c} is over 10%, consider starting insulin and referring the patient to an internist.

- Administer the flu vaccine every fall and the pneumococcal vaccine every 6 years.

ADA, American Diabetic Association; HgA_{1c}, hemoglobin A_{1c}; CBC, complete blood count; ECG, electrocardiogram; FSG, fasting serum glucose.
Adapted from The Expert Committee on the Diagnosis and Classification of Diabetes Mellitus. Report of the Expert Committee on the Diagnosis and Classification of Diabetes Mellitus. *Diabetes Care* 2000;23: S4–S42.

uncontrolled, yearly dilated retinal examination by an ophthalmologist, and a yearly comprehensive foot exam.
Reference: Table 9.10; Page 221

9. **D**

The only way to determine if a patient is taking an adequate amount of thyroid replacement therapy is to measure the thyrotropin and T_4. A low thyrotropin and high T_4 level indicates hyperthyroidism and the dosage must be decreased because of the risk of atrial fibrillation, cardiac hypertrophy, and decreased bone mineral density. The dose of thyroxine in hypothyroidism should be adjusted at 6- to 8-week intervals after measuring the thyrotropin and T_4.
Reference: Pages 222–225

10 Family Planning

Phillip G. Stubblefield

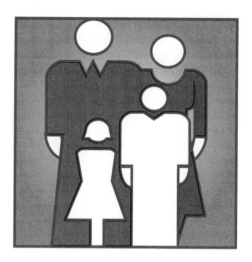

Learning Objectives

1. Describe the pattern of use of fertility control methods in the United States.

2. Discuss the mechanism of action contraceptive methods.

3. Describe the efficacy of contraceptive methods under best-results and usual-results conditions.

4. List the health risks of each method and describe the evidence.

5. List the health benefits of each and describe the evidence.

6. Describe the common methods for inducing legal abortion, their complications, and prevention and management of complications.

7. Describe male and female methods of sterilization and their complications.

8. Be able to adequately counsel couples as to choice of and method of use of contraception, abortion, and sterilization.

Questions

Match the type of intrauterine device (IUD) to the statement. Each statement may have more than one correct answer.

A. *ParaGard (Copper T380A)*
B. *Progestasert* (T with natural *progesterone*)
C. *Mirena (levonorgestrel T)*

1. U.S. Food and Drug Administration (FDA)–approved for 10 years:

2. Must be replaced every year:

3. Blocks ovulation in some women:

4. Pregnancy rates are less than 0.2 per 100 women years:

5. Pregnancy rates are about 3 per 100 women years:

6. Is an effective treatment for menorrhagia and has replaced hysterectomy for some women:

7. May increase the risk for ectopic pregnancy:

8. Reduces the risk of ectopic pregnancy by 80% to 90%:

Which are true statements about oral contraceptives (OCs) and vascular disease?

9. The apparent increase in risk of thrombosis with combination OCs containing the new progestins may be the result of several types of bias and not real risk.

10. The most common identifiable predisposing factor to venous thrombosis in a white population is antithrombin III deficiency.

11. Risk for myocardial infarction (MI) is increased for users of low-dose OCs even after adjusting for age, illness, smoking, ethnicity and body habitus.

12. Benefits of combination OCs include: reduced risk for ovarian cancer, reduced risk for endometrial cancer, and reduced risk for cervical cancer.

13. Your 25-year-old patient, G2P1, presents with last menstrual period 7 weeks ago. She has a *Progestasert* IUD that she has worn for 3 years with no problem. She wants to continue the pregnancy. What should you do?

    A. Reassure her that problems from the IUD are not likely, because it has been in place 3 years with no trouble.
    B. If the strings are visible, discuss the alternatives with her, but suggest removal of the IUD at this visit immediately.
    C. Advise frequent visits, reporting of any pain, bleeding or fever, and allow the pregnancy to continue with the IUD in place.
    D. Strongly recommend termination of the pregnancy because of the high risk for infection.

14. Your healthy 23-year-old patient, G1P1, is in her third month of contraception with *depomedroxyprogesterone acetate (DMPA)*. She reports spotting and staining almost every day. Your plan?

    A. Suggest she discontinue this form of contraception immediately.

    B. Reassure her that this is very common, that the abnormal bleeding usually subsides over time, though it may take many months and offer her short-term treatment with a low dose of estrogen.

    C. Perform laboratory tests for gonorrhea and *Chlamydia*.

    D. Perform a pregnancy test.

15. It is 1:00 a.m. Your 18-year-old patient just paged you to report that she was making love around 4 p.m., the condom broke, and she is so worried she cannot sleep. She is using no other contraceptive now, but she used *Levlen,* a combination oral contraceptive containing *levonorgestrel* and *ethinyl estradiol,* until 6 months ago. Her last menstrual period started 12 days ago. What is the best advice you can give her?

    A. She should wait and see if she missed a period and then come in for a pregnancy test.

    B. She should see you in the office tomorrow afternoon for a pregnancy test, an examination, and a discussion of emergency contraception.

    C. If she still has some *Levlen* tablets, she should take four right now and four more 12 hours later.

    D. You will call a prescription to her pharmacy for Plan B (*levonorgestrel*) tomorrow morning. She should pick up the prescription and immediately take one tablet, then one more 12 hours later.

Which of these statements about female tubal sterilization are true?

16. The pregnancy rate increases almost fourfold if fewer than three sites are coagulated on each tube.

17. Pregnancy after bipolar sterilization is usually not ectopic.

18. The Hulka clip appears to have a higher pregnancy rate than the tubal ring or the Filshie clip.

19. Having had a tubal sterilization procedure has no effect on risk for developing ovarian cancer later.

20. Which statement is a correct comparison of maternal mortality risk from legal abortion in the United States to maternal mortality from childbirth.

    A. Abortion is always more dangerous for the mother.

    B. The death rate from legal abortion in the United States is about 4 per 100,000 abortions while the death rate from childbirth is about 8 per 100,000 live births.

    C. The death rate from legal abortion in the United States is less than 1 per 100,000 abortions while the death rate from childbirth is about 8 per 100,000 live births.

    D. The death rate from legal abortion in the United States 30 per 100,000 abortions while the death rate from childbirth is about 50 per 100,000 live births.

Answers

1. A

See discussion under Question 8.

2. B

See discussion under Question 8.

3. C

See discussion under Question 8.

4. A and C

See discussion under Question 8.

5. B

See discussion under Question 8.

6. C

See discussion under Question 8.

7. B

See discussion under Question 8.

8. A and C

IUDs are very important worldwide but play a minor role in contraception for the U.S. population because of a fear of infection that is no longer justified. The high-dose copper IUD sold in the Unites States (*TCU380,* or ParaGard) provides safe, long-term contraception with an effectiveness equivalent to tubal sterilization. Three IUDs are now in use in the United States. These are the *Copper T380A (ParaGard),* the progesterone-releasing T (*Progestasert*), and the *levonorgestrel*-releasing T (*Mirena*). The *Copper T380A* has bands of copper on the cross-arms of the T in addition to copper wire around the stem, providing a total surface area of 380 mm of copper, almost double the surface area of copper of earlier copper devices (see Fig. 10.6). The *Copper T380A* is approved for up to 10 years of continuous use. The *Progestasert* must be replaced every year. The *Mirena* (see Fig 10.7) is approved in the United States for 5 years, although studies through 7 years show no loss of efficacy.

IUDs cause the formation of a "biologic foam" within the uterine cavity that contains strands of fibrin, phagocytic cells, and proteolytic enzymes. Copper IUDs continuously release a small amount of the metal, producing an even greater inflammatory response. All IUDs stimulate the formation of prostaglandins within the uterus, consistent with both smooth muscle contraction and inflammation. Scanning electron microscopy studies of the endometrium of women wearing IUDs show alterations in the surface morphology of cells, especially of the microvilli of ciliated cells. There are major alterations in the composition of proteins within the uterine cavity, and new proteins and proteinase inhibitors are found in washings from the uterus. The altered intrauterine environment interferes with sperm passage through the uterus, preventing fertilization. The natural progesterone in the Progestasert induces endometrial atrophy. The levonorgestrel in the Mirena is much more potent than natural progesterone. Blood levels of the hormone are about half that seen with the *levonorgestrel* subdermal implant (*Norplant*), and are sufficient to block ovulation in many women.

The IUD is not an abortifacient. The contraceptive effectiveness does not depend on interference with implantation, although this phenomenon also occurs and is the basis for using copper IUDs for emergency contraception. Sperm can be obtained via laparoscopy in washings from the fallopian tubes of control women at midcycle, whereas no sperm are present in the tubal washings from women wearing IUDs. Ova flushed from the tubes at tubal sterilization showed no evidence of fertilization in women wearing IUDs, and studies of serum β-human chorionic gonadotropin (β-hCG) do not indicate pregnancy in women wearing IUDs.

The *Copper T380A* and the *levonorgestrel T* have remarkably low pregnancy rates, less than 0.2 per 100 women-years. Total pregnancies over a 7-year period were only 1.1 per 100 for the *levonorgestrel T* and 1.4 for the *Copper T380A* in a comparative study. Twelve-year data for the *Copper T380A* showed a cumulative pregnancy rate of only 1.9 per 100 women. The *Progestasert* has a higher failure rate, about 3 per 100 women per year.

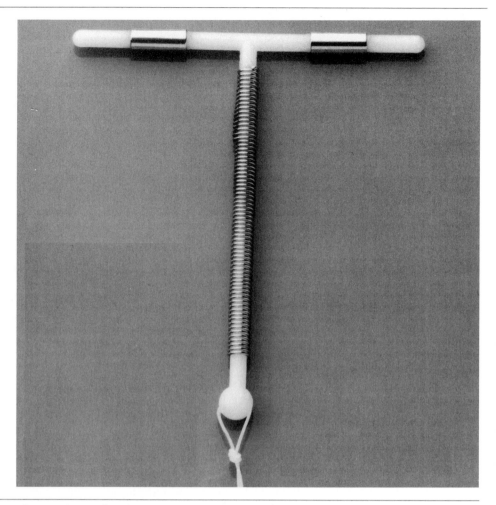

Figure 10.6   The Copper T380A (ParaGard) intrauterine device. (From Gynopharma, Inc., with permission.)

Modern IUDs provide excellent contraception, independent of coitus, without continued effort by the user. Both the *ParaGard* and the *Mirena* protect against ectopic pregnancy (see below). The *Progestasert* and *Mirena,* by releasing progesterone or levonorgestrel, reduced menstrual bleeding and cramping. The *Mirena* has been used extensively to treat heavy menstrual bleeding and is used in Europe and the United Kingdom as an alternative to hysterectomy for menorrhagia.

The Women's Health study found the *Dalkon Shield* device (now withdrawn from the market) to increase the risk of pelvic inflammatory disease (PID) by eightfold when women hospitalized for PID were compared to control women hospitalized for other illnesses. In contrast, risk from the other IUDs was markedly less: relative risk (RR) of PID was 2.2 for the *Progestasert;* 1.9 for the *Copper 7;* 1.3 for the *Saf-T-Coil;* and 1.2 for the *Lippes Loop.* Increased risk was detectable only within 4 months of insertion of the IUD. A larger, prospective World Health Organization (WHO) study revealed that PID increased only during the first 20 days after insertion. Thereafter, the rate of diagnosis of PID was about 1.6 cases per 1000 women per year, the same as in the general population.

Exposure to sexually transmitted pathogens is a more important determinant of PID than the wearing of an IUD. In the Women's Health Study, women who were currently married or cohabiting and who said they had only one sexual partner in the past 6 months had no increase in PID. In contrast, previously married or single women had marginal

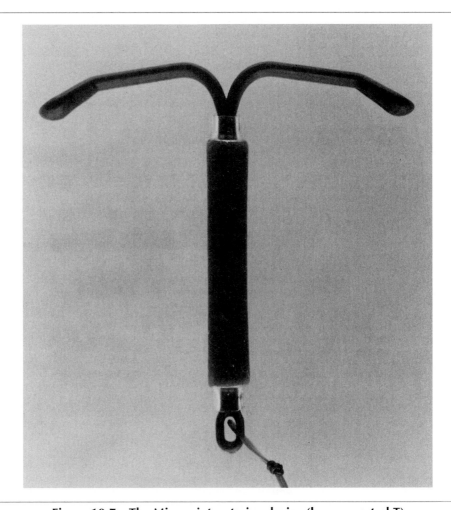

Figure 10.7   The Mirena intrauterine device (levonorgestrel T).

increase in risk, even though they had only one partner in the previous 6 months. The only pelvic infection that has been unequivocally related to IUDs is actinomycosis. It appears that PID with actinomycosis has been reported only in women wearing IUDs. Rates of colonization with actinomycosis increase with duration of use for plastic devices but appear to be much less for copper-releasing IUDs.

When PID is suspected in an IUD-wearing woman, the IUD should be immediately removed, appropriate cultures should be taken, and high-dose antibiotic therapy should be started. Pelvic abscess should be suspected and ruled out by ultrasound examination.

If pregnancy occurs in an IUD wearer, it will be ectopic in about 5% of cases. This is because the fallopian tubes are less well protected against pregnancy than the uterus. Compared with women using no contraception, however, women wearing either the *Copper T380A* or the *levonorgestrel T* have an 80% to 90% reduction in the risk of ectopic pregnancy, which is a greater reduction than that seen for users of barrier methods. Women using OCs have a 90% reduction of risk. In contrast, the *Progestasert* increases risk slightly, probably because the progesterone affects tubal motility and does not inhibit ovulation. Rossing and colleagues reported an increased risk for ectopic among past users of older IUDs, but the study did not include the current higher dose copper IUD (*ParaGard*) or the *levonorgestrel T (Mirena)*.

Case-control studies of infertile women in the United States have revealed that a history of IUD use is associated with a twofold increase in the risk of tubal infertility. The risk

applies to methods other than the copper IUD, for which there is no increased risk. Risk was not increased among women who reported only one sexual partner. The Oxford Study found that women gave birth just as promptly after IUD removal as they did after discontinuing use of the diaphragm.
Reference: Pages 242–247

9. True

Several studies have found a modest increased risk of venous thrombosis when users of OCs containing new progestins, *desogestrel,* or *gestodene* were compared to users of older progestins. Physiologically this was hard to understand because the estrogen and its dose are the same, and a 1993 review of *desogestrel*-containing OCs found only minimal changes in coagulation and fibrinolysis. Lewis and colleagues concluded that the biases "attrition of susceptibles" and "adverse selection" explain the apparent increase in thrombosis. Most cases of venous thrombosis attributable to OCs occur during the initial months of use. Hence, comparing new users to women already on OCs for some time without incident will demonstrate an apparent increase with the new product that is artificial. Also, physicians may presume that newer drugs are safer, and prescribe them selectively for women with risk factors. Analysis of data from a large European study of thrombosis with different OCs has shown that apparent risk of thrombosis was least for the first low dose pills introduced and greatest for those recently introduced, even though the newest pill had the lowest estrogen dose (see Figure 10.11).
Reference: Pages 247–249

10. False

The most common identifiable factor in a white population is factor V Leiden. Women with inherited deficiencies of antithrombin III, protein C, or protein S are at very high

Figure 10.11   Risk ratios of oral contraceptives for thrombosis by year of market introduction for women aged 25 to 44 years. LNG, levonorgestrel with 30 μg ethinyl estradiol; GES, gestodene with 30 μg ethinyl estradiol; NORG, norgestimate with 35 μg of ethinyl estradiol; DES20, desogestrel with 20 μg of ethinyl estradiol. (From **Lewis MA, Heinemann LAJ, MacRae KD, et al.** The increased risk of venous thrombosis and the use of third generation progestagens: role of bias in observational research. *Contraception* 1996;54:5–13, with permission.)

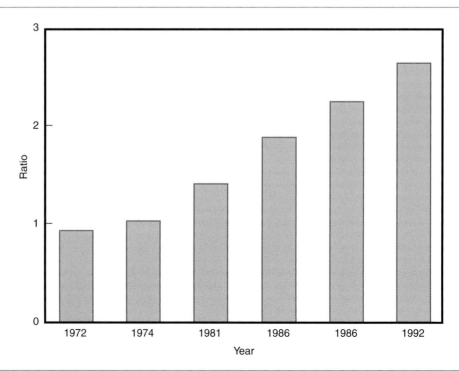

risk for thrombosis with pregnancy or estrogen therapy, but they make up a very small proportion of potential OC users. A much more common variation has been identified, factor V Leiden. This genetic variation exists in 3% to 5% of the white population. It codes for a one amino acid mutation in the factor V protein, inhibiting cleavage of the protein by activated protein C, an essential step in maintaining the balance between coagulation and fibrinolysis. A study of risk for a first thromboembolic episode among women using OCs found it to be 2.2 per 10,000 women years for women without the factor V mutation and 27.7 per 10,000 women years for women with the mutation. For women homozygous or heterozygous for factor V Leiden who do not use OCs, the risk is estimated to be 4.9 per 10,000 women years. The effect of estrogen dose was not examined. Cigarette smoking did not affect this risk. There are pronounced ethnic differences in the presence of this mutation. The Leiden allele is found in 5% of whites, but is rare in Africans, Asians, Amerindians, Inuits, and Polynesians. A similar mutation is found in the prothrombin gene at position 20210, and is described as prothrombin G20210A. It is found in 3% of a European population, and is strongly associated with venous thrombosis on OCs.
Reference: Pages 250–253

11. **False**

In a large U.S. study, no risk for MI was found after adjustment for these factors. A very large U.S. study confirms the safety of OCs as currently prescribed. One hundred eighty-seven women, aged 15 to 44 years, with confirmed MI were identified during 3.6 million women-years of observation in the Kaiser Permanente Medical Care Program in California between 1991 and 1994, a rate of 3.2 per 100,000 women-years. Nearly all current users took OCs with less than 50 mcg of *ethinyl estradiol*. After adjusting for age, illness, smoking, ethnicity and body mass index, risk of MI was **not** increased (odds ratio [OR], 1.14; 95% confidence interval [CI], 0.27–4.72). Sixty-one percent of heart attack victims were smokers; only 7.7% were current OC users. In a later study, the same investigators pooled results from the California study with a similar study from Washington State. The results were the same. Current users of low dose OCs had no increased risk for MI, after adjustment for major risk factors and sociodemographic factors. That past use of OCs does not increase risk for MI later is already clearly established.
Reference: Pages 253–254

12. **False**

OC use has not been found to decrease cervical cancer risk, and may increase risk. Combination OCs reduce the risk for subsequent endometrial cancer and ovarian cancer. A recent study found that as little as 1 year of OC use was protective (OR, 0.57; 95% CI, 0.87–1.03) and continued use reduced risk by 7% per year. Benefit persisted for 15 years after last use, with little diminution. A 50% reduction in ovarian cancer risk was observed for women who took OCs for 3 to 4 years, and an 80% reduction was seen with 10 or more years of use. There was some benefit from as little as 3 to 11 months of use. The benefit continues for at least 15 years since last use, and it does not diminish even at 15 years from use. National vital statistics data from England support these observations. Ovarian cancer mortality is declining in England and Wales for women younger than 55 years of age, and this decline has been attributed to OC use. Use of OCs after 1980 when low dose pills predominated provides protection equivalent to older, higher dose OCs.

There may be a weak association between OC use and squamous cancer of the cervix. Important risk factors are early sexual intercourse and exposure to human papilloma virus (HPV). Women who have used OCs typically started sexual relations at younger ages than women who have not used OCs and, in some studies, report more partners. This is the same pattern of behavior that increases one's chance of acquiring sexually transmitted HPV, the most important risk factor for cervical cancer. Because barrier contraceptives reduce risk for cervical cancer, use of alternatives for contraception can compound the difficulty in establishing an association with OC use alone. Presence of HPV types 16 or 18 is associated with a 50-fold increase in risk for preneoplastic lesions of the cervix. If a woman already has HPV, OCs produces no further increase in her risk for cervical neoplasia, but among women who are HPV-negative, OC use doubles the risk of having such a lesions. This apparent adverse effect could be explained entirely by OC users being less likely to use barrier contraception. Adenocarcinomas of the cervix are rare, but they are not as easily detected as other lesions by screening cervical cytology and the incidence appears to be increasing. A 1994 study found a doubling of risk of adenocarcinoma with OC use that increased with duration of use, reaching a RR of 4.4 if total use of OCs exceeded 12 years. This study adjusted for history of genital warts, number of sexual partners, and age at first intercourse. Because adenocarcinoma of the cervix is rare, absolute risk is low. If this apparent association is real, the cumulative risk of long-term OC use to 55 years of age would be about one in 1000 patients. Use of OCs is, at most, a minor factor in causation of cervical cancer; however, women who have used OCs should have annual Papanicolaou (Pap) tests. To reduce risk, women who are not in monogamous relationships should be advised to use barriers in addition to hormonal contraception. Reference: Pages 255–257

13. B

A woman who presents with an IUD in place and amenorrhea should have a pregnancy test and physical examination. If an intrauterine pregnancy is diagnosed and the IUD strings are visible, the IUD should be removed as soon as possible in order to prevent later septic abortion, premature rupture of the membranes, and premature birth. Reference: Page 246

14. B

DMPA, a suspension of microcrystals of a synthetic progestin, was approved for contraception in 1992. A single 150-mg intramuscular dose will suppress ovulation in most women for 14 weeks or longer. The regimen of 150 mg every 3 months is highly effective, producing pregnancy rates of approximately 0.3 per 100 women per year. Probably because of the high blood levels of the progestin, efficacy appears not to be reduced by administration of other drugs and is not dependent on the patient's weight. Women treated with *DMPA* experience disruption of the menstrual cycle and have initial spotting and bleeding at irregular intervals. Eventually, total amenorrhea develops in most women who take *DMPA;* with continued administration, amenorrhea develops in 50% of women by 1 year and in 80% by 3 years (see Fig. 10.14). Treat persistent irregular bleeding by adding low-dose estrogen temporarily; for example, conjugated estrogens, 1.25 mg per day, can be given for 10 to 21 days at a time. *DMPA* persists in the body for several months in women who have used it for long-term contraception and return to fertility may be delayed; however, in a large study, 70% of former users desiring pregnancy had conceived within 12 months and 90% conceived within 24 months. Reference: Pages 263–265

15. C or D

Plan B was found more effective than the Yuzpe method for emergency contraception in the large WHO trial; however, both work better the sooner they are taken. If the patient can start the *Levlen* right now, it may work as well as starting Plan B 10 to 12 hours from now.

High-dose estrogen was largely replaced the combination of *ethinyl estradiol* 0.200 mg and *dl-norgestrel* 2 mg (two *Ovral* tablets followed by two more 12 hours later) as first described by Yuzpe. The average pregnancy rate with this method is 1.8% but is 1.2% if treatment is started within 12 hours of intercourse. Nausea and vomiting are common with both regimens and an antiemetic is usually prescribed. A comparable dosing of *ethinyl estradiol* and *levonorgestrel* is provided by taking four tablets of *LoOvral, Nordette, Levlen, Triphasil* or *TriLevlen,* or 5 tablets of *Allese,* instead of two tablets of *Ovral.* A kit containing four tablets, each containing 0.050 mg of *ethinyl*

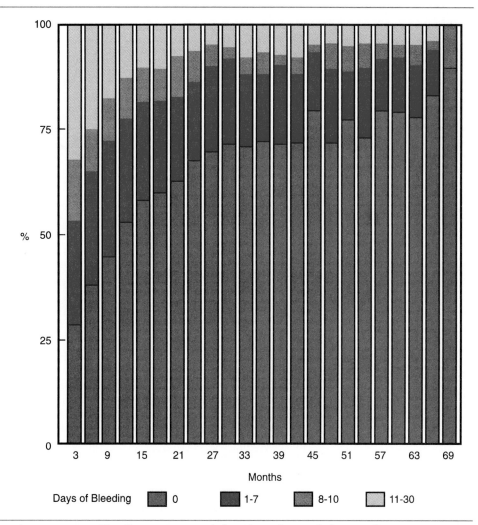

Figure 10.14   Bleeding pattern and duration of use of *depomedroxyprogesterone acetate (DMPA)*: percent of women who have bleeding, spotting, or amenorrhea while taking DMPA 150 mg every 3 months. (From **Schwallie PC, Assenzo JR.** Contraceptive use-efficacy study utilizing *medroxyprogesterone acetate* administered as an intramuscular injection once every 90 days. *Fertil Steril* 1973;24:331, with permission.)

estradiol and 0.250 mg of *levonorgestrel* is marketed in the United States under the name Preven specifically for emergency contraception.

A new and better alternative is *levonorgestrel* alone, 0.75 mg initially, followed by 0.75 mg 12 hours later. This preparation is sold in the United States as Plan B. The WHO carried out a randomized trial with 1998 women assigned to the Yuzpe method or to *levonorgestrel* alone, started within 72 hours of intercourse. The pregnancy rate was 3.2% with the Yuzpe method, and only 1.1% with *levonorgestrel* alone (RR for pregnancy, 0.32; CI, 0.18–0.70). Nausea and vomiting was much less with *levonorgestrel* alone (23.1% vs. 50.5% and 5.6% vs. 18.8%) (190). The efficacy of both methods declines as time increases since intercourse. However, even at 49 to 72 hours, the pregnancy rate with the *levonorgestrel* treatment was only 2.7% and it is likely that considerable efficacy would be found beyond 72 hours (see Fig. 10.15). Because of greater efficacy and less nausea, *levonorgestrel* alone appears to be the best hormonal method for emergency contraception currently available in the U.S. Reference: Pages 267–268

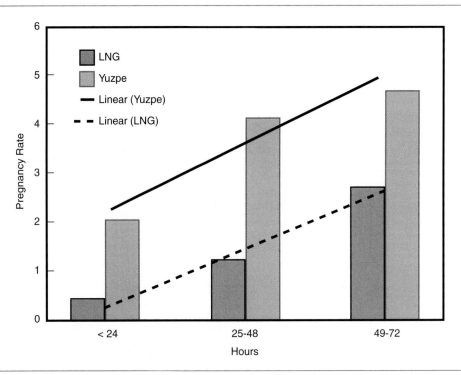

Figure 10.15 Emergency contraception: pregnancy rates by treatment group and time since unprotected coitus. LNG, levonorgestrel 0.75 mg × 2; Yuzpe method, *ethinyl estradiol* 0.100 mg + *levonorgestrel* 0.50 mg × 2, 12 hours later. (From Task Force on Postovulatory Methods of Fertility Regulation. *Lancet* 1998;352: 430, with permission.)

16. True

An important later analysis of the Center for Disease Control and Prevention's Collaborative Review of Sterilization (CREST) data found that bipolar sterilization could have a very low long-term failure rate if an adequate portion of the tube is coagulated. CREST study subjects who were sterilized with bipolar electrosurgery from 1985 to 1987 had lower failure rates than those sterilized earlier (1978–1985). The important difference was in the technique of application of the electric energy to the tubes. Women whose bipolar procedure involved coagulation at three sites or more had low 5-year failure rates (3.2 per 1,000 procedures) while women who had fewer than three sites of tubal coagulation had a 5-year failure rate of 12.9 per 1,000 ($P = .01$). Reference: Pages 274–275

17. False

Failures of the Falope ring, or the clips generally result from misapplication, and pregnancy, if it occurs, is usually intrauterine. Pregnancy after bipolar sterilization may occur from tuboperitoneal fistula and is ectopic in more than 50% of cases. Reference: Pages 274–275

18. True

The *Filshe clip* and the *Hulka clip* were compared in two trials. A total of 2,126 women were studied. 878 had either clip placed by minilaparotomy and 1,248 had either clip placed by laparoscopy and were then evaluated at up to 24 months after the procedure. Pregnancy rates were 1.1 per 1,000 women with the *Filshie clip* and 6.9 per 1,000 with the *Hulka clip* at 12 months, a difference in rates that was close to statistical significance ($P = .06$). This same group compared the *Filshie clip* to the silastic tubal ring in a similar study of 2,746 women. Nine hundred fifteen had the devices placed at minilaparotomy and 1,831 had laparoscopy. Pregnancy rates at 12 months were the same for the *Filshie clip* and the tubal ring: 1.7 per 1,000 women.

Table 10.12. Death to Case Rates for Legal Abortion Mortality by Weeks of Gestation, United States, 1972–1987

Weeks of Gestation	Deaths	Abortions	Rate[a]	Relative Risk
≤8	33	8,673,759	0.4	1.0
9–10	39	4,847,321	0.8	2.1
11–12	33	2,360,768	1.4	3.7
13–15	28	962,185	2.9	7.7
16–20	74	794,093	9.3	24.5
≥21	21	175,395	12.0	31.5

[a] Legal abortion deaths per 100,000 procedures; excludes deaths from ectopic pregnancies or pregnancy with gestation length unknown.
From **Lawson HW, Frye A, Atrash HK, et al.** Abortion mortality, United States, 1972–1987. *Am J Obstet Gynecol* 1994;171:1365–1372, with permission.

The ring was judged more difficult to apply, but three women spontaneously expelled the *Filshie clip* during the 12 months of follow-up.
Reference: Pages 274–275

19. False

In addition to providing excellent contraception, tubal ligation is associated with reduced risk for ovarian cancer that persists for as long as 20 years after surgery.
Reference: Page 274

20. C

The risk of death from legal abortion was 0.7 per 100,000 induced abortions in 1996. In contrast, total maternal mortality is approximately 7 to 8 per 100,000 live births. The risk of death from legal abortion prior to 16 weeks is tenfold less than that from continuing the pregnancy on to delivery. As shown in Table 10.12, the risk of death increases with gestational age.
Reference: Pages 276–278

11 Sexuality, Sexual Dysfunction, and Sexual Assault

David A. Baram

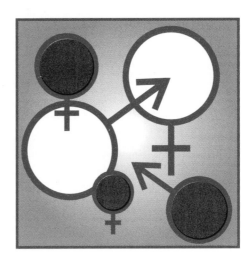

Learning Objectives

1. Understand the rationale for and barriers to obtaining an adequate sexual history.

2. Be able to identify the variations in sexual practices of men and women.

3. Understand the sexual response cycle in women.

4. Enumerate the factors affecting sexual response.

5. Understand the types and causes of sexual dysfunction.

6. Be able to evaluate and treat sexual assault in children and adults.

Questions

1. Compared to the sexual response cycle in women, the unique feature of the sexual response cycle in men is the presence of the

   A. Desire phase
   B. Arousal phase
   C. Plateau phase
   D. Resolution phase
   E. Refractory phase

2. Vaginal lubrication formed during the arousal phase of the sexual response cycle in women comes from the

   A. Bartholin glands
   B. Skene glands
   C. Transudate from the walls of the vagina
   D. Cervix
   E. Periurethral glands

3. Correct statements regarding the effect of aging on sexuality in women include each of the following **except**

   A. Vaginal lubrication in older women takes longer to appear.
   B. Orgasmic contractions in older women are less intense and less frequent.
   C. Frequency of intercourse decreases as women age.
   D. Older women are more likely to experience dyspareunia.
   E. Women lose interest in sex at an earlier age than men.

4. A 27-year-old woman has never been able to insert a tampon or have a pelvic examination. She has no difficulty becoming sexually aroused. She is orgasmic, but has never been able to have intercourse. When she and her partner attempt intercourse, she becomes anxious and experiences involuntary spasmodic contractions of the muscles surrounding her introitus. This conditions is known as

   A. Vaginismus
   B. Dyspareunia
   C. Inhibited sexual desire
   D. Phobic avoidance of sex
   E. Impaired arousal

5. Adult survivors of childhood sexual abuse, when compared to women who have not been sexually abused, are at increased risk for each of the following conditions **except**

   A. Depression
   B. Eating disorders
   C. Schizophrenia
   D. Sexual dysfunction
   E. Chronic pelvic pain

6. A woman who has been raped is most likely to have been raped by

   A. A stranger
   B. Her teacher
   C. An acquaintance
   D. Her minister
   E. Her husband

7. A 25-year-old woman presents to the emergency department 5 hours after she was sexually assaulted. The assailant ejaculated in her vagina. Which of the following antibiotic regimens would be most effective in treating this patient for sexually transmitted diseases (STDs) that may have been acquired during the assault?

A. *Ampicillin, metronidazole,* and *doxycycline*
B. *Metronidazole* and *doxycycline*
C. *Ceftriaxonek, metronidazole,* and *azithromycin*
D. *Ampicillin, metronidazole,* and *doxycycline*
E. *Ceftriaxone sodium* and *metronidazole*

8. A 20-year-old woman presents to her family physician 30 hours after she was sexually assaulted. The assailant ejaculated in her vagina. She uses no birth control. Her last menstrual period started 2 weeks ago. The most appropriate way to prevent pregnancy in this patient is to

A. Insert a copper-containing intrauterine device
B. Administer a tablet containing 0.75 mg of *levonorgestrel* followed by a second tablet 12 hours later
C. Administer of two tablets of a combination oral contraceptive containing 0.05 mg of *ethinyl estradiol* and 0.5 mg of *norgestrel*
D. Administer *depomedroxyprogesterone acetate (DMPA)*
E. Administer *misoprostol* suppositories

9. The percentage of women who will be raped during their lifetime is

A. 1%
B. 3%
C. 13%
D. 20%
E. 25%

10. Each of the following medications interferes with sexual functioning **except**

A. Antihypertensives
B. Antidepressants
C. Oral contraceptives
D. Antihistamines
E. Antidiabetic agents

11. The best predictor of sexual functioning and satisfaction following surgery for breast cancer is

A. The type of mastectomy
B. Precancer sexual functioning
C. The presence or absence of metastatic disease
D. The size of the scar
E. The degree of postsurgical pain

12. A woman presenting with the recent onset of inhibited sexual desire should have which of the following laboratory tests performed?

A. Thyrotropin and prolactin
B. Thyrotropin and testosterone
C. Testosterone and prolactin
D. Estrogen and follicle-stimulating hormone (FSH)
E. FSH and prolactin

13. A 52-year-old woman noted the recent onset of hot flashes and dyspareunia. Her last menstrual period was 6 months ago. Which of the following is the most likely cause of her dyspareunia?

    A. Vulvar vestibulitis
    B. Bacterial vaginosis
    C. Atrophic vaginitis
    D. Infected Bartholin gland
    E. Episiotomy scar

Answers

1. E

Orgasm is a myotonic response mediated by the sympathetic nervous system and is experienced as a sudden release of the tension that has built up during the arousal and plateau stages. Orgasm is the most intensely pleasurable of the sexual sensations. Orgasm consists of multiple (3–15) 0.8-second reflex rhythmic contractions of the muscles surrounding the vagina, perineum, anus, and orgasmic platform. Many women who are orgasmic prefer to have orgasms before intercourse, during the time when clitoral stimulation is most intense. Unlike men, who are relatively unresponsive to sexual stimulation after orgasm (refractory period), women are potentially multiorgasmic and capable of experiencing more than one orgasm during a single sexual cycle. Thus, they can experience orgasms both before and during intercourse, provided enough clitoral stimulation is provided.
Reference: Pages 297–299

2. C

The arousal phase is mediated by the parasympathetic nervous system and is characterized by erotic feelings and the appearance of vaginal lubrication. Sexual arousal increases blood flow to the vagina, and the resulting vasocongestion and possible changes in capillary permeability create a condition that increases the capillary filtration fraction. The filtered capillary fluid transudates between the intercellular spaces of the vaginal epithelium causing droplets of fluid to form on the walls of the vagina.
Reference: Pages 297–299

3. E (see Tables 11.1 and 11.2)

Aging and the cessation of ovarian function accompanying menopause has a significant effect on the sexual response cycle of women. Sexual desire and the frequency of intercourse decrease as women age, although women retain interest in sex and continue to have the potential for sexual pleasure for their entire lives. The need for closeness, love, and intimacy does not change with age. The way women function sexually as they grow older is largely dependent on partner availability and how frequently they had sex and how much they enjoyed sex when they were younger. Anatomic changes that accompany aging include reduced vaginal size, thinning and decreased elasticity of the vaginal walls, shrinkage of the labia majora and thinning of the labia minora, decreased clitoral sensitivity and size, reduced perineal muscle tone, and a thinner orgasmic platform. Breast atrophy, decreased breast engorgement during arousal, and sensory changes in the nipple and areola are also noted. These physiologic changes predispose women to more frequent episodes of vulvovaginitis and urinary tract infections, which, along with decreased vaginal lubrication, may cause dyspareunia. As they age, women require more time to become sexually aroused, take longer to lubricate, produce less vaginal lubrication, have less intense orgasms, and need more stimulation to become orgasmic. The ability to have orgasms does not change significantly with aging, but older women are less likely to be multiorgasmic. Interestingly, women who remain coitally active after menopause have less vulvar and vaginal atrophy than abstinent women.
Reference: Pages 299–300

Table 11.1. Anatomic Changes of Aging

Reduced pubic hair
Loss of fat and subcutaneous tissue from the mons pubis
Reduced vaginal size
Thinning of vaginal walls
Decreased elasticity of vaginal walls
Shrinkage of the labia majora
Thinning of the labia minora
Decreased clitoral sensitivity
Decreased clitoral size
Reduced uterine size
Cervical atrophy
Reduced ovarian size and weight
Reduced perineal muscle tone
Thinner orgasmic platform
Breast atrophy
Decreased breast engorgement during arousal
Sensory changes in the nipple and areola

From **Meston CM.** Aging and sexuality. *West J Med* 1997;167:285–290, with permission.

4. A

Vaginismus is the recurrent or persistent involuntary contraction of the perineal muscles surrounding the outer third of the vagina when vaginal penetration with a penis, finger, tampon, or speculum is attempted. Vaginismus is an involuntary reflex precipitated by real or imagined attempts at vaginal penetration and can be *global* (the woman is unable to place anything inside her vagina) or *situational* (she is able to use a tampon and can tolerate a pelvic examination but cannot have intercourse). Many women with vaginismus have normal sexual desire, experience vaginal lubrication, and are orgasmic but are unable to have intercourse. Vaginismus can be *primary* (the woman has never been able to have intercourse) or *secondary* (often due to acquired dyspareunia). Some couples may cope with this situation for years before they decide to seek help. They usually seek treatment because they desire children or decide they would like

Table 11.2. Sexual Physiology—Effects of Aging

Decreased sexual desire
Increased time required to become sexually aroused
Longer time needed to lubricate
Production of less vaginal lubrication
Less intense orgasms
Increased need for stimulation to become orgasmic
No change in the ability to have orgasms
Less likely to be multiorgasmic

From **Mooradian AD, Greiff V.** Sexuality in older women. *Arch Intern Med* 1990;150:1033–1038, with permission.

to consummate their relationship. Vaginismus is relatively rare, affecting approximately 1% of women.
Reference: Pages 307–308

5. C

Women who have been sexually abused as children or sexually assaulted as adults often experience sexual dysfunction and difficulty with intimate relationships and parenting. Compared with women who have not been sexually assaulted, they are more likely to experience depression, chronic anxiety, anger, substance abuse problems, multiple personality disorder, borderline personality disorder, fatigue, low self-esteem, feelings of guilt, and sleep disturbance. They often experience social isolation, phobias, and feelings of vulnerability and loss of control. Survivors of sexual assault represent a disproportionate number of patients with chronic headaches and chronic pelvic pain. They may develop posttraumatic stress disorder and are more likely to commit suicide. The cognitive sequelae include flashbacks, nightmares, disturbances in perception, and dissociative experiences. These women may not be able to tolerate pelvic examinations and may avoid seeking routine gynecologic care, yet they are more likely to utilize the medical care system for nongynecologic concerns. They are at greater risk for being overweight and for having gastrointestinal disturbances.
Reference: Pages 310–312

6. C (see Table 11.5)

There are many myths about rape. Perhaps the most common is that women are raped by strangers. In fact, only about 20% to 25% of women are raped by someone they do not know. Most women are raped by a relative or acquaintance (9% by husbands or ex-husbands, 11% by father or stepfather, 10% by boyfriend or ex-boyfriend, 16% by other relatives, and 29% by other nonrelative). Although acquaintance rape may seem to be less traumatic than stranger rape, survivors of acquaintance rape often take longer to recover.
Reference: Pages 312–314

7. C (see Table 11.6)

The risk of acquiring an STD is difficult to assess, because the prevalence of preexisting sexually transmitted diseases is high (43%) in rape survivors. STD prophylaxis should be offered to all survivors and should cover infections with *Neisseria gonorrhoeae, Chlamydia trachomatis, Trichomonas,* and incubating syphilis. Current recommendations include (a) *ceftriaxone sodium* 125 mg intramuscularly (if allergic to *cephalosporins, spectinomycin* 2 mg intramuscularly or *ciprofloxacin* 500 mg orally may be used), (b) *metronidazole* 2 g orally, and (c) *azithromycin* 1 g orally or *doxycycline* 100 mg orally twice a day for 7 days.
Reference: Page 314

Table 11.5. Physician Responsibilities in Treating Sexual Assault Survivors

1. Obtaining an accurate gynecologic history, including a recording of the sexual assault

2. Assessing, documenting, and treating physical injuries

3. Obtaining appropriate cultures (including samples for forensic tests), treating any existing infection, and providing prophylaxis for sexually transmitted diseases

4. Providing therapy to prevent unwanted pregnancy

5. Providing counseling for the patient and her partner and/or family

6. Arranging for follow-up medical care and counseling

7. Reporting to legal authorities as required by state law

From **American College of Obstetricians and Gynecologists.** *Sexual assault. Technical bulletin.* Washington, DC: ACOG, 1997:242, with permission.

Table 11.6. Laboratory Studies in the Evaluation of Sexually Assaulted Adults

Cultures of the cervix, mouth, and rectum for:

   Neisseria gonorrhoeae

   Chlamydia trachomatis

   Herpes simplex

Serologic test for syphilis

Wet prep for trichomonas

Hepatitis B surface antigen

Human immunodeficiency virus antibody

Pregnancy test

8. B

Approximately 5% of fertile rape survivors will become pregnant. Options include (a) awaiting the next expected menses, (b) repeating the serum pregnancy test in 1 to 2 weeks, and (c) emergency contraception. If the patient desires emergency contraception, a preexisting pregnancy can usually be ruled out by performing a sensitive human chorionic gonadotropin assay. Pregnancy prophylaxis is best provided by the immediate administration of one tablet containing 0.75 mg of *levonorgestel* followed by a second tablet of *levonorgestrel* 12 hours later (Plan B). Other regimens for emergency contraception include (a) combination oral contraceptives (two tablets, each containing 0.05 mg of *ethinyl estradiol* and 0.5 mg *norgestrel* [i.e., *Ovral* birth control pills], followed by two more tablets 12 hours later or four tablets of a combination birth control pill containing 0.035 mg of *ethinyl estradiol* and a progesterone followed by 4 more tablets 12 hours later); (b) placement of a copper-containing intrauterine device; or (c) *mifepristone* as a single 600-mg dose. These regimens will be most effective if administered within 72 hours after the sexual assault. Some investigators believe that emergency contraception can be effective up to 5 days after unprotected intercourse. Some patients experience nausea and vomiting when given combination oral contraceptives for emergency contraception. Nausea can be controlled with an antiemetic agent like *promethazine hydrochloride,* 12.5 mg every 4 to 6 hours. Emergency contraception has a small failure rate (about 1%) and potential teratogenicity, which should be discussed with the patient.

9. C

The National Women's Study provides the best statistics about the incidence of forcible rape in the United States. This study found that 13%, or one of eight adult women, are survivors of at least one completed rape during their lifetime. Of the women they surveyed, 0.7% had been raped in the past year, equating to an estimated 683,000 adult women who were raped during a 12-month period. Thirty-nine percent of the women they surveyed were raped more than once. Most disturbing, however, is their finding that most rapes occurred during childhood and adolescence, with 29% of all forcible rapes occurring when the survivor was younger than 11 years, and 32% occurring between the ages of 11 and 17. Indeed, rape in the United States is a tragedy of youth. Twenty-two percent of rapes occurred between the ages of 18 and 24, 7% between the ages of 25 and 29, and only 6% when the survivor was older than 30.

10. E (see Table 11.3)

Drugs that interfere with sexual functioning include the following:

- Antihypertensives
- Thiazide diuretics
- Antidepressants

Table 11.3. Drugs that Can Interfere with Sexual Functioning

Antihypertensives
Thiazide diuretics
Antidepressants
Lithium
Antipsychotics
Antihistamines
Barbiturates
Narcotics
Benzodiazepines
Hallucinogens
Amphetamines
Cocaine
Oral contraceptives
Anticonvulsants
Cimetidine
Danazol
Digoxin
Levodopa

- *Lithium*
- Antipsychotics
- Antihistamines
- Barbiturates
- Narcotics
- Benzodiazepines
- Hallucinogens
- Amphetamines
- *Cocaine*
- Oral contraceptives
- Anticonvulsants
- *Cimetidine*
- *Digoxin*
- *Danocrine*

Reference: Pages 301–302

11. B

Breast cancer diagnosis and treatment affect women's sexuality. However, most women cope well with the stress of treatment and do not develop major psychiatric disorders or significant sexual dysfunction. A number of studies have compared women who undergo mastectomies to women who have conservative surgery with breast conservation, and have found little difference between the two groups in postoperative marital satisfaction, psychological adjustment, frequency of sex, or incidence of sexual dysfunction. The frequency of breast stimulation with sexual activity does decrease after mastectomy. Women who undergo lumpectomy have more positive feelings about their bodies, especially their appearance in the nude, than do women who have mastectomies. The strongest predictor of postcancer sexual satisfaction is not the extent of

Table 11.4. Assessment of Dyspareunia

Behavior: Faulty technique

Affect: Guilt, anger, fear, and shame

Sensation: Where is the pain?

Imagery: Do intrusive thoughts or negative images disrupt sexual enjoyment?

Cognition: Are there dysfunctional beliefs or misinformation that play a role in undermining sexual participation?

Interpersonal: How do the partners communicate and relate in both sexual and nonsexual settings?

Drugs: Is the patient on any medication that would diminish vaginal lubrication?

From **Lazarus AA.** Dyspareunia: a multimodal psychotherapeutic perspective. In: **Leiblum SR, Rosen RC,** eds. *Principles and practice of sex therapy,* 2nd ed. New York: The Guilford Press, 1989:89–112, with permission.

surgery but rather the woman's overall psychological health, relationship satisfaction, and precancer sexual functioning.
Reference: Pages 301–302

12. C

Physiologic causes of hypoactive sexual desire include medications, chronic medical illnesses, depression, stress, substance abuse, aging, and hormonal alterations. Any patient presenting with the recent onset of a desire phase disorder should have serum testosterone and prolactin titers evaluated, because an elevated prolactin titer (from a pituitary adenoma) or a low testosterone titer (noted with aging and following natural or surgical menopause) could be responsible.
Reference: Pages 305–306

13. C (see Table 11.4)

Causes of pain on stimulation of the external genitalia include chronic vulvitis and clitoral irritation and hypersensitivity. Pain at the introitus caused by penile entry can be caused by a rigid hymenal ring, scar tissue in an episiotomy repair, a müllerian abnormality, vaginitis caused by one of the many common vaginal pathogens such as *Candida, Trichomonas,* or *Gardnerella,* or by irritation from over-the-counter vaginal sprays, douches, or contraceptive devices. Vaginal infection is one of the most common causes of successfully treated dyspareunia in premenopausal women. Another common cause of dyspareunia is friction due to inadequate sexual arousal. This can be treated by counseling the couple to spend more time with foreplay, ensuring that the woman has adequate lubrication before intercourse. Use of a water-soluble lubricant such as KY Jelly is also helpful. Vaginal atrophy resulting from hypoestrogenic states (menopause and lactation) can be treated with systemic or vaginal estrogen replacement.
Reference: Pages 308–310

12 Common Psychiatric Problems

Nada L. Stotland

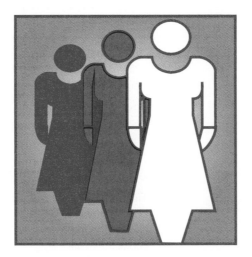

Learning Objectives

1. Be able to identify the indications and techniques of psychiatric referral.

2. Be able to identify the signs and symptoms of depression.

3. Understand the pitfalls in the diagnosis and treatment of premenstrual dysphoria.

4. Recognize the characteristics and dangers of anorexia nervosa.

Questions

1. Gynecologists' attitudes toward gender issues are clinically significant because

   A. Patients select physicians on the basis of gender
   B. Patients demand to know whether their physicians have gender prejudices
   C. They can lead to misdiagnosis
   D. Patients' and physicians' attitudes should be congruent

2. Compared with psychiatric diagnostic systems used in the past, *the Diagnostic and Statistical Manual of Mental Disorders, Fourth Edition (DSM-IV)*:

   A. Contains more diagnostic options
   B. Is based on laboratory evidence
   C. Describes a diagnosis for every person
   D. Is comparable in accuracy to other medical diagnoses

3. A psychiatric referral should be explained on the basis of

   A. The patient's signs and symptoms
   B. Danger to self or others
   C. Negative workup
   D. Personality traits

4. The expertise that distinguishes social workers from other mental health professionals is

   A. Testing cognitive function
   B. Performing psychotherapy
   C. Talking to patients' families
   D. Identifying social resources

5. Patients with manic depression, also called bipolar illness, often resist treatment because

   A. They enjoy the hypomanic state.
   B. They fear antidepressant treatment.
   C. Their relatives discourage it.
   D. It is too time-consuming.

6. A common reason women discontinue treatment with selective serotonin reuptake inhibitors is (SSRIs)

   A. Weight gain
   B. Anticholinergic side effects
   C. Lack of efficacy
   D. Sedation

7. The diagnosis of premenstrual dysphoric disorder requires

   A. First ruling out a diagnosis of depression
   B. A decrease in circulating premenstrual hormone levels
   C. A trial of lifestyle changes
   D. Two months of prospective daily mood ratings

8. SSRIs differ from other antidepressants in

   A. Efficacy in clinical use
   B. Efficacy in research studies
   C. Onset of action
   D. In-class interchangeability

9. Panic attacks are most frequently confused with which general medical condition?

   A. Thyroid storm
   B. Pituitary adenoma
   C. Adrenal hyperplasia
   D. Myocardial infarction

10. The major risk associated with the use of benzodiazepines is

   A. Fatal overdose
   B. Drug–drug interactions
   C. Oversedation
   D. Drug dependence

11. The somatizing disorder characterized by preoccupation with a conviction one is ill is

   A. Hypochondria
   B. Malingering
   C. Conversion
   D. Pain disorder

Answers

1. C
Few patients have either the interest or the assertiveness to demand information about their physicians' attitudes toward men and women, and few medical encounters allow time for this kind of discussion. Some patients have preferences about the genders of their physicians, but this preference is not directly related to the physicians' attitudes about genders. The attitudes of physicians are by no means determined by gender alone; those attitudes are significantly affected by individual experiences, circumstances, and training. Neither is it necessary for a gynecologist's attitudes to be the same as a patient's. It is not realistic to expect that kind of congruence, nor would it be possible for each physician and patient to explain his or her attitudes to one another. There is evidence, however, that physicians who believe that women report symptoms more readily than men have failed to diagnose serious conditions in female patients.
Reference: Pages 323–324

2. D
Although no psychiatric diagnoses can be made on the basis of laboratory findings alone, the *DSM-IV* criteria for each diagnosis are as valid and reliable as those of diagnostic algorithms in other areas of medicine. Because each illness is described in terms of specific signs and symptoms, duration, and effects on the patient's life, there are fewer, not more, options for the diagnostician than when diagnostic process was driven by each clinician's interpretation of the unconscious meaning of the patient's behaviors and feelings and their derivation from childhood experience. The belief that mental health professionals have a diagnostic label for every individual, whether symptomatic or not, if ever true, is not accurate today.
Reference: Pages 323–324

3. A
The social stigma against psychiatric illnesses and psychiatrists makes some gynecologists feel awkward about referring a patient to a psychiatrist. They fear patients may be insulted or wounded. Not having had specialty mental health training, they are not sure how to present the suggestion. A mental health referral should not be explained as an avenue of last resort, when all tests and examinations have failed to reveal a gynecologic diagnosis underlying a patient's somatic symptoms. Such a referral conveys to the

patient the idea that the gynecologist does not believe her symptoms are real, or finds her a bother, and does not wish to care for her in the future. Referrals are not made on the basis of personality traits alone. Although very occasionally a patient may present to a gynecologist in the midst of a suicidal or homicidal episode, it is certainly not wise to wait until things become that serious for the patient with depression, anxiety, or multiple somatic symptoms in many organ systems. A psychiatrist should never be called in before the patient has been informed and has agreed, unless there is a life-threatening psychiatric emergency. Even in that case, the patient should be informed.

Psychiatric referral is made on the basis of the patient's signs and symptoms, and explained to her in just those terms. The gynecologist expresses concern about the patient's nervousness, sleep problems, poor mood, or loss of concentration and pleasure. For patients with multiple unexplained somatic symptoms in several organ systems, the referral can be based on the distress caused by these unexplained symptoms, not on a conclusion that they must have a psychological basis. When the gynecologist has articulated the signs and symptoms that are apparent to both physician and patient, he or she can add that there is a member of the medical team who specializes in those problems. The gynecologist should make it clear that he or she intends to follow the patient through the psychiatric consultation and treatment, if indicated.
Reference: Pages 324–326

4. D

Among mental health professionals, it is nearly always Ph.D.-level psychologists who are trained to administer and interpret psychological tests, including tests of cognitive function. All mental health practitioners should be prepared to discuss issues with patients' families. Training in psychotherapy varies not only among, but also within, mental health disciplines. Although an intensive psychotherapy program is required in psychiatric residency training, and knowledge about it is required for psychiatric board examinations, some training programs emphasize psychopharmacology and some psychiatrists specialize in pharmacologic treatment. Social workers may choose various concentrations during their 2 years of master's-level training; these concentrations include social policy and may be very weak in psychotherapy training. However, social workers in a clinical setting should be prepared to provide information and some degree of practical help for patients and their families in need of social support systems including support groups and assistance with housing, employment, or child care problems.
Reference: Pages 326–327

5. A

Hypomania, which generally precedes a full-blown manic episode, is characterized by a sense of self-confidence, increased energy, decreased need for sleep, and decreased appetite. All of these experiences are highly prized by many women, and, in fact, envied by their friends and colleagues. Their families, on the other hand, after the ramifications of the diagnosis are clear, desperately want the patients to be treated so that the dire consequences of mania and depression do not recur. The depressive episodes are aversive to the patient; patients in the depressed state will generally accept treatment willingly. Treatment for manic depression is not particularly time-consuming; finding the effective medication or combination of medications can be a challenge, and concomitant psychotherapy to help patients cope with their disease is useful, but taking the time for treatment is seldom, if ever, a barrier to care.
Reference: Page 327

6. A

Anticholinergic side effects are a major problem for elderly patients and others taking other medication with similar side effects. The lack of anticholinergic side effects is a major advantage of SSRIs over tricyclic antidepressants. Although patients do need to be counseled about the need to allow 3 to 4 weeks for SSRIs to take effect, rates of symptom relief are high. The common side effects of SSRIs include headache, anxiety, tremor, and gastrointestinal upset—either diarrhea or constipation. These side effects generally dissipate within a few days; residual tremor is not clinically significant.

A given patient may react differently to each SSRI; these effects are not predictable upon first use. Recurrences are best treated with an agent that has been successful in the past. There is a spectrum of relatively calming to relatively activating effects, with *paroxetine hydrochloride* most calming and *fluoxetine hydrochloride* most activating. Although effects may be idiosyncratic, these generalizations are useful as a guide for the clinician choosing an SSRI for patients on the basis of the most prominent manifestations of their depressions: anxiety/agitation or exhaustion/loss of energy. Many women fear weight gain so much that they are willing to give up an effective medication. Data about the relationship between SSRIs and weight gain are mixed. It is impossible to rule out the effect of increased appetite and food intake caused by the relief of depression in the studies in which modest weight gain was noted.
Reference: Pages 331–333

7. D

Premenstrual dysphoric disorder (PMDD) is a condition still under study that is estimated to affect 3% to 5% of menstruating women. Unlike premenstrual syndrome, a catchall term to which over 100 signs and symptoms have been attributed, PMDD is defined as a constellation of mood symptoms very similar to those of depression, including irritability, which peak before the menstrual period and cease within hours after the onset of bleeding. Patients must be symptom-free for part of the month. Although PMDD is said to interfere significantly with a woman's domestic relationships and effectiveness at work, convincing evidence of disability, especially in the workplace, is lacking.

The diagnosis of PMDD is complicated by the fact that most women who seek care for premenstrual symptoms turn out, after completing prospective daily mood ratings, to have symptoms unrelated to the menstrual cycle. The belief in premenstrual morbidity is so strong in our culture that there is a strong tendency to attribute any mood and behavioral symptoms to premenstrual syndrome or PMDD. The problem is complicated by social expectations that women suppress anger and social realities, including the stresses of poverty, domestic violence, and responsibility for dependent children and disabled adult relatives while engaging in paid employment. In addition, because of the stigma of mental illness, many women fail to recognize or accept the fact that they have clinical depression. It is much more acceptable to blame symptoms on "hormones." It is crucial, therefore, that patients complete two cycles of prospective daily mood ratings, entered on a different calendar than they use to record their menstrual cycles, before the condition is diagnosed. It is possible to have both depression and PMDD; in this case, the diagnosis is best expressed as "depression with premenstrual exacerbation." The gynecologist should reassure patients that the 2 months of record keeping, while it may delay treatment, ensure that treatment is based on an accurate diagnosis.
Reference: Page 329

8. A

No antidepressant has been demonstrated in scientific studies to be more efficacious than another in relieving depressive signs and symptoms. Onset of action is 2 to 3 weeks for all antidepressants. The advantages of SSRIs over older preparations become apparent in actual clinical use, where the once-a-day dosing schedule and relatively milder side effects result in greater patient compliance and the relative lack of anticholinergic side effects make them safer to use with elderly patients and those on other medications. Monoamine oxidase inhibitors require strict dietary limitations and can cause hypertensive crises. Tricyclic antidepressants are extremely dangerous in overdose; therefore, their use in patients who are or who may become suicidal must be intensely supervised. SSRIs are not fatal even in very large doses, including a month or more's supply of medication.

Although all antidepressants, including SSRIs, are equally effective in clinical trials, there is considerable variability in their effectiveness in individual patients. They have different side effects, and even those side effects vary from patient to patient. Some are more activating (*fluoxetine hydrochloride*) and some more sedating (*paroxetine hydrochloride*). Despite manufacturers' claims, there is no SSRI currently on the market that does not have a high incidence of sexual side effects, including decreased libido and interference with orgasm. SSRIs have different half-lives, a factor significant for patients who occasionally forget a dose, run out of medication, or discontinue treatment without tapering. Lastly, for unknown reasons, many patients respond to one SSRI and not to another. This may be related to the fact that they affect neurotransmitters in different proportions. It is generally advisable to treat a patient with an agent to which she has responded in the past or one to which a close family member has responded.
Reference: Pages 331–333

9. D

The signs and symptoms of panic disorder closely resemble those of a myocardial infarction. The patient experiences an overwhelming terror, without a reasonable precipitant, and symptoms including palpitations, diaphoresis, trembling, shortness of breath, a choking sensation, and chest pain. Unlike myocardial infarctions, however, panic attacks are most common in otherwise healthy young women. In contrast with cardiovascular or endocrine disease, each attack lasts approximately 15 minutes and then resolves. The chronic complications are behavioral, not somatic; the patient becomes preoccupied with fear of having more attacks and begins to constrict her activities in hopes of avoiding any imagined precipitant and situations in which the attack will be noticed by other people. She wants to remain close to an environment in which she feels safe, such as her home, and may avoid travel in which return to home is restricted, such as taking airplanes or driving over a bridge or through a tunnel where traffic may jam, trapping her in her car.

Although patients who have panic attacks can also have endocrine and cardiovascular disease—and there is a documented tendency for women's cardiovascular events to be underdiagnosed—extensive workups are rarely necessary if a complete history is taken and the above characteristics are reported. Not only can costly and time-consuming laboratory studies be avoided, but specific and effective treatment for the panic disorder can then be initiated.
Reference: Pages 335–336

10. D

Although patients may attempt to use them in suicide gestures or attempts, benzodiazepines are not highly dangerous in overdose. It is not a good idea to mix them with alcohol or other central nervous system depressants, but drug–drug interactions are not a major problem. Patients who take more than the suggested dose can become groggy, but oversedation is not a major problem. The major risk of benzodiazepines is dependence, both psychological and physical. Patients require higher and higher doses to achieve the same therapeutic effect. They may try to alleviate any anxiety that occurs in the course of ordinary living with a medication rather than mastering and using other self-soothing techniques such as concentrating on an absorbing task, taking a warm bath, calling a friend, or exercising. Benzodiazepines should not be an automatic therapeutic response to a patient's difficult situation and the natural emotions it provokes, such as when a pregnancy is lost. On the other hand, fear of these longer-term effects should not deter the physician from prescribing benzodiazepines for the short-term, such as 1 to 5 days, for a patient in an inordinately stressful, time-limited situation.
Reference: Pages 337–338

11. A

Somatizing disorders are those in which emotional conflicts are expressed through physical symptoms. Conversion is the modern term for what used to be called hysteria. Conversion causes paralysis or anesthesia of one or more limbs, or loss of a special sense: hearing or sight. In pain disorder, medically unexplained pain is the sole symptom. In neither of these disorders is the patient aware of the psychogenic origin of her symptoms or using them to attain some tangible end. The malingerer, on the other hand, deliberately presents symptoms solely for clear personal benefit, such as relief from military duty, release from prison, or obtaining a large damage award in court. Secondary gain accrues to any disease, whether medically defined or not; disease entitles a patient to extra attention, physical care, and relief from ordinary duties. Secondary gain can prolong illness in vulnerable patients, but its presence is not a major diagnostic clue to the nature of a somatizing disorder. The hypochondriacal patient is more preoccupied with the sense that she has a serious, possibly fatal, disease, than with the specific symptoms she experiences. She is not reassured by normal findings on physical examinations and medical tests; if one disease is definitively ruled out, she may either persist in her anxiety or become worried about some other condition. She interprets normal bodily sensations as signs of disease.

Reference: Pages 338–341

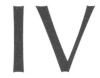

GENERAL GYNECOLOGY

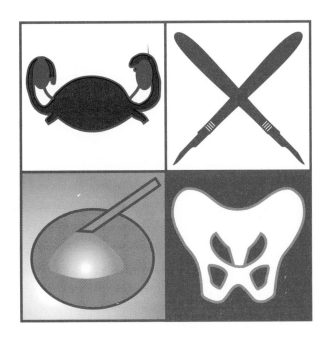

13

Benign Diseases of the Female Reproductive Tract: Symptoms and Signs

Paula A. Hillard

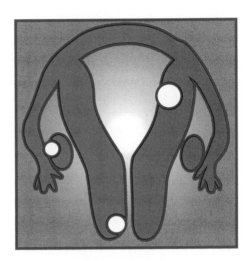

Learning Objectives

1. Be able to state two causes of abnormal bleeding in each of the following age groups: prepubertal girls, adolescents, reproductive age women, perimenopausal women, and postmenopausal women.

2. Be able to state two causes of a pelvic mass in each of the following age groups: prepubertal girls, adolescents, reproductive age women, perimenopausal women, and postmenopausal women.

3. Be able to describe the technique of office endometrial sampling.

4. Be able to describe the technique of office vulvar biopsy.

Questions

1. A 3-year-old girl is brought to the office because of a foul-smelling vaginal discharge. Common causes of this symptom that should be investigated include each of the following **except**

   A. Bacterial infection
   B. Candidal vaginitis
   C. Vaginal foreign body
   D. Sexual abuse

2. A 12-year-old girl is brought to the emergency department because of very heavy vaginal bleeding, with the onset of her first menstrual period. Her hemoglobin level is 9.0 mg/dL. Each of the following diagnoses should be considered **except**

   A. Anovulatory, dysfunctional bleeding
   B. Coagulopathy
   C. Pregnancy
   D. Endometrial polyps
   E. Thyroid dysfunction

3. A 27-year-old woman is found to have a 5-cm, left adnexal mass during a routine pelvic examination. She denies symptoms. She is sexually active, but is not using any method of contraception. Her last menstrual period was 13 days earlier. A urine pregnancy test is negative. The most likely diagnosis is

   A. Follicular cyst
   B. Corpus luteal cyst
   C. Ectopic pregnancy
   D. Pedunculated leiomyoma
   E. Pelvic kidney

4. Which of the following characteristics is considered abnormal in a 14-year-old girl who underwent menarche at age 12?

   A. Cycle length of 38 days
   B. Cycle length of 23 days
   C. Bleeding for 8 days
   D. Blood loss of 65 mL per cycle
   E. Bleeding for 3 days

5. The first line of treatment for cystic glandular hyperplasia is

   A. Hysterectomy
   B. Endometrial ablation
   C. Progestin therapy
   D. Estrogen therapy
   E. Antifibrinolytic therapy

6. A 6-year-old girl comes to your office with lower abdominal pain. Ultrasonography reveals an enlarged ovary on the right side. The most likely diagnosis is

   A. Benign epithelial neoplasm
   B. Malignant germ cell tumor
   C. Benign germ cell tumor
   D. Malignant epithelial neoplasm
   E. Follicular cyst

7. In which of the following situations is surgery for uterine leiomyomata *not* indicated?

   A. Anemia, abnormal uterine bleeding, unresponsive to hormonal management
   B. Asymptomatic, uterus enlarged to 14-week size
   C. Asymptomatic, hydronephrosis on intravenous pyelogram (IVP)
   D. Urinary frequency and a 14-week-size uterus
   E. Prolapsing submucosal myoma

8. A 23-year-old woman presents to your office with a small, raised area on her vulva. You perform a biopsy. The most likely diagnosis is

   A. Epidermal inclusion cyst
   B. Lentigo
   C. Carcinoma *in situ*
   D. Melanocytic nevi
   E. Hidradenoma

Answers

1. B

Vulvovaginitis is the most common gynecologic problem in prepubertal girls. Girls are often unable to adequately describe their symptoms, but parents may notice that the child cries during urination, scratches herself repeatedly, or complains of vague symptoms in the genital area. Consideration should be given to a possible urinary tract infection or pinworms, because these can lead to vulvar symptoms. Chronic skin conditions such as lichen sclerosus can occur in prepubertal girls, but the symptoms are usually vulvar symptoms of itching or burning, rather than a *vaginal* discharge. Vulvovaginal symptoms of any sort in a young child should prompt the consideration of possible sexual abuse. Evaluation should include questioning the child; parents rarely object if an appropriate explanation is given before questioning. If the child answers negatively, the opportunity can be used as a "teachable moment" to ensure that the child knows what she should do if she encounters inappropriate touching. A vaginal discharge in a prepubertal child should be cultured for sexually transmitted diseases (STDs). The most common cause of vaginal discharge in this age group is that of a multibacterial origin due to the presence of perineal organisms, the proximity of the anus to the vaginal introitus, and hormonal factors rendering the hypoestrogenic vagina and vestibule more susceptible to infection. *Candida* vaginitis is uncommon in prepubertal children who are out of diapers. A foreign body may cause a foul-smelling discharge that is persistent in spite of appropriate therapy with topical estrogen cream and a broad-spectrum antibiotic. The most common foreign body is a small piece of toilet paper within the vagina. Irrigation can be performed in the office using a small catheter, flushing small foreign bodies from the vagina.
Reference: Pages 352–355

2. D

Anovulatory cycles are common during the first 1 to 2 gynecologic years. The mechanism relates to a failure of the feedback mechanism in which rising estrogen levels result in a decline of follicle-stimulating hormone (FSH) with subsequent decline of estrogen levels. Thus, estrogen secretion continues, resulting in endometrial proliferation with subsequent unstable growth and incomplete shedding. The clinical result is irregular, prolonged, and heavy bleeding. Dysfunctional bleeding is a diagnosis of exclusion, and testing for other causes of abnormal bleeding should be performed. The possibility of a pregnancy-related complication must be considered when an adolescent presents with abnormal bleeding. A pregnancy test is indicated in all adolescents with excessive bleeding, regardless of her statements about whether she has had intercourse. The medical consequences of failing to diagnose a pregnancy are too severe to risk

missing the diagnosis. Exogenous hormone usage may be a cause of abnormal bleeding and should be excluded by history. In the adolescent age group, the possibility of a hematologic cause of abnormal bleeding must be considered. Several studies have shown that coagulopathies such as von Willebrand's disease or idiopathic thrombocytopenic purpura (ITP) may be causative, particularly in the youngest age group or those presenting at menarche. Patients who present with menorrhagia have been found to have a higher incidence of STDs, and subclinical endometritis may be causative. Structural lesions such as endometrial polyps or uterine leiomyomata are rare in adolescents.
Reference: Pages 357–360

3. A

It is difficult to determine the frequency of diagnoses of pelvic mass in women of reproductive age because many pelvic masses are not ultimately treated with surgery. Nonovarian or nongynecologic conditions should be considered and excluded, although a pelvic kidney is an infrequent diagnosis. Pedunculated leiomyoma may be asymptomatic, but an isolated pedunculated fibroid is uncommon in the absence of fibroids palpable within the uterine wall. Nonneoplastic functional ovarian masses are common, and comprise follicular cysts, corpus luteum cysts, and theca lutein cysts. All are benign, and the most common functional cyst is the follicular cyst, which is usually found incidentally during the pelvic examination; however, these cysts may rupture, causing pain and peritoneal signs. Corpus luteum cysts are less common than follicular cysts and are typically a complex mass, rather than a simple, unilocular cyst. Given the sensitivity of the currently available urine pregnancy tests, a negative urine pregnancy virtually excludes the possibility of ectopic pregnancy.
Reference: Pages 380–398

4. C

To assess vaginal bleeding during adolescence, it is necessary to have an understanding of the range of normal menstrual cycles. During the first 2 years after menarche, most cycles are anovulatory. Despite this, they are somewhat regular, within a range of approximately 21 to 40 days. In more than one fourth of girls, a pattern of +10 days and a cycle length of 20 to 40 days are established within the first three cycles; in one half of girls, the pattern is established by the seventh cycle; and, in two thirds of girls, such a pattern is established within 2 years of menarche.

The mean duration of menses is 4.7 days; 89% of cycles last 7 days or less. The average blood loss per cycle is 35 mL, and the major component of menstrual discharge is endometrial tissue. Recurrent bleeding in excess of 80 mL per cycle results in anemia. The transition from anovulatory to ovulatory cycles takes place during the first several years after menarche. It results from the so-called "maturation of the hypothalamic–pituitary–ovarian axis," characterized by positive feedback mechanisms in which a rising estrogen level triggers a surge of luteinizing hormone and ovulation. Most adolescents have ovulatory cycles by the end of their second year of menstruation, although most cycles (even anovulatory ones) remain within a rather narrow range of 21 to 42 days.

Cycles that are longer than 42 days, cycles that are shorter than 21 days, and bleeding that lasts more than 7 days should be considered out of the ordinary, particularly after the first 2 years from the onset of menarche. The variability in cycle length is greater during adolescence than adulthood; thus, greater irregularity is acceptable if significant anemia or hemorrhage is not present. However, consideration should be given to an evaluation of possible causes of abnormal menses (particularly underlying causes of anovulation such as androgen excess syndromes) for girls whose cycles are consistently outside normal ranges.
Reference: Page 358

5. C (see Fig. 13.10)

The terminology that has been used to describe endometrial hyperplasia is confusing, and the clinician must consult with the pathologist to ensure an understanding of the diagnosis. The following lesions are considered to be benign: anovulatory, proliferative, cystic glandular hyperplasia, simple cystic hyperplasia, simple hyperplasia, and adenomatous hyperplasia without atypia. These terms reflect and describe an exaggerated proliferative response of the endometrium. In most cases, benign endometrial hyperplasia is resolved with dilatation and curettage (D & C) or progestin therapy. Repeated surveillance with endometrial biopsy may be warranted.

The presence of atypia with abnormal proliferation, including features of "back-to-back" crowding of the glands, with epithelial activity demonstrated by papillary projections into the glands, is associated with an increased risk of progression to endometrial carcinoma. These architectural abnormalities may be associated with individual cellular atypia (enlarged, irregular nuclei; chromatin clumping; and prominent nucleoli). The presence of mitotic activity also can be variable.

The management of endometrial hyperplasia rests on an understanding of the natural history of the lesion involved. In one study, only 2% of 122 patients with hyperplasia without cytologic atypia progressed to carcinoma, whereas 23% of those with atypical hyperplasia subsequently developed carcinoma. Architectural complexity and crowding appear to place patients at greater risk for progression than does the presence of cytologic atypia alone.

These data suggest that most women with endometrial hyperplasia will respond to progestin therapy and are not at increased risk of developing cancer. Patients who do not respond are at a significantly increased risk of progressing to invasive cancer and should be advised to have a hysterectomy. Patients who are unlikely to respond can be identified on the basis of cytologic atypia.
Reference: Pages 372–375

6. B

Fewer than 5% of ovarian malignancies occur in children and adolescents. Ovarian tumors account for approximately 1% of all tumors in these age groups. Germ cell tumors make up one half to two thirds of ovarian neoplasms in individuals younger than 20 years of age. A review of studies conducted from 1940 through 1975 concluded that 35% of all ovarian neoplasms occurring during childhood and adolescence were malignant. In girls younger than 9 years, approximately 80% of the ovarian neoplasms were found to be malignant. Germ cell tumors account for approximately 60% of ovarian neoplasms in children and adolescents, compared with 20% of these tumors in adults. Epithelial neoplasms are rare in the prepubertal age group.
Reference: Pages 373–374

7. B

Determining potential indications for surgical treatment requires careful judgment and assessment of the degree of associated symptoms. Asymptomatic leiomyomas do not usually require surgery. Some indications for surgery include the following:

1. Abnormal uterine bleeding with resultant anemia, unresponsive to hormonal management
2. Chronic pain with severe dysmenorrhea, dyspareunia, or lower abdominal pressure and/or pain
3. Acute pain, as in torsion of a pedunculated leiomyoma, or prolapsing submucosal fibroid
4. Urinary symptoms or signs such as hydronephrosis after complete evaluation
5. Rapid enlargement of the uterus during the premenopausal years, or any increase in

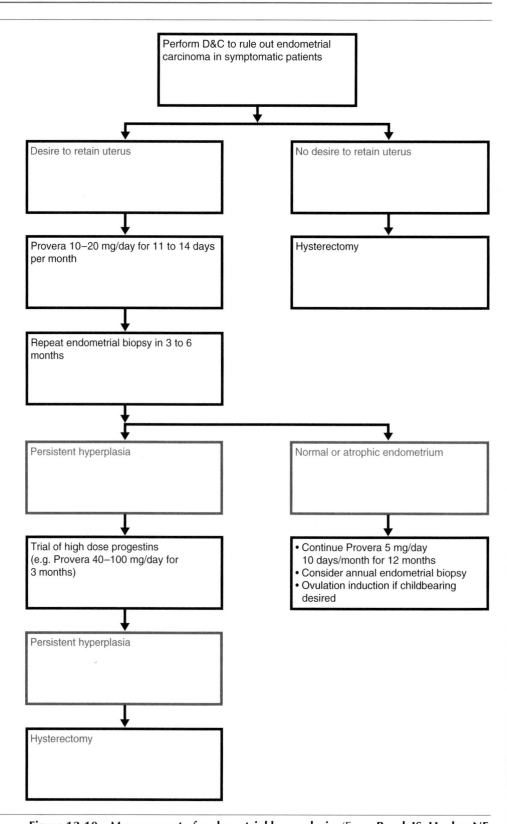

Figure 13.10   Management of endometrial hyperplasia. (From **Berek JS, Hacker NF.** *Practical gynecologic oncology,* 3rd ed. Philadelphia: Lippincott Williams & Wilkins, 2000:422, with permission.)

uterine size in a postmenopausal woman, because of inability to exclude a uterine sarcoma

6. Infertility, with leiomyomas as the only abnormal finding
7. Enlarged uterine size with compression symptoms or discomfort

Reference: Pages 380–382

8. **A**
A vulvar biopsy is essential in distinguishing benign from premalignant vulvar lesions, especially because many lesions may have a somewhat similar appearance. Vulvar biopsies should be performed liberally to ensure that these lesions are diagnosed and treated appropriately. A prospective study of vulvar lesions biopsied in a gynecologic clinic found lesions occurring in the following order of frequency: epidermal inclusion cyst, lentigo, Bartholin duct obstruction, carcinoma *in situ,* melanocytic nevi, acrochordon, mucous cyst, hemangiomas, postinflammatory hyperpigmentation, seborrheic keratoses, varicosities, hidradenomas, verruca, basal cell carcinoma, and unusual tumors such as neurofibromas, ectopic tissue, syringomas, and abscesses. Clearly, the frequency with which a lesion would be reported on biopsy is related to the frequency with which all lesions of a given pathology are biopsied. Thus, the above listing probably underrepresents such common lesions as condylomas.
Reference: Pages 404–405

14 Pelvic Pain and Dysmenorrhea

Julie A. Jolin
Andrea J. Rapkin

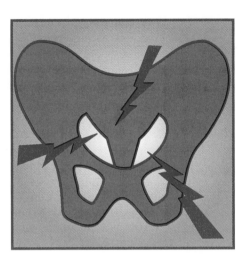

Learning Objectives

1. Know the differential diagnosis of acute pelvic pain.

2. Be aware of the pathophysiologic mechanisms of acute pelvic pain.

3. Understand the causes and treatments of dysmenorrhea.

4. Know the definition and differential diagnosis of chronic pelvic pain.

5. Be aware of the method of evaluation for chronic pelvic pain.

6. Understand the causes and treatments of chronic pelvic pain.

7. Be able to define vulvar vestibulitis syndrome.

Questions

1. A patient presents with amenorrhea for 7 weeks with occasional spotting and acute, localized right lower quadrant pain. Which of the following is *not* typically consistent with her presentation:

   A. Low progesterone concentration
   B. Relief of local pain, replaced by generalized pelvic and abdominal pain
   C. Less than a 66% rise in human chorionic gonadotropin (hCG) level over 48 hours
   D. Double–decidual sac sign

2. Characteristic symptoms or signs of irritable bowel syndrome include

   A. Decreased pain after bowel movement
   B. Excessive flatulence
   C. Increased pain during menses
   D. Palpable, tender sigmoid colon
   E. All of the above

3. The *Minnesota Multiphasic Personality Inventory* (MMPI) studies of women with chronic pelvic pain reveal

   A. Low prevalence of a convergence "V" profile
   B. Indistinguishable profiles between women who have pain and no pathology and women who have endometriosis-related pain
   C. Higher prevalence of hysteria and lower prevalence of depression
   D. No improvement in personality profile with treatment resulting in increased activity level

4. Diagnostic laparoscopy for pelvic pain should be performed to

   A. Evaluate women with cyclic pelvic pain who respond to nonsteroidal antiinflammatory agents or oral contraceptives
   B. Initially evaluate women with chronic noncyclic pelvic pain
   C. Biopsy endometriotic lesions
   D. Lyse all adhesions

5. What percentage of women presenting to pain clinics have already undergone hysterectomy without experiencing pain relief?

   A. 5%
   B. 15%
   C. 30%
   D. 50%

Answers

1. **D**

   The patient likely has an ectopic pregnancy, which probably developed in the fallopian tube, where 95% of ectopic pregnancies occur. Symptoms of ectopic pregnancy include amenorrhea, vaginal bleeding, and pain, of which the severity and nature varies widely from unilateral to bilateral, dull and continuous, or sharp and intermittent. Many patients experience temporary relief of pain when rupture occurs, followed by generalized pelvic pain and abdominal pain as hemoperitoneum develops. Abnormal hCG level doubling time (<66% rise in hCG over 48 hours) and low serum progesterone level (<5.0 ng/mL) highly suggest ectopic pregnancy. In conjunction with hCG levels, ultrasonographic findings aid in diagnosing ectopic pregnancy. The double–decidual

sac sign differentiates true sacs from pseudosacs, which may occur in 8% to 29% of patients with ectopic pregnancy.
Reference: Pages 421–425

2. E

It is important to understand gastrointestinal causes of pain because the uterus, cervix, and adnexa share the same visceral innervation with the lower ileum, sigmoid colon, and rectum, and pain from gynecologic and gastrointestinal causes may be difficult to distinguish. Irritable bowel syndrome (IBS) may account for up to 60% of referrals to gynecologists for chronic pelvic pain. Symptoms of IBS include abdominal pain, which is usually intermittent but occasionally constant, abdominal distention, excessive flatulence, alternating diarrhea and constipation, increased pain before a bowel movement, decreased pain after a bowel movement, and pain exacerbated by high-fat diet, stress, anxiety, depression, and menses. Signs of IBS include a palpable tender sigmoid colon; discomfort on rectal examination; and hard feces in rectum.
Reference: Pages 442–443

3. B

The MMPI studies of women with chronic pelvic pain reveal a high prevalence of a convergence "V" profile that correlates with elevated scores on the hypochondriasis, hysteria, and depression scales. Studies have shown that women who have pain and no pathology and women who have endometriosis-related pain have similar MMPI profiles, although both pain groups differed from controls. It has also been shown that treatment resulting in subjective improvement in pain severity and increased activity level produces significant improvement in the personality profile.
Reference: Pages 446–447

4. C

Evaluating patients with pelvic pain by diagnostic laparoscopy is most helpful for women with disabling cyclic pain nonresponsive to nonsteroidal antiinflammatory agents or oral contraceptives, or for women with chronic noncyclic pelvic pain when other nongynecologic somatic or visceral causes have been excluded. When performing diagnostic laparoscopy, endometriotic lesions should be biopsied and cultures should be obtained if infection is suspected. Although visible adhesions may be lysed, there is little evidence to support complete lysis of adhesions in relieving pelvic pain, and many adhesions reform after adhesiolysis.
Reference: Pages 447–448

5. D

Although hysterectomy has been often performed to relieve pelvic pain, many women suffering from pelvic pain experience little relief until the underlying cause of pain is appropriately identified, evaluated, and treated.
Reference: Page 448

15 Genitourinary Infections and Sexually Transmitted Diseases

David E. Soper

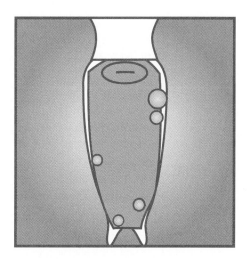

Learning Objectives

1. Be able to identify the causes, diagnosis, and treatment of vaginal infections.

2. Know the causes, diagnosis, and treatment of pelvic inflammatory disease.

3. Be aware of the differential diagnosis of genital ulcers.

4. Understand the impact of human immunodeficiency virus infection in women.

5. Be able to consider the differential diagnosis of acute dysuria.

Questions

1. The normal vaginal flora is predominantly

   A. Aerobic, pH less than 4.5
   B. Aerobic, pH higher than 4.5
   C. Anaerobic, pH less than 4.5
   D. Mixed aerobic/anaerobic, pH higher than 4.5

2. A 21-year-old woman complains of vaginal discharge that she states has a fishy odor. It is particularly noticeable following coitus. You examine her and find the pH is 5. The most likely diagnosis is

   A. *Candida albicans*
   B. Bacterial vaginosis
   C. *Trichomonas vaginalis*
   D. Normal postcoital discharge

3. A 28-year-old complains of a "cottage cheese" discharge associated with vulvar irritation. The net amount of the vaginal secretions fails to confirm fungal elements. The most appropriate next step in this patient's treatment is to

   A. Empirically treat with a topical antifungal
   B. Perform a vaginal culture for yeast
   C. Treat for bacterial vaginosis
   D. Educate the patient concerning normal vaginal flora

4. A 22-year-old woman presents with a purulent vaginal discharge 1 week after having sexual intercourse for the first time with a new boyfriend. She states that he informed her in retrospect that he had felt burning with urination. She is asymptomatic. At the time of pelvic examination, cervical cultures are taken for *Neisseria gonorrhea* and *Chlamydia trachomatis*. The gonorrhea culture is positive. She has no known allergies. You should prescribe

   A. *Doxycycline*
   B. *Erythromycin*
   C. *Azithromycin*
   D. *Cefixime*
   E. *Gentamicin*

5. A 25-year-old woman presents with diffuse acute pelvic and lower abdominal pain, fever, chills, and nausea. There is lower abdominal guarding and cervical motion tenderness. A "fullness" in the pelvis is appreciated, and therefore, a tuboovarian abscess is suspected. The diagnosis of acute salpingitis (pelvic inflammatory disease) is made. The patient is admitted to the hospital for antibiotic therapy. Of the following, which is the most appropriate antibiotic therapy:

   A. *Cefoxitin* and *doxycycline*
   B. *Ceftriaxone sodium* and *erythromycin*
   C. *Amoxicillin* and *trimethoprim*
   D. *Clindamycin* and *clotrimazole*

6. A 34-year-old woman presents with a painful vulvar ulceration. The ulcer has irregular margins and is deep with undermined edges. The ipsilateral inguinal lymph nodes are swollen and tender. The most likely diagnosis is

   A. Syphilis
   B. Herpes

C. Chanchroid
D. Lymphogranuloma venereum

7. The most common human papillomavirus (HPV) subtypes associated with genital warts are

A. HPV-1 and -2
B. HPV-4 and -7
C. HPV-6 and -11
D. HPV-18 and -24
E. HPV-22 and -33

8. A 22-year-old woman presents with symptoms of dysuria. She has a new sex partner. The physical examination reveals some mucopurulent discharge of the cervix. Urinalysis shows some pyuria, but no hematuria. Urinary cultures are negative. The most likely diagnosis is

A. Cystitis with false-negative culture
B. Ureterolithiasis and pyelitis
C. Urethritis associated with *Chlamydia*
D. Vulvovaginitis caused by fungi

Answers

1. A

The normal vaginal flora is predominately aerobic, with an average of six different species of bacteria, the most common of which is hydrogen peroxide–producing lactobacilli. The pH of the normal vagina is lower than 4.5, which is maintained by the production of lactic acid. Estrogen-stimulated vaginal epithelium is rich in glycogen. Vaginal epithelial cells break down glycogen to monosaccharides, which can then be converted by the cells themselves and lactobacilli to lactic acid.
Reference: Pages 453–454

2. B

Bacterial vaginosis (BV) has previously been called "nonspecific vaginitis" or *Gardnerella* vaginitis. The condition is an alteration of the normal vaginal flora that results in the loss of normal lactobacilli and the associated hydrogen peroxide production. This situation encourages the overgrowth of the anaerobic bacteria, which normally account

---

Table 15.2. Treatment Regimens for Gonococcal and Chlamydial Infections

Neisseria gonorrhoeae **endocervicitis**

Cefixime, 400 mg orally (single dose), *or*
Ceftriaxone, 125 mg intramuscularly (single dose), *or*
Ciprofloxacin, 500 mg orally (single dose)*, *or*
Ofloxacin, 400 mg orally (single dose)*, *or* levofloxacin 250 mg orally in a single dose
   (quinolones should not be used for infections acquired in Asia or the Pacific, including
   Hawaii)

Chlamydia trachomatis **endocervicitis**

Azithromycin, 1 g orally (single dose), *or*
Doxycycline, 100 mg orally twice daily for 7 days, *or*
Ofloxacin, 300 mg orally twice daily for 7 days, *or* levofloxacin, 500 mg orally for 7 days
Erythromycin base, 500 mg orally 4 times a day for 7 days, *or*
Erythromycin ethylsuccinate, 800 mg orally 4 times a day for 7 days

From **Centers for Disease Control and Prevention.** *The sexually transmitted diseases treatment guidelines.* Washington, DC: Centers for Disease Control and Prevention, 2002, with permission.

Table 15.3. Clinical Criteria for the Diagnosis of Pelvic Inflammatory Disease

Symptoms

None necessary

Signs

Pelvic organ tenderness
Leukorrhea and/or mucopurulent endocervicitis

Additional criteria to increase the specificity of the diagnosis

Endometrial biopsy showing endometritis
Elevated C-reactive protein or erythrocyte sedimentation rate
Temperature higher than 38°C
Leukocytosis
Positive test for gonorrhea or chlamydia

Elaborate criteria

Ultrasound documenting tuboovarian abscess
Laparoscopy visually confirming salpingitis

---

for less than 1% of normal vaginal flora, and produces the infection. It is the most common form of vaginitis in the United States. The fishy odor and the exacerbation of the condition by coitus are characteristic of the infection. The vaginal pH is typically between 4.7 and 5.7. The treatment is typically *metronidazole* or *clindamycin*. The infection can be distinguished for the other conditions by the use of a vaginal

---

Table 15.4. CDC Guidelines for Treatment of Pelvic Inflammatory Disease

Outpatient Treatment

Regimen A

Ofloxacin, 400 mg orally 2 times daily for 14 days, or
Levofloxacin, 500 mg orally once daily for 14 days
   With or Without:
Metronidazole, 500 mg orally 2 times daily for 14 days

Regimen B

Cefoxitin, 2 g intramuscularly, plus *probenecid,* 1 g orally concurrently, or
Ceftriaxone, 250 mg intramuscularly, or
Equivalent cephalosporin
   Plus:
Doxycycline, 100 mg orally 2 times daily for 14 days
   With or Without:
Metronidazole, 500 mg orally twice a day for 14 days

Inpatient Treatment

Regimen A

Cefoxitin, 2 g intravenously every 6 hours, *or*
Cefotetan, 2 g intravenously every 12 hours,
   Plus:
Doxycycline, 100 mg orally or intravenously every 12 hours

Regimen B

Clindamycin, 900 mg intravenously every 8 hours
   Plus:
Gentamicin, loading dose intravenously or intramuscularly (2 mg/kg of body weight)
   followed by a maintenance dose (1.5 mg/kg) every 8 hours

From **Centers for Disease Control and Prevention.** *The sexually transmitted diseases treatment guidelines.* Washington, DC: Centers for Disease Control and Prevention, 2002, with permission.

"wet mount," because trichomonads are seen in normal saline and *Candida* species are seen in potassium hydroxide.
Reference: Pages 455–456

3. B

Most patients with irritative vulvovaginal symptoms and a negative microscopy for fungal elements do not have yeast vaginitis. A vaginal culture for yeast is crucial in sorting out those patients with yeast vaginitis from those with a hypersensitivity reaction or alternative explanation for their symptoms.
Reference: Pages 456–457

4. D

As presented in Table 15.2, the standard treatment for asymptomatic women with a positive culture for *N. gonorrhea* is a single oral dose of *cefixime.*

Alternatively, *ofloxacin, ceftriaxone sodium,* or *ciprofloxacin* are recommended. *Doxycycline* or *azithromycin* would be appropriate if *Chlamydia* organisms were identified.
Reference: Pages 460–462

Figure 15.2   Showing the appearance of the ulcers of chancroid (A), herpes (B), and syphilis (C). The ulcer of chancroid has irregular margins and is deep with undermined edges. The syphilis ulcer has a smooth, indurated border and a smooth base. The genital herpes ulcer is superficial and inflamed. (From **Schmid GP, Shcalla WO, DeWitt WE. Chancroid.** In: **Morse SA, Moreland AA, Thompson SE,** eds. *Atlas of sexually transmitted diseases.* Philadelphia: JB Lippincott, 1990, with permission.)

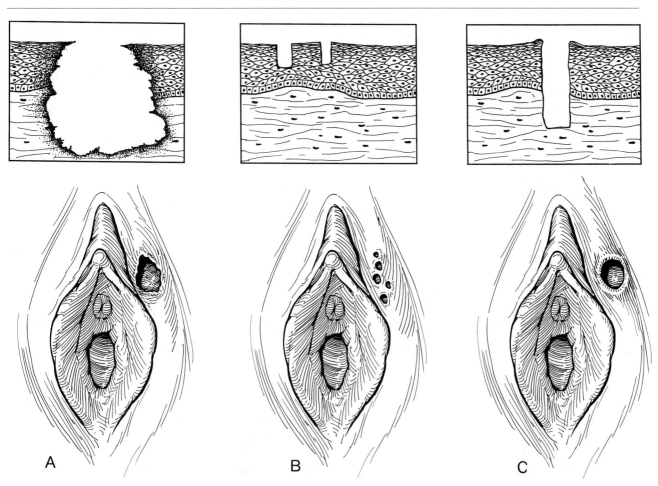

A   B   C

5. A (see Tables 15.3 and 15.4)

The appropriate treatment of pelvic inflammatory disease with a suspected tuboovarian abscess is combination antibiotic therapy administered in the hospital. The Centers for Disease Control recommends treatment with either *cefoxitin* plus *doxycycline* or *clindamycin* plus *gentamicin.*
Reference: Pages 462–463

6. C (see Fig. 15.2)

The differential diagnosis of genital ulcers is often difficult without appropriate tests. Although the pattern described is most likely to be chanchroid, syphilis must be excluded by the performance of VDRL, fluorescent treponemal antibody absorption (FTA-ABS), and/or dark-field tests. The appropriate treatment of the condition is *azithromycin, ceftriaxone sodium,* or *erythromycin.*
Reference: Pages 463–464

7. C

The most common subtypes of HPV associated with genital warts are HPV-6 and HPV-11. Most often, these are nononcogenic. They tend to occur in the areas most directly affected by coitus. Exophytic genital warts are highly contagious.
Reference: Page 465

8. C

In patients with a negative urine culture, pyuria, and no hematuria, the most likely diagnosis is urethritis associated with a sexually transmitted disease. Appropriate tests of the cervix should identify the specific organism that should be treated as discussed above in Question 4.
Reference: Pages 466–467

16 Intraepithelial Disease of the Cervix, Vagina, and Vulva

Jonathan S. Berek

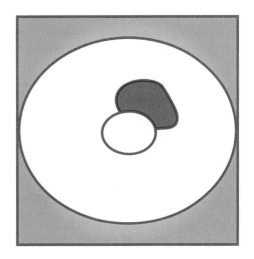

Learning Objectives

1. Understand the pathophysiology of cervical intraepithelial neoplasia.

2. Know the role of diagnostic methods for cervical intraepithelial neoplasia.

3. Have an algorithm for the evaluation, treatment, and follow-up of an abnormal Pap test.

4. Know the treatment options for cervical intraepithelial neoplasia.

5. Know the diagnosis and treatment of vaginal intraepithelial neoplasia.

6. Be able to identify vulvar intraepithelial disease and know its differential diagnosis.

Questions

1. Which of the following statements regarding cervical intraepithelial neoplasia (CIN) is incorrect?

   A. CIN 1 refers to the situation in which immature or dysplastic cells are present in the lower one third of the epithelium.
   B. CIN is more likely to develop in the anterior lip of the cervix than in the posterior lip.
   C. The transformation zone refers to the zone between the active squamocolumnar junction (SCJ) and the columnar epithelium.
   D. Nabothian cysts may be useful in determining the location of the original SCJ.
   E. In neonates, the SCJ is located on the exocervix.

2. Which of the following human papillomavirus (HPV) types is most common in patients with invasive cervical cancer, CIN 3, and CIN 2?

   A. HPV-6
   B. HPV-11
   C. HPV-16
   D. HPV-18
   E. HPV-31

3. Which of the following HPV types is most common in women with normal cervical cytology?

   A. HPV-6
   B. HPV-11
   C. HPV-16
   D. HPV-18
   E. HPV-31

4. Which of the following statements regarding the Bethesda system is false?

   A. The category "atypical squamous cells of undetermined significance" (ASC-US) refers to cells described as reactive, inflammatory, or reparative.
   B. The "high-grade squamous intraepithelial" (HSIL) category includes cells consistent with carcinoma *in situ* (CIS) by the CIN system.
   C. Ideally, when standardized diagnostic criteria are used, the rate of ASC cytology should be 3% to 5%.
   D. Cellular changes associated with HPV (koilocytosis and CIN 1) should be classified as "low-grade squamous intraepithelial lesion" (LSIL).

5. Which of the following situations are appropriate to treat with a loop electrosurgical excision procedure (LEEP) procedure?

   A. High-grade lesions such as CIN 3
   B. Large lesion size
   C. Positive endocervical curettage (ECC)
   D. Endocervical glandular involvement
   E. All of the above

6. Which of the following situations provide indications for cervical conization?

   A. ECC positive for CIN 2 to 3
   B. Lack of correlation between cytology, biopsy, and colposcopy with persistent HSIL cytology
   C. Suspicion for microinvasion

D. Inadequate colposcopy in the setting of persistent HSIL

E. All of the above

7. Which of the following statements regarding glandular cell abnormalities is false?

    A. AGC (atypical glandular cells) is more predictive of significant underlying disease than is ASC.

    B. Microinvasive adenocarcinoma of the cervix is a well-established phenomenon.

    C. Fifty percent of women with adenocarcinoma *in situ* (AIS) will also have squamous CIN.

    D. A patient with negative margins after conization for AIS should be counseled that there is a significant chance she may still have residual AIS.

    E. Any patient with AIS and positive margins after conization should undergo repeated cone biopsy at a minimum and should be offered hysterectomy if fertility is not desired.

8. The most appropriate initial treatment for a 70-year-old woman diagnosed with vaginal intraepithelial neoplasia 3 (VAIN 3) near the vaginal cuff is

    A. Cryosurgery

    B. Fulguration with the electrosurgical ball under colposcopic guidance

    C. Surgical excision

    D. Laser therapy

    E. *5-Fluorouracil* (*Efudex* cream)

9. Histologically, Paget's disease of the vulva

    A. is primarily a squamous cell lesion.

    B. arises in melanocytes.

    C. is a type of sarcoma of the vulva.

    D. arises primarily in Bartholin gland.

    E. is a disease of the apocrine sweat glands.

10. Which of the following statements regarding vulvar intraepithelial disease is true?

    A. The malignant potential of vulvar intraepithelial neoplasia (VIN) is similar to that of CIN.

    B. VIN lesions should always be treated by superficial vulvectomy.

    C. Most cases of Paget's disease of the vulva are intraepithelial.

    D. Mucicarmine staining may assist in differentiating melanoma from Paget's disease, because melanocytes stain positive.

    E. Paget's disease of the vulva is primarily a disease of premenopausal women.

Answers

1. C

The transformation zone is an area established as metaplasia advances from the original SCJ inward toward the external os and over the columnar villi. The transformation zone extends from the original SCJ to the physiologically active SCJ.

In the neonatal period, the SCJ is indeed located on the ectocervix and the SCJ at this time is termed the original SCJ. During menarche, metaplasia occurs inward over the columnar cells and new or active SCJ forms (see Fig. 16.2). The transformation zone actually refers to the area between the original SCJ and the physiologically active SCJ. Nabothian cysts may aid in the identification of the original SCJ. The importance of the transformation zone is that this is the area in which CIN is likely to develop. The anterior cervix is twice as likely as the posterior lip to develop CIN. CIN rarely develops

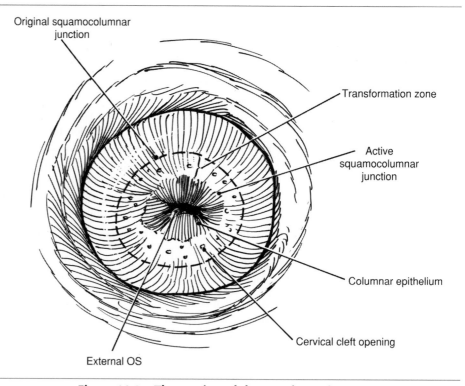

Original squamocolumnar junction

Transformation zone

Active squamocolumnar junction

Columnar epithelium

Cervical cleft opening

External OS

Figure 16.2   The cervix and the transformation zone.

in the lateral angles. CIN 1 refers to the situation in which immature cells are present in the lower one third of the epithelium whereas CIN 2 and CIN 3 refer to involvement of the middle and upper thirds, respectively, in addition to the lower one third (see Fig. 16.1).
Reference: Pages 472–473

2. C
See answer to Question 3.

Figure 16.1   Diagram of the different grades of cervical intraepithelial neoplasia (CIN).

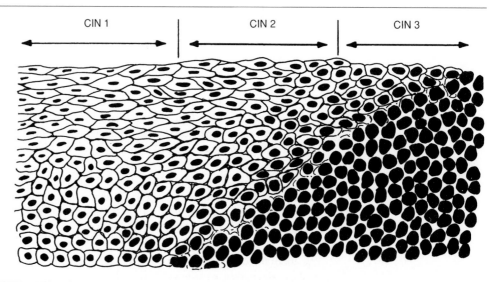

CIN 1   CIN 2   CIN 3

3. C

The percent of intraepithelial neoplasia associated with HPV infection approaches 90%. The number of known genital HPV types is greater than 20 but certain subtypes account for the majority of high-grade and cancerous lesions of the cervix: HPV types 16, 18, 31, 33, 35, 39, 45, 51, 52, 56, and 58. Type 16 is the most common subtype found in CIN 2, CIN 3, and invasive carcinoma, and is present in nearly 50% of women with these lesions. Interestingly, it is also the most common subtype found in women with normal cytology and it is, therefore, not very specific. By contrast, HPV type 18 is found in 23% of women with invasive cancers and in only 5% of women with CIN 1, CIN 2, and CIN 3. It is found in less than 2% of women with normal cytology and is, therefore, more specific than HPV 16 for invasive lesions. Most women exposed to HPV do not subsequently develop CIN. Any factor (such as cigarette smoking) that influences incorporation of HPV-DNA into the host genome may contribute to the development of CIN and ultimately to the development of invasive cancer.
Reference: Pages 475–476

4. A (see Table 16.1)

In 1989, the Bethesda System for cervical cytology was developed in an attempt to standardize the reporting of cytology. A recent revision (2001), the Bethesda III, had been adopted. According to this system, premalignant conditions of the cervix fall into three categories: ASC, LSIL, and HSIL.

The ASC category is further broken down into ASC-US (undetermined significance, and ASC-H (exclude high-grade intraepithelial lesion). The determination and follow-up of these two subcategories can be assisted by the performance of HPV-testing. In general, the former group should be managed expectantly, and in the absence of oncogenic HPV, the Pap smear is simply repeated in 1 year, whereas with the second category or when oncogenic HPV is present, the patient should undergo colposcopy and biopsy. Cytologic smears that exhibit reactive, reparative, or inflammatory changes alone are not classified as ASC and, in fact, are reported separately. Ideally, ASC cytologic

Table 16.1. Comparison of Cytology Classification Systems

Bethesda System	Dysplasia/CIN System	Papanicolaou System
Within normal limits	Normal	I
Infection (organism should be specified)	Inflammatory atypia (organism)	II
Reactive and reparative changes		
Squamous cell abnormalities		
Atypical squamous cells (1) of undetermined significance (**ASC-US**)	Squamous atypia / HPV atypia, exclude **LSIL**	IIR
(2) exclude high-grade lesions (**ASC-H**)	Exclude **HSIL**	
Low-grade squamous intraepithelial lesion (**LSIL**)	HPV atypia / Mild dysplasia	CIN 1 — III
High-grade squamous intraepithelial lesion (**HSIL**)	Moderate dysplasia	CIN 2
	Severe dysplasia / Carcinoma *in situ*	CIN 3 — IV
Squamous cell carcinoma	Squamous cell carcinoma	V

CIN, cervical intraepithelial neoplasia.
Updated from **Berek JS, Hacker NF,** eds. *Practical gynecologic oncology,* 2nd ed. Baltimore: Williams & Wilkins, 1994:205, with permission.

cervical Pap smears should comprise approximately 3% to 5% of all cytologic smears within a given laboratory.

LSIL lesions include those classified as CIN 1 by the "CIN" system as well as those which exhibit changes consistent with HPV infection such as koilocytosis. Lesions that fall into the category of CIN 2, CIN 3, and CIS by the CIN system are grouped together under the category of HSIL by the Bethesda system. The reason for incorporating most abnormal Pap smears into two broad categories (HSIL and LSIL) is that all lesions falling into one or the other category will be managed similarly depending on the particular category. High-risk HPV subtypes such as 16 and 18 are not limited to HSIL lesions and, in fact, may be associated with CIN 1.
Reference: Pages 483–484

5. E (see Fig. 16.13)

LEEP is most appropriate for high-grade lesions (e.g., CIN 2–3). If there is a positive ECC for high-grade dysplasia or if there is documented endocervical glandular involvement, LEEP is appropriate. Most important, however, given the high rate (up to 60%–80%) of spontaneous resolution of low-grade cervical lesions (HPV/CIN 1), expectant management is quite appropriate as an alternative to the use of LEEP for these patients, even when CIN 1 only is in the canal.
Reference: Pages 489–491

6. E

All of the above scenarios are situations in which cervical conization should be performed. Conization provides a pathologic specimen for review and, therefore, is preferable over the ablative therapies in the evaluation and treatment of higher grade lesions or if an occult carcinoma is suspected. All of these situations should raise a concern for microinvasion, or possibly invasive cancer, and cervical cone biopsy should be performed to exclude these diagnoses. A conization can be performed with a LEEP or a scalpel (so-called, "cold knife" conization), and the technique recommended depends on the clinical circumstance. If one is suspicious of microinvasive carcinoma or adenocarcinoma, in general a more traditional approach (using a scalpel) is recommended in order to ensure that the surgical margins of the biopsy are adequate and that the geometry of the cone is appropriate.
Reference: Pages 491–492

7. A

The Bethesda system has a separate category for reporting glandular cell abnormalities. AGC is more likely than ASC to reflect significant underlying pathology. In a recent study of 63 patients with AGC, approximately 50% were found to have significant abnormalities, including two patients with invasive adenocarcinoma. Therefore, a Pap smear read as AGC should be given serious consideration and appropriate biopsies taken depending on the patient's age and clinical scenario. The phenomenon of microinvasive adenocarcinoma of the cervix has been proposed but has not been proven to exist. Therefore, the term should be avoided and such tumors should be classified as AIS or invasive adenocarcinoma. Several recent publications have addressed the issue of conization margins in the setting of AIS. Negative margins are not necessarily reassuring because a high percentage of patients may have residual AIS. A scant 40% of patients with positive margins after cone biopsy are found to have residual disease at repeated conization or hysterectomy. Treatment of AIS should be individualized and hysterectomy should be considered if fertility is not desired.
Reference: Pages 492–493

8. C

Patients with VAIN 1 need not be treated, because these lesions will often regress spontaneously. VAIN 2 lesions are usually treated with simple excision or possibly

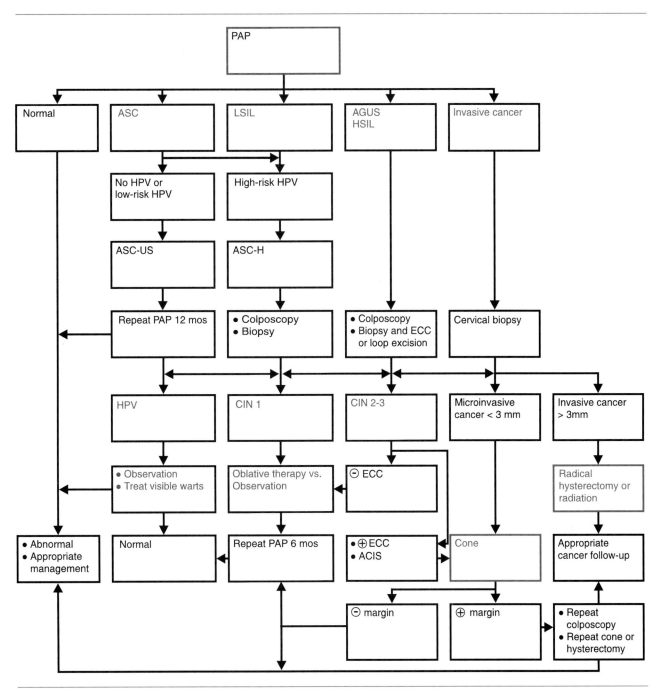

Figure 16.13   An algorithm for the evaluation, treatment, and follow-up of an abnormal Pap test.

with laser vaporization. The malignant potential of VAIN appears to be less than that of CIN but VAIN 3 lesions have a significant chance of harboring an occult invasive lesion. Therefore, surgical excision, as opposed to one of the ablative procedures, should be undertaken initially to rule out an invasive carcinoma. Once invasion has been ruled out, consideration may be given to treating VAIN 3 with laser ablation. In postmenopausal women, some VAIN 2 and VAIN 3 lesions respond to improved estrogenization and thus, the use of topical estrogen preparations are recommended.
Reference: Pages 494–495

9. E
See answer to Question 10.

10. C

Paget's disease of the vulva is an intraepithelial lesion involving cells of the apocrine sweat glands but may be associated with an underlying adenocarcinoma. This disease must be differentiated from superficial spreading melanoma. Mucicarmine stains may assist in this determination, because melanocytes stain negative. Interestingly, a synchronous or metachronous primary neoplasm is associated with extramammary Paget's disease in 30% of patients. Treatment is wide surgical excision, because this disease frequently extends beyond the gross lesion, and positive margins are associated with a significant chance of recurrence. Paget's disease is seen primarily in postmenopausal white women.

The malignant potential of VIN is believed to be significantly lower than that of CIN and progression to invasive carcinoma is uncommon. Smaller lesions may be treated with simple excision or recurrent VIN.
Reference: Pages 500–501

17

Early Pregnancy Loss and Ectopic Pregnancy

Thomas G. Stovall
Jonathan S. Berek

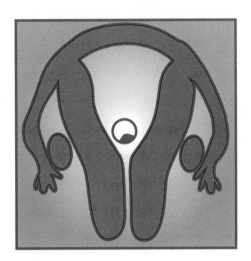

Learning Objectives

1. Know the different types of abnormal intrauterine pregnancy, including their definitions and sequelae.

2. Know the epidemiology of ectopic pregnancy, including risk factors.

3. Understand the methods of diagnosis of ectopic pregnancy, and be able to provide an algorithm for diagnosis.

4. Know the medical and surgical treatment options for ectopic pregnancy, including the relative merits of each.

Questions

1. If one uses serial human chorionic gonadotropin (hCG) measurements to detect early subclinical pregnancy losses, the percentage of pregnancies that terminate in spontaneous abortion is

   A. 5%
   B. 10%
   C. 20%
   D. 30%
   E. 50%

2. After an ectopic pregnancy, there is an increased risk of subsequent ectopic pregnancy. The risk is increased by how many fold?

   A. 2
   B. 5
   C. 10
   D. 20
   E. 50

3. A 27-year-old woman presents with a copper-T intrauterine device (IUD) in place, right lower quadrant abdominal pain, and an adnexal mass. The hCG is positive, and an ultrasound documents a right tubal pregnancy. Compared with the risk of ectopic pregnancy in patients without the IUD, the risk is

   A. Higher
   B. Lower
   C. The same

4. A 19-year-old woman who is known to have an early pregnancy presents with some vaginal "spotting." She is suspected of having either a threatened abortion or an ectopic pregnancy. At the time of initial presentation 5 weeks from her last menstrual period, the hCG level is just less than 2,000 mIU/mL. The ultrasound does not yet document an intrauterine pregnancy. An ectopic pregnancy is not seen. After 48 hours, the patient remains asymptomatic. In order to distinguish an intrauterine pregnancy from an ectopic pregnancy, the change in the hCG over 48 hours is observed. The hCG is now 2,450 mIU/mL. What percentage rise in hCG represents the lower limit of normal values for viable intrauterine pregnancies?

   A. 33%
   B. 50%
   C. 66%
   D. 80%
   E. 100%

5. The earliest ultrasonographic sign of an intrauterine pregnancy is

   A. A small fluid space and the gestational sac surrounded by a thick echogenic ring
   B. A fetal heart with evidence of pulsatile activity
   C. A large decidual sac with a very thick concentric ring
   D. A fetal neural tube sign

6. At what level of hCG will essentially all intrauterine pregnancies be identifiable by transvaginal ultrasonography?

   A. 6,500 mIU/mL
   B. 500 mIU/mL

C. 2,000 mIU/mL

D. 8,500 mIU/mL

7. A 31-year-old woman presents with vaginal bleeding 6 weeks from her last menstrual period. Her hCG is 4,860 mIU/mL. An ultrasonogram of the pelvis shows a tubal gestation measuring 4 cm, with cardiac activity. The surgical treatment of choice for this tubal pregnancy, which cannot be treated with *methotrexate* is

   A. Salpingectomy
   B. Salpingostomy
   C. Salpingotomy
   D. Salpingoplasty

8. A good candidate for the use of *methotrexate* to treat an ectopic pregnancy is

   A. No intrauterine gestational sac or fluid collection, hCG levels higher than 2,000 mIU/mL, ectopic smaller than 3.5 cm
   B. Equivocal intrauterine sac, hCG levels 2,000 to 4,500 mIU/mL, ectopic smaller than 5 cm
   C. No intrauterine gestational sac, ectopic 3 to 5 cm, with cardiac activity, regardless of hCG level
   D. Any patient with an unruptured ectopic

9. A 28-year-old woman presents with a positive pregnancy test and vaginal bleeding 6 weeks from her last menstrual period. On pelvic examination, the uterus feels small and the cervix is expanded. On ultrasound, the cervix appears to contain a gestational sac. The best management of this presumed case of cervical pregnancy is

   A. Dilatation and curettage (D & C)
   B. Hysterectomy
   C. Embolization
   D. *Methotrexate*

10. A 24-year-old G1P0 presents with a positive urine pregnancy test and vaginal spotting for the last 12 hours. The pelvic examination is essentially within normal limits. Ultrasound shows no intrauterine gestational sac, and the quantitative hCG level is 1,250 mIU/mL. The next step in the treatment of this patient should be

   A. D & C for a failed intrauterine pregnancy
   B. Laparoscopy to rule out an ectopic gestation
   C. Repeat the hCG level in 48 hours
   D. Repeat the ultrasound using a transabdominal probe

Answers

1. **D (see Table 17.1)**
   Although 15% to 20% of known pregnancies terminate in spontaneous abortion, if the serial follow-up with hCG is added, the percentage increases to 30%, as there are many losses that otherwise go undetected. About 80% of spontaneous abortions occur in the first trimester, and the incidence decreases with each gestational week. Spontaneous pregnancy losses include anembryonic gestations, inevitable abortions, and incomplete abortions.
   Reference: Page 507

2. **C**
   After an ectopic pregnancy, there is a 7- to 13-fold increase in the risk of subsequent ectopic pregnancy. The chance that a subsequent ectopic pregnancy will be intrauterine is

Table 17.1. Definitions of Types of Abnormal Intrauterine and Extrauterine Pregnancies

Extrauterine Pregnancy

Tubal pregnancy	A pregnancy occurring in the fallopian tube—most often these are located in the ampullary portion of the fallopian tube
Interstitial pregnancy	A pregnancy that implants within the interstitial portion of the fallopian tube
Abdominal pregnancy	Primary abdominal pregnancy—the first and only implantation occurs on a peritoneal surface. Secondary abdominal pregnancy—implantation originally in the tubal ostia, subsequently aborted, and then reimplanted onto a peritoneal surface
Cervical pregnancy	Implantation of the developing conceptus in the cervical canal
Ligamentous pregnancy	A secondary form of ectopic pregnancy in which a primary tubal pregnancy erodes into the mesosalpinx and is located between the leaves of the broad ligament
Heterotopic pregnancy	A condition in which ectopic and intrauterine pregnancies coexist
Ovarian pregnancy	A condition in which an ectopic pregnancy implants within the ovarian cortex

Abnormal Intrauterine Pregnancy

Incomplete abortion	Expulsion of some but not all of the products of conception before 20 completed weeks of gestation
Complete abortion	Spontaneous expulsion of all fetal and placental tissue from the uterine cavity before 20 weeks of gestation
Inevitable abortion	Uterine bleeding from a gestation of less than 20 weeks' gestation, accompanied by cervical dilation but without expulsion of placental or fetal tissue through the cervix
Anembryonic gestation	An intrauterine sac without fetal tissue present at more than 7.5 weeks of gestation
First-trimester fetal death	Death of the fetus in the first 12 weeks of gestation
Second-trimester fetal death	Death of the fetus between 13 and 24 weeks of gestation
Recurrent spontaneous abortion	The loss of more than three pregnancies before 20 weeks' gestation

50% to 80%, and the chance that the pregnancy will be tubal is 10% to 25%; the remaining patients will be infertile. However, many variables make the accurate assessment of the risk very difficult.
Reference: Page 510

3. A

Women who conceive with an IUD in place are 0.4 to 0.8 times more likely to have a tubal pregnancy than those not using contraceptives. However, because IUDs prevent implantation more effectively in the uterus than in the tube, a woman conceiving with an IUD is 6 to 10 times more likely to have a tubal pregnancy than if she conceives without contraception.
Reference: Pages 511–512

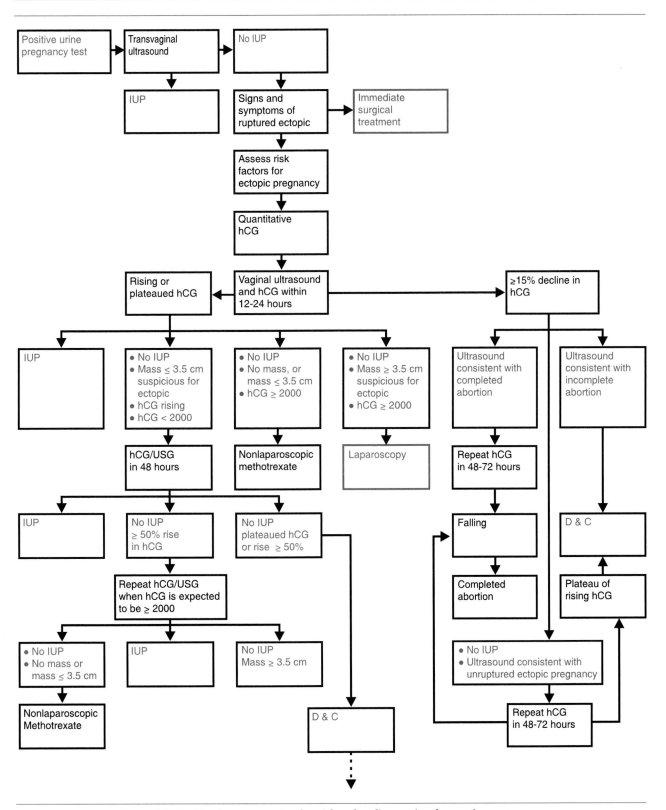

Figure 17.4   Nonlaparoscopic algorithm for diagnosis of ectopic pregnancy.

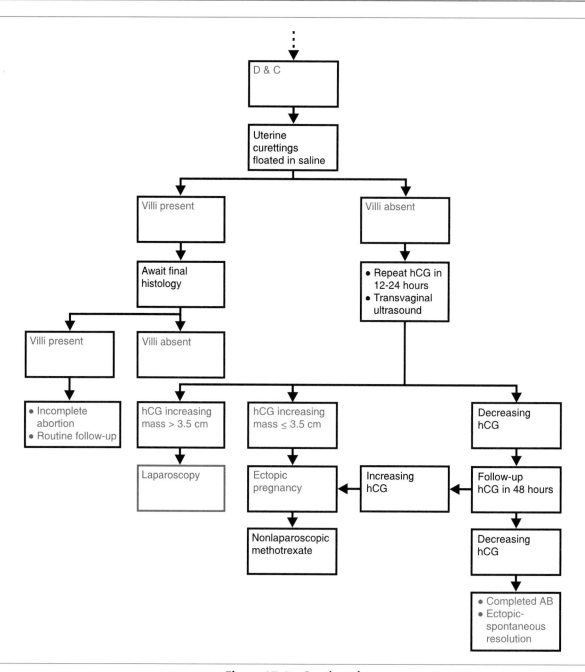

Figure 17.4   Continued

4. **C (see Fig. 17.4)**

    A 66% rise in the hCG level over 48 hours (85% confidence level) represents the lower limit of normal values for viable intrauterine pregnancies. Approximately 15% of patients with viable intrauterine pregnancies will have a rise in hCG level less than 66% over 48 hours, and a similar percentage with an ectopic pregnancy will a have rise of more than 66%. The hCG pattern most predictive of an ectopic pregnancy is one that has reached a plateau over 1 week. These serial measurements are usually required when the initial ultrasound examination is indeterminate.
    Reference: Pages 516–517

5. **A**

    The earliest ultrasonographic finding of an intrauterine pregnancy is usually located eccentrically within the endometrial cavity. The earliest normal gestational sac is seen at

Table 17.3. Single-dose Methotrexate Protocol for Ectopic Pregnancy

Day	Therapy *
0	D & C, hCG
1	CBC, SGOT, BUN, creatinine, blood type and Rh
4	*Methotrexate* 50 mg/m^2 IM
7	hCG

CBC, complete blood count; SGOT, serum glutamic-oxaloacetic transaminase; BUN, blood urea nitrogen; IM, intramuscularly.
* If less than a 15% decline in human chorionic gonadotropin (hCG) level between days 4 and 7, give second dose of *methotrexate,* 50 mg/m^2, on day 7.
If more than a 15% decline in hCG level between days 4 and 7, follow weekly until hCG is below 10 mIU/mL.
In patients not requiring dilation and curettage (D & C) (hCG > 2,000 mIU/mL and no gestational sac on transvaginal ultrasonography), days 0 and 1 are combined.

5 weeks of gestation with transabdominal ultrasonography and at 4 weeks of gestation with transvaginal ultrasonography. As the gestational sac grows, a yolk sac is seen within it, followed by an embryo with cardiac activity.
Reference: Pages 518–520

6. C

Accurate interpretation of ultrasonographic findings to determine the location of a pregnancy (intrauterine versus extrauterine), requires a correlation with the hCG level. This is called the "discriminatory zone." All viable intrauterine pregnancies can be visualized by transabdominal sonography correlated with serum hCG levels of greater than 6,500 mIU/mL. This number is reduced to 2,000 mIU/mL with the use of transvaginal ultrasound Nonvisualization at that level indicates an abnormal pregnancy, either an ectopic or an incomplete spontaneous abortion. Intrauterine sacs seen at lower levels of hCG are abnormal and represent aborting intrauterine pregnancies or the pseudo-gestational sac of an ectopic pregnancy.
Reference: Page 520

Table 17.4. Initiation of Methotrexate: Physician Checklist and Patient Instructions

Physician Checklist

Obtain hCG level.
Perform transvaginal ultrasound within 48 hours.
Perform endometrial curettage if hCG level is less than 2,000 mIU/mL.
Obtain normal liver function (SGOT), normal renal function (BUN, creatinine), and a normal CBC (WBC < 2,000/mL and platelet count > 100,000)
Administer *Rhogam* if patient is Rh-negative.
Identify unruptured ectopic pregnancy smaller than 3.5 cm.
Obtain informed consent.
Prescribe FeSO$_4$, 325 mg PO bid if hematocrit is less than 30%.
Schedule follow-up appointment on days 4, 6, and 7.

Patient Instructions

Refrain from alcohol use, multivitamins containing folic acid, and sexual intercourse until hCG level is negative.
Call your physician:
    If you experience prolonged or heavy vaginal bleeding.
    The pain is prolonged or severe (lower abdomen and pelvic pain is normal during the first 10–14 days of treatment).
    Use oral contraception or barrier contraceptive methods.

About 4%–5% of women experience unsuccessful *methotrexate* treatment and require surgery.
hCG, human chorionic gonadotropin; SGOT, serum glutamic-oxaloacetic transaminase; BUN, blood urea nitrogen; CBC, complete blood count; WBC, white blood cell.

Table 17.5. Ultrasound Criteria for Cervical Pregnancy

1. Echo-free uterine cavity or the presence of a false gestational sac only
2. Decidual transformation of the endometrium with dense echo structure
3. Diffuse uterine wall structure
4. Hourglass uterine shape
5. Ballooned cervical canal
6. Gestational sac in the endocervix
7. Placental tissue in the cervical canal
8. Closed internal os

From **Hofmann HMH, Urdl W, Hofler H, et al.** Cervical pregnancy: case reports and current concepts in diagnosis and treatment. *Arch Gynecol Obstet* 1987;241:63–69, with permission.

7. B

Linear salpingostomy is currently the procedure of choice when the patient has an unruptured ectopic pregnancy and wishes to retain her potential for future fertility. It can be accomplished either via the laparoscope or via laparotomy. The salpingostomy is left open to heal spontaneously.
Reference: Pages 523–526

8. A

Based on current data, a conservative approach to the use of medical therapy is warranted. *Methotrexate* is best used in women whose ectopic pregnancies are small and have no cardiac activity. The treatment protocol for such patients is presented in Table 17.3, and a method for the initiation of *methotrexate* is presented in Table 17.4.
Reference: Pages 527–529

9. D

Cervical pregnancy is rare (reported incidence ranges from 1:2,400 to 1:50,000 pregnancies), and therefore, optimal management has not been clearly defined. However, the surgical manipulation of the cervix (e.g., with dilation) can be risky because of the chance of hemorrhage.

Methotrexate offers the chance to treat the condition nonsurgically and hopefully to avoid hysterectomy. Ultrasonographic criteria for the diagnosis of cervical pregnancy are presented in Table 17.5.
Reference: Pages 531–532

10. C

When evaluating a patient for a possible abnormal pregnancy, a single hCG level is not generally helpful. This is especially true when the hCG level is below the discriminatory zone for transvaginal scanning. A D & C is not indicated because, most likely, this patient has a normal intrauterine pregnancy. The next step in the patient's care should be to repeat the quantitative hCG measurement in 48 hours to determine if it is rising appropriately. Because the hCG level should be above 2,000 mIU/mL at this time, a repeated transvaginal ultrasound should also be helpful.
Reference: Pages 522–523

18 Benign Breast Disease

Baiba J. Grube
Armando E. Giuliano

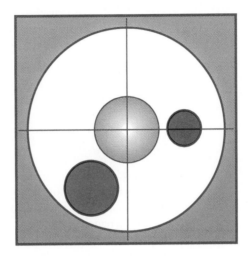

Learning Objectives

1. Know the methods of detection of breast disease.

2. Be aware of the recommendations for breast cancer screening.

3. Be able to provide an algorithm for the management of breast masses in premenopausal and postmenopausal women.

4. Know the benign breast conditions that can and do occur and their differential diagnoses.

5. Be able to identify which breast conditions require evaluation.

Questions

1. A 20-year-old woman presents for evaluation of a mass in her left breast. The mass has been present for approximately 1 year. When questioned, she is vague about change in size of the mass or fluctuation with menstrual cycles and denies the presence of any nipple discharge. She is not currently taking medications. There is no family history of breast cancer, and she is not sexually active. On physical examination, a palpable mass measuring 2 cm is detected in the left lower outer breast quadrant. The mass is smooth and mobile with no associated skin changes or retraction. Your initial recommendation is

   A. Mammography
   B. Ultrasound examination
   C. Excision of the mass
   D. Reassurance

2. Of the following statements, which is true regarding breast tumors, especially cancerous ones?

   A. They are asymptomatic and are discovered only by physical examination or screening mammography.
   B. They are typically symptomatic and, therefore, are more likely to be discovered by the patient.
   C. They are most likely to be discovered by routine palpation by the physician at the time of an annual physical examination, but not by mammography.
   D. They are most likely to go undetected until disease has spread and they produce symptoms in other organs.

3. A 37-year-old woman presents for a baseline clinical examination and mammography. There is a strong family history of breast cancer in multiple first- and second-generation relatives. She denies having any nipple discharge and would like to get pregnant. The clinical breast examination results are negative. The report of the screening mammography states that the results are Breast Imaging Reporting and Data System (BI-RADS) 0. You inform the patient that

   A. There are no suspicious findings on the mammography.
   B. Her next mammography examination should be done at age 40.
   C. She can proceed with her plans for pregnancy.
   D. The cancer detection rate for screening mammography is 5 per 1000.

4. A 45-year-old woman undergoes annual screening mammography. The mammography reveals new calcifications in the left upper outer quadrant. Magnification views are obtained that reveal pleomorphic calcifications, and the mammogram is interpreted as a BI-RADS 4. The results of the clinical breast examination are benign. You recommend a biopsy for diagnosis and offer the patient either needle localization excisional biopsy or stereotactic core biopsy. The patient prefers stereotactic core biopsy. The results of the biopsy reveal normal breast tissue with no calcifications present. You discuss the findings with the patient and tell her

   A. The histology is benign and she does not have to worry.
   B. She can resume her annual clinical breast examination and mammography.
   C. She should undergo needle localization excisional biopsy.
   D. She should undergo magnetic resonance imaging (MRI).

5. A 65-year-old postmenopausal woman presents with a 1.5-cm breast mass in the left upper outer quadrant. The most appropriate management is

   A. Lumpectomy and axillary node dissection based on a suspicious mammographic finding

    B. Observation based on a negative fine-needle aspiration cytology

    C. A 2-week period of observation

    D. Lumpectomy and axillary node dissection based on a fine-needle aspiration cytology

    E. Fine-needle aspiration followed by mammography

6. A 45-year-old woman with a history of right breast carcinoma 2 years ago who was treated with a lumpectomy and sentinel node biopsy noted spontaneous left nipple discharge. The patient has serous, straw-colored nipple discharge that tests guaiac-positive. Mammography performed 4 months previously had negative results except for the postoperative changes in the right breast. Clinical breast examination reveals no skin changes, nipple retraction, breast masses, or adenopathy. You proceed as follows:

    A. Reassure her that because there are no suspicious findings on breast examination and her recent mammography results were negative, the most likely cause of her nipple discharge is a benign process and that she can return for a follow-up in 6 months.

    B. Recommend assessment of prolactin levels because she is perimenopausal and the discharge is most likely related to hormonal changes.

    C. Recommend a diagnostic mammography examination with magnification views of the subareolar area.

    D. Recommend ductal lavage for assessment of cytology.

7. A 35-year-old woman presents with a 2-cm breast mass in the left lower outer quadrant. She complains of breast pain that varies with her menstrual cycle. The lesion has not changed in size for the past 3 months. The most appropriate management is

    A. Decrease intake of caffeine and start Vitamin E (400 IU daily)

    B. Take *danazol* (100–200 mg twice daily orally)

    C. Observation through two menstrual cycles

    D. Biopsy the lesion

    E. Mammography

8. A 48-year-old woman develops a new right breast mass. She noted the mass 2 months ago and followed it through two menstrual cycles with no change in size noted. She reports pain associated with the mass, but no nipple discharge. She does not drink coffee or black tea, nor does she consume chocolate. There is no family history of breast cancer and she is not taking any medications. On examination, the patient has a 3-cm mass in the right upper outer quadrant that is mobile and firm but not attached to the skin or underlying pectoralis muscle. Mammography reveals a density and an ultrasound is performed. The mass is a cyst, which is aspirated. Dark fluid is aspirated and there is a residual mass. You tell the patient that

    A. The fluid can be discarded because it is always benign.

    B. There is a residual mass that needs to undergo tissue diagnosis.

    C. The fluid was tested for blood and, because it was negative, she can be reassured that the cyst was benign.

    D. She should return in 6 weeks for a reexamination because cysts frequently recur.

9. A 50-year-old woman presents with severe breast pain with the absence of nipple discharge. She does not consume coffee, black tea, or chocolate. There is no family history of breast cancer. She has taken vitamin E, 400 units twice a day, for the past 6 months without resolution of her symptoms. On clinical breast examination, the breast parenchyma is moderately nodular and bilaterally symmetrical with diffuse tenderness. There is no evidence of skin dimpling, nipple retraction, or peau d'orange. Mammography results are BI-RADS 2. You obtain serum blood level measurements of thyrotropin releasing hormone (TRH) and prolactin, and they are normal. You discuss the etiology of her symptoms and recommend all of the following options for consideration except

    A. Good supportive bra 24 hours a day

    B. Oral evening primrose oil

C. *Danazol*

D. *Bromocriptine mesylate*

10. A 45-year-old woman presents with an increase in size of a known breast mass. Core biopsy had previously been performed on this mass and the pathology was consistent with a fibroadenoma. The patient denies nipple discharge, breast trauma, redness, or swelling. Her menstrual cycles are normal and there is no family history of breast cancer. Her last mammography examination was 1 year ago and revealed the stable mass. The patient undergoes diagnostic mammography that reveals a significant increase in the size of the lesion. An ultrasound examination is performed and reveals a smooth mass that is suggestive of a fibroadenoma, but a phyllodes tumor cannot be excluded. You recommend

A. Mastectomy

B. Repeated core biopsy

C. Excision

D. Observation

11. A 36-year-old woman presents with a tender swollen breast. The symptoms occurred acutely. She has a swollen left breast that is warm, tender, and red. She is unable to tolerate mammography. An ultrasound examination is performed, which reveals a multiloculated mass. The best recommendation is

A. Excision of mass

B. Fine-needle aspiration, cytology, culture, and antibiotics if purulent

C. Neoadjuvant chemotherapy

D. Incision and drainage of an abscess

12. A 36-year-old, nonlactating woman presents with a 2-month history of bloody nipple discharge from her left breast. No mass is palpable on physical examination. The most appropriate management is

A. Measure serum prolactin and TRH levels

B. Obtain cytologic examination of the bloody nipple discharge

C. Obtain ductography

D. Observation alone

E. Excision of the involved duct

Answers

1. **B**

   The most likely cause of a breast mass in a 20-year-old woman is a cyst or a fibroadenoma. The first step in treatment should be an ultrasound examination that can distinguish a solid from cystic lesion. At this age, the breast tissue is dense and mammography is unlikely to be helpful as a first step. A cyst can be drained with fine-needle aspiration and does not require excision. A solid mass requires definitive histologic assessment either by fine-needle aspiration or core biopsy. If the core biopsy shows malignant cells, a mammogram would be performed even in a 20-year-old to rule out other findings in the breast, although it will most likely demonstrate dense breast tissue. Excision of a mass without determining whether the lesion is solid or cystic is inappropriate. Reassurance in the absence of a histologic diagnosis of a new breast mass is dangerous, even in a 20-year-old, because breast cancer has been reported to occur in all age groups. (See sections on mammography, ultrasonography, and breast biopsy.) Reference: Pages 546–556

2. **A**

   Most tumors of the breast, particularly those that are malignant, are asymptomatic and are detected either by physical examination or by screening mammography. While

the value of breast self-examination is controversial, some lesions are detected by the patient, undoubtedly before they have a chance to metastasize.
Reference: Pages 544–545

3. D

A **BI-RADs** 0 mammography is an incomplete study, not one with no findings. An incomplete mammography report means that further evaluation with additional mammographic views or other diagnostic modalities such as ultrasound or MRI are needed. The American Cancer Society recommends that an average-risk woman start annual mammography at age 40. In women with a high risk, guidelines are modified to begin approximately 10 years earlier than the youngest age at which breast cancer has been diagnosed. Mammography before the age of 30 must take into consideration the risk of exposure of breast tissue to ionizing radiation and the benefits of detecting a lesion. The patient should not proceed with conception until her mammographic findings are evaluated and, if indicated, treated. The treatment of breast cancer after conception is much more difficult, medically and psychologically. (See sections on mammography, mammographic reports, ultrasonography, MRI, PET scan, sestamibi, and mammographic screening.)
Reference: Pages 548–549

4. C

The patient's mammogram reveals new pleomorphic calcifications that are considered suspicious (BI-RADS 4). Tissue diagnosis is mandatory. The tissue diagnosis must be concordant with the physical findings and mammographic findings (triple test concordance). In this case, no calcifications are visible in the core biopsy specimen, indicating insufficient tissue sampling. Further evaluation with needle localization biopsy is mandatory to obtain tissue that contains representative calcifications.

The presence of calcifications should be noted on a specimen mammography and in the pathology report. There is no role for MRI in this situation. Negative MRI results would not preclude excisional biopsy. Positive MRI results would only support the need for a tissue diagnosis that is already mandated by the discordant histologic and mammographic findings. (See sections on mammography, mammographic reports, mammographic abnormalities, and triple test.)
Reference: Pages 548–549

5. D (see Fig. 18.5)

A breast mass in a 65-year-old postmenopausal woman is cancer until proven otherwise. A tissue diagnosis must be made before undertaking a definitive operative procedure. There is no role for observation in the patient described. Fine-needle aspiration cytology is a useful technique whereby cells from a breast tumor are aspirated with a small (usually 22-gauge) needle and examined by a pathologist. However, it requires the availability of a pathologist skilled in the cytologic diagnosis of breast cancer to interpret the results and it is subject to sampling problems, particularly when lesions are deep. The incidence of false-positive diagnosis is only about 1% to 2%, but the rate of the false-negative is as high as 10% in some series. Mammography should be performed before biopsy so other suspicious areas can be noted and the contralateral breast can be checked. (See section on breast biopsy.)
Reference: Pages 551–555

6. C

The most common cause of bloody nipple discharge in a perimenopausal woman is a benign process—intraductal papilloma or duct ectasia. However, new-onset, unilateral bloody discharge must be evaluated by definitive triple testing plus examination to rule out a malignancy. The patient should undergo a repeat diagnostic mammography with magnification views of the nipple areolar complex to rule out any suspicious finding in the subareolar area. Most intraductal papillomas occur within 2 cm of the nipple. Nipple discharge associated with hyperprolactinemia is usually bilateral, milky, and

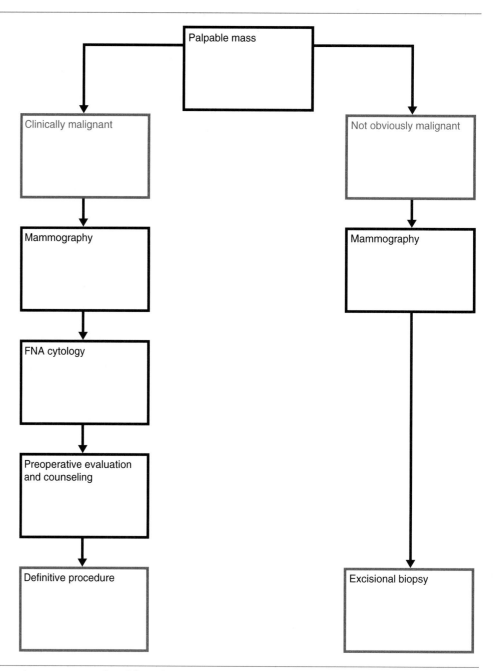

Figure 18.5 Algorithm for management of breast masses in postmenopausal women. (From **Giuliano AE.** Breast disease. In: **Berek JS, Hacker NF,** eds. *Practical gynecologic oncology.* 2nd ed. Baltimore: Williams & Wilkins, 1994:493, with permission.)

guaiac-negative. This would not be the first test to undertake in this circumstance. Ductal lavage is a new technology that may prove effective as a diagnostic tool. It should not however precede breast-imaging studies to identify an occult lesion. It may be considered as an adjunct after diagnostic imaging studies are performed. (See sections on BSE, nipple discharge, and nipple lavage.)
Reference: Page 555

7. D (see Fig. 18.4)
Pain, fluctuation in size, and multiplicity of lesions are the features most helpful for differentiating fibrocystic change from carcinoma. However, if a dominant mass

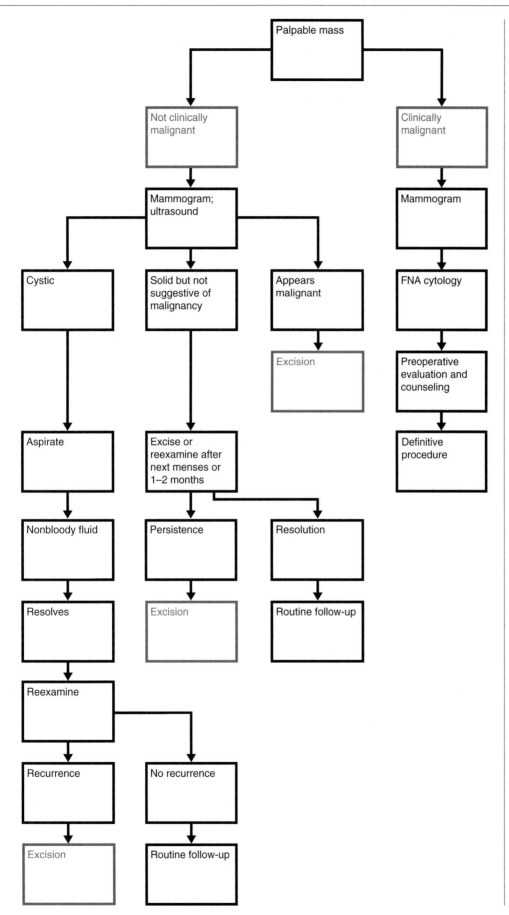

Figure 18.4 Algorithm for management of breast masses in premenopausal women. (From **Giuliano AE**. Breast disease. In: **Berek JS, Hacker NF,** eds. *Practical gynecologic oncology* 3rd ed. Philadelphia: Lippincott Williams & Wilkins, 2000:553, with permission.)

is present, as in this patient, the diagnosis of cancer should be suspected until it is disproved by biopsy. Final diagnosis of the mass usually depends on biopsy. Mammography may be helpful, but there are no mammographic signs diagnostic of fibrocystic change. *Danazol*, a synthetic androgen, has been used for patients with severe pain. This treatment suppresses pituitary gonadotropins, and its androgenic effects (acne, edema, hirsutism) are usually intolerable; therefore, it probably should not be used. The role of caffeine consumption in the development and treatment of fibrocystic change is controversial. Observations about these effects have been difficult to confirm and are anecdotal. (See sections on breast biopsy.)
Reference: Pages 553–557

8. B

The presence of a mass after cyst aspiration requires further diagnostic evaluation. A simple cyst, when aspirated, results in complete collapse and, if the aspirate is negative for blood, it can be discarded. In the absence of a residual mass, a short-interval follow-up to evaluate reaccumulation of the cyst is important. A recurrent cyst can be subjected to reaspiration and result in complete collapse. In the current situation, however, a residual mass suggests a pathologic process that requires definitive tissue diagnosis. (See Fig. 18.4 and sections on BSE, fine needle aspiration, and fibrocystic change.)
Reference: Pages 552–556

9. D

Mastalgia can be a severe debilitating problem and one that 70% of women experience to some degree in their lives. Cyclic mastalgia is more easily treated than noncyclic breast pain. A good supportive bra is fundamental to therapy. Avoidance of methyl-xanthines has been reported to be effective in some cases. Evening primrose oil has been associated with improvement of symptoms in women who have low levels of essential fatty acids. *Danazol* has been used but has significant side effects including acne, edema, and hirsutism. A recent report on luteal phase–only *danazol* use seems to indicate there is a significant improvement in symptoms without the associated negative side effects. *Bromocriptine mesylate* is an effective agent in cases where there is elevation of thyrotropin level. In this case, the patient had normal levels and is better suited for one of the other treatment interventions. (See section on mastalgia.)
Reference: Pages 557–558

10. C

A known fibroadenoma that is increasing in size is a worrisome sign of a phyllodes tumor. Phyllodes tumors can be benign or malignant. A repeat core biopsy will not prevent definitive removal of the mass and may potentially seed the biopsy track if the tumor is a malignant. Observation of a mass that is increasing in size, even with a previous core biopsy of benign fibroadenoma, is not appropriate. In rare situations, fibroadenomas have the potential to undergo transformation to phyllodes tumors. If excision of the mass reveals a phyllodes tumor, wide excision is recommended. Mastectomy is not indicated as the first line of therapy unless clear margins cannot be obtained. (See sections on fibroadenoma and phyllodes tumor.)
Reference: Pages 558–560

11. B

The patient presents with acute symptoms of a breast infection. Although an inflammatory breast carcinoma cannot be ruled out completely, the progression of symptoms in the present ultrasound findings that demonstrate a multiloculated mass is suggestive of an abscess. Excision of the mass in the absence of a diagnosis is inappropriate. If it is an abscess, removal of benign breast tissue will leave a deformed breast. If it is inflammatory carcinoma, the first line of treatment is neoadjuvant chemotherapy, but a tissue diagnosis must be determined before initiation of neoadjuvant chemotherapy.

Incision and drainage of an abscess is not appropriate. The first approach to breast abscesses is aspiration of abscess contents. Repeat aspirations may be performed. Administration of antibiotics is recommended. If the abscess cannot be successfully treated by percutaneous aspiration and antibiotics, incision and drainage should be undertaken. (See section on breast abscess.)
Reference: Pages 561–562

12. E

Unilateral, spontaneous, bloody, or serosanguinous discharge from a single duct is usually caused by an intraductal papilloma or, rarely, by an intraductal cancer. Cytologic examination is usually of no value but may identify malignant cells. Negative findings do not rule out cancer, which is more likely in women older than 50 years. In any case, the involved duct—and the mass, if present—should be excised. Although ductography may identify a filling defect prior to excision of the duct system, this study is of little value. Serum prolactin and TRH levels should be obtained to search for a pituitary tumor or hypothyroidism. In this case, a milky discharge would be present (See section on nipple discharge.)
Reference: Pages 560–561

19

Preoperative Evaluation and Postoperative Management

Daniel L. Clarke-Pearson
Angeles A. Alvarez
Laura J. Havrilesky
Johnathan Lancaster

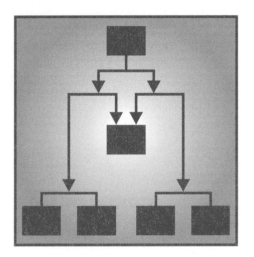

Learning Objectives

1. Provide cost-effective treatment of postoperative deep-vein thrombosis.

2. Identify the level of thromboembolism prophylaxis required in high-risk patient populations.

3. Identify patients at high risk for necrotizing fasciitis and describe appropriate management.

4. Understand the appropriateness, as well as the risks, of preoperative imaging studies in patients with potential gynecologic malignancies.

5. Understand which preoperative factors are independently related to increased rates of postoperative myocardial infarction.

Questions

1. The principal purpose of the preoperative consent is

    A. To establish a trust relationship with the patient
    B. To clarify the goals of the proposed procedure
    C. To outline the expected outcome of the procedure
    D. To outline the risks, benefits, and alternatives to the procedure

2. Weight loss prior to surgery potentially can have an adverse affect on outcome. Below what percentage of ideal body weight is a patient at risk for higher postoperative morbidity?

    A. 6%
    B. 12%
    C. 18%
    D. 24%

3. The normal daily fluid requirement in the average adult is

    A. 1 to 1.5 L
    B. 2 to 3 L
    C. 3 to 4 L
    D. 4 to 5 L

4. The most common fluid and electrolyte disorder in the postoperative period is

    A. Hypovolemia from too little fluid
    B. Hypernatremia
    C. Fluid overload
    D. Hyperkalemia

5. The most common electrolyte problem seen in the immediate postoperative period is

    A. Acidosis
    B. Alkalosis
    C. Hyperkalemia
    D. Hyponatremia

6. The best means of maintaining postoperative pain control is to keep the level of pain reliever above the MEAC (minimum effective analgesic concentration) by using

    A. Intermittent intramuscular injections
    B. Scheduled intravenous bolus infusions
    C. Scheduled oral administration
    D. Patient-controlled analgesia (PCA)

7. Antibiotic prophylaxis should be used in

    A. Vaginal hysterectomy
    B. Abdominal hysterectomy
    C. Vaginal and abdominal hysterectomy
    D. Vaginal and selected abdominal hysterectomy

8. Febrile morbidity is defined as

    A. Temperature higher than or equal to 38°C on two occasions 4 hours apart after first 24 hours
    B. Temperature higher than or equal to 39°C on two occasions 4 hours apart after first 24 hours

C. Temperature higher than 39.5°C at any time after 24 hours
D. Temperature higher than 40°C.

9. The most common source of postoperative infection is the

    A. Urinary tract
    B. Incision
    C. Lung
    D. Vaginal cuff

10. Wound infection rates can be decreased by all of the following, **except**

    A. Shaving the wound site
    B. Shortening the postoperative stay
    C. Meticulous surgical technique
    D. *Hexachlorophene* showers prior to surgery
    E. Bringing drains out through sites other than the incision

11. The most common infectious agent responsible for necrotizing fasciitis is

    A. *Hemolytic streptococcus*
    B. *Clostridium perfringens*
    C. *Staphylococcus aureus*
    D. *Escherichia coli*

12. The primary purpose of a preoperative "intestinal preparation" is to

    A. Empty the contents of the bowel
    B. Accelerate postoperative bowel recovery
    C. Reduce the postoperative infectious morbidity
    D. Minimize the risk of intraoperative colorectal injury

13. The principal thrust of management of postoperative ileus is

    A. Instillation of hypertonic radiologic contrast material to stimulate function
    B. Administration of pharmacologic agents to stimulate gastrointestinal function
    C. Gastrointestinal decompression and intravenous fluids
    D. Surgical intervention to correct intestinal blockage

14. Immediate surgical decompression of the colon is warranted if the diameter of the cecum reaches

    A. 4 to 5 cm
    B. 6 to 8 cm
    C. 10 to 12 cm
    D. 13 to 14 cm

15. Of the following techniques for the prevention of deep-vein thrombosis, which one is preferable for most patients undergoing major gynecologic operations?

    A. Elastic stockings
    B. Low-dose *heparin*
    C. Standard-dose *heparin*
    D. External pneumatic compression

16. When acute deep-vein thrombosis of the lower extremity has been diagnosed, the optimal number of days of therapeutic levels of heparin is

    A. 3
    B. 5
    C. 7
    D. 10

17. Of the following, which is most likely to predispose to a postoperative myocardial infarction?

    A. Emergency surgery
    B. Age older than 70 years
    C. Poor general medical condition
    D. Myocardial infarction in the preceding 6 months

18. In the management of perioperative congestive heart failure, the measurement of which variable with a pulmonary artery catheter is most helpful in guiding fluid management?

    A. Left ventricular pressure (LVP)
    B. Right ventricular filling pressure (RVFP)
    C. Left ventricular end-diastolic pressure (LVEDP)
    D. Pulmonary capillary pressure (PCP) during systole

19. The standard regimen for prophylactic antibiotics to prevent subacute bacterial endocarditis in patients with any valvular abnormality is

    A. *Ampicillin/gentamicin*
    B. *Vancomycin hydrochloride/gentamicin*
    C. *Amoxicillin* alone
    D. *Vancomycin hydrochloride* alone

20. In patients with extensive intraoperative blood loss, in addition to the replacement of red blood cells, replacement with which of the following will most likely be necessary?

    A. Albumin
    B. Cryoprecipitate
    C. White blood cells
    D. Fresh-frozen plasma

21. The greatest risk factor for the development of postoperative pulmonary complications is the presence of underlying

    A. Asthma
    B. Malignancy
    C. Bronchiectasis
    D. Chronic obstructive pulmonary disease

22. The most common postoperative pulmonary complication is

    A. Atelectasis
    B. Pneumothorax
    C. Pulmonary edema
    D. Bronchopneumonia

23. A pulmonary complication of septicemia, which is the result of damage to the capillary side of the alveolar–capillary membrane resulting in an increase in pulmonary capillary permeability, is known as

    A. Pulmonary edema
    B. Pulmonary hypertension
    C. Respiratory permeability defect
    D. Adult respiratory distress syndrome (ARDS)

24. A 45-year-old woman without other complicating medical conditions undergoes abdominal hysterectomy and bilateral salpingo-oophorectomy for stage II ovarian carcinoma. On the fifth postoperative day, she develops femoral, deep-vein thrombosis. What is the proper medical management of this patient?

A. Intravenous *streptokinase* for 72 hours followed by oral *coumadin* for 3 months

B. Intravenous *heparin* therapy for 24 hours followed by oral *coumadin* therapy for 3 months

C. Intravenous *heparin* therapy for 10 days followed by oral *coumadin* for 3 months

D. Intravenous *heparin* for 5 days followed by oral *coumadin* for 3 months

E. Bed rest with leg elevation and immediate initiation of oral *coumadin* therapy for 3 months

25. A 65-year-old woman with clinical stage I, grade 3 endometrial adenocarcinoma is being prepared for surgical therapy to include total abdominal hysterectomy, bilateral salpingo-oophorectomy, and pelvic and periaortic lymphadenectomy. What is the most cost-effective prophylactic regimen available to prevent postoperative venous thromboembolic complications?

A. Low-dose *heparin* (5,000 units preoperatively and every 12 hours postoperatively)

B. Low-dose *heparin* (5,000 units preoperatively and every 8 hours postoperatively)

C. Intermittent pneumatic leg compression intraoperatively and for 24 hours postoperatively

D. Intermittent pneumatic leg compression intraoperatively and for 5 days postoperatively

E. Graded-compression stockings intraoperatively and for 2 weeks postoperatively

26. A 65-year-old obese woman, with hypertension and insulin-dependent diabetes mellitus, has undergone a total abdominal hysterectomy and bilateral salpingo-oophorectomy for a benign pelvic mass. After an unremarkable initial postoperative course, the patient develops a fever of 39.4°C (102.8°F) on postoperative day 3. On physical examination, the patient appears ill. Vital signs include a blood pressure of 95/60 mm Hg and heart rate of 108 beats per minute. Physical examination findings are remarkable for cold and clammy skin. The patient's wound is very tender. On palpation, the incision is intact but has some purulent drainage. The left aspect of the incision has a brown discoloration and significant erythema with edema of the superficial skin that fades gradually into the normal surrounding skin. Upon opening the incision, purulent material is evacuated and digital palpation of the wound reveals an intact fascia. The subcutaneous fat overlying the fascia can easily be undermined. Which of the following regimens is most appropriate?

A. Evacuation of the purulent material, irrigation with half-strength peroxide, reapproximation of the skin edges using staples or sutures, and initiation of broad-spectrum antibiotic therapy.

B. Initiation of wound care including three times daily irrigation with half-strength peroxide and packing of the wound with saline-soaked gauze, and initiation of broad-spectrum antibiotic therapy.

C. Same as answer B, but no antibiotic therapy is required because this wound abscess has been adequately drained.

D. Aggressive intravenous hydration, initiation of broad-spectrum antibiotic therapy, aggressive surgical debridement in the operating room to remove all necrotic and infected tissue until healthy skin margins are achieved, and consideration of postoperative hyperbaric oxygen therapy.

27. A 60-year-old black woman with a long-standing history of hypertension and insulin-dependent diabetes presents to your office with a history of stage IV ovarian carcinoma. She initially presented at an outside medical center approximately 5 months earlier with a large left-sided malignant pleural effusion, massive intraabdominal ascites, and a relatively small asymptomatic 5- to 6-cm left adnexal mass, but no other soft-tissue or retroperitoneal abnormalities. After a paracentesis was performed, which revealed cells suspicious for papillary serous adenocarcinoma with psammoma bodies (likely of ovarian origin), she was treated with six cycles of *cisplatin* and *paclitaxel*. Her ascites and pleural effusion resolved and her CA125, previously over 2,000 μ/mL is now in the normal range. A computed tomography (CT) scan (without contrast) was normal after the third cycle of chemotherapy with the exception of a solid pelvic mass. Unfortunately, her pelvic mass had persisted on examination and she presents to your office at this time for consideration of an interval debulking surgery. Her physical examination is unremarkable with the exception of the solid pelvic mass, which is compressing the rectum. You have discussed with her the palliative role of the surgery but in your discussion, you explain your concern about the compression on the rectum and the probable need for continued chemotherapy if cancer is still present in the abdominal cavity. Her medical oncologist has taken the liberty of ordering her preoperative admission tests, which include a CT scan of the abdomen and pelvis with contrast. The only remarkable study on her serum chemistry reveals a creatinine of 1.2 mg/dL. The next most appropriate step would be:

A. Have the patient complete the studies and schedule her for an exploratory laparotomy

B. Discontinue the order for the CT scan and order a pelvic ultrasound instead

C. Obtain a radiolabeled *lasix* renal scan to estimate the creatinine clearance in each kidney

D. Order a magnetic resonance imaging (MRI) study of the abdomen and pelvis

E. Cancel the CT scan and schedule the patient for an exploratory laparotomy

28. Which of the following is not an independent risk factor for postoperative myocardial infarction?

A. Significant aortic valvular stenosis

B. Hypertension

C. Evidence of congestive heart failure (S_3 gallop or jugular venous distention)

D. More than five premature ventricular contractions (PVCs) per minute preoperatively

E. Myocardial infarction within the last 6 months

Answers

1. D

While the process of obtaining preoperative "informed consent" includes the establishment of a relationship with the patient and a clarification of the goals and specifics of the proposed operation, the principal purpose (from a legal standpoint) is to document that you have informed the patient regarding the risks, benefits, and alternatives to the operation.
Reference: Pages 571–573

2. B

Preoperative nutritional status is an important correlate of postoperative outcome. Although no single test accurately predicts the outcome in malnourished surgical patients, those whose weight is 12% or more below their ideal body weight are at higher risk for complications.
Reference: Pages 573–574

3. B

The body adjusts to higher and lower volumes of intake by changes in plasma tonicity. However, the typical intake that a patient without significant insensible losses is about 2 to 3 L per day. Patients with high fever can have increased pulmonary and skin loss of free water, sometimes in excess of 2 to 3 L per day. In patients with bowel obstruction, 1 to 3 L of fluid per day can be sequestered in the gastrointestinal tract.
Reference: Page 578

Table 19.3. Acid-Base Disorders and Their Treatment

Primary Disorder	Defect	Common Causes	Compensation	Treatment
Respiratory acidosis	Carbon dioxide (hypoventilation)	Central nervous system depression Airway and lung impairment	Renal excretion of acid salts Bicarbonate retention Chloride shift into red blood cells	Restoration ventilation Control of excess dioxide production
Respiratory alkalosis	Hyperventilation	Central nervous excitation system Excess ventilator support	Renal excretion of sodium, potassium bicarbonate Absorption of hydrogen and chloride ions Lactate release from red blood cells	Correction hyperventilation
Metabolic acidosis	Excess loss of base Increased nonvolatile acids	Excess chloride versus sodium Increased bicarbonate loss Lactic, ketoacidosis Uremia Dilutation acidosis	Respiratory alkalosis Renal excretion of hydrogen and chloride ions Resorption of potassium bicarbonate	Increase sodium load give bicarbonate for pH <7.2 Restore buffers, protein, hemoglobin
Metabolic acidosis	Excess loss of chloride and potassium Increased bicarbonate	Gastrointestinal losses of chloride Excess intake of bicarbonate Diuretics Hypokalemia Extracellular fluid volume contraction	Respiratory acidosis May be hypoxia Renal excretion of bicarbonate and potassium Absorption of hydrogen and chloride ions	Increased chloride content Potassium replacement Acetazolamide (Diamox) to waste bicarbonate Vigorous volume replacement Occasional 0.1 NaHCl as needed

NaHCl, sodium hydrochloride.

4. C

The most common problem seen in patients is iatrogenic (i.e., too much fluid given). The fluid excess can occur with normal or decreased sodium because large amounts of isotonic fluids will remain in the extracellular space. Simple fluid restriction will correct the problem. When necessary, diuretics can be used to increase urinary water excretion.
Reference: Page 582

5. B (see Table 19.3)

Alkalosis is usually of no clinical significance and resolves spontaneously. The most common etiologic factors are hyperventilation associated with pain; posttraumatic transient hyperaldosteronism, which results in a decrease in bicarbonate excretion; nasogastric suction, which removes hydrogen ions; infusion of bicarbonate with transfusions; and the use of diuretics. Alkalosis can usually be promptly reversed by removing the inciting cause.
Reference: Pages 582–583

6. D

The best way to control pain in the immediate postoperative period after major abdominal surgery is probably patient controlled analgesia (PCA), because a relative steady state of drug can be maintained above the MEAC threshold. In this manner, peaks and valleys above and below this threshold can be minimized. This approach produces the best pain relief. Guidelines for the use of intravenous analgesics are presented in Table 19.4.
Reference: Pages 584–586

Table 19.4. Guidelines for Front-Loading IV Analgesics for Relief of Postoperative Pain

Drug	Total Front-Loaded Dose	Increments	Cautions
Morphine	0.08–0.12 mg/kg	0.03 mg/kg q 10 min	Histaminergic effects; nausea; biliary colic; reduce dose for elderly
Meperidine	1.0–1.5 mg/kg	0.30 mg/kg q 10 min	Reduce dose or change drug for impaired renal function
Codeine	0.5–1.0 mg/kg	1/3 of total q 15 min	Nausea
Fentanyl	0.4–1.0 μg/kg	0.2–0.5 μg/kg q 6 min	Bradycardia; minimal hemodynamic alterations

7. D

The benefit of prophylactic antibiotics in vaginal hysterectomy has been clearly established. However, the benefit in abdominal hysterectomy is controversial. Some data do indicate a benefit in the latter case, especially in obese women, the presence of malignancy, surgery that lasts longer than 2 hours, and low socioeconomic status.
Reference: Pages 588–589

8. A

This definition has now been well accepted. Within 24 hours, higher temperatures often occur and the correlation with infection is low. If the fever cutoff is set higher than 38°C, significant morbidity is missed, especially in elderly patients who are less likely to mount a febrile response to infection.
Reference: Page 590

9. A

The urinary tract has been the most common site of infection in surgical patients. However, this risk is substantially reduced in gynecologic patients who have received prophylactic antibiotics. Recent literature has indicated a urinary tract infection rate as low as 4% in women who have received prophylactic therapy. Most urinary tract infections occur in the lower urinary tract, and very few patients develop serious pyelonephritis.
Reference: Pages 591–592

10. A

One should minimize the shaving of the incision site, because shaving, particularly when it is done hours prior to the surgery instead of immediately before the incision, increases the rate of wound infection. All of the other parameters are associated with lower infection rates.
Reference: Pages 592–593

11. A

Although *hemolytic Streptococcus* is responsible for many of these cases, it is not the only organism. Furthermore, this infection may predispose to other infections and a polymicrobial infection often exists. Other organisms, including other gram-positive organisms, coliforms, and anaerobes are often cultured in addition to the *hemolytic Streptococcus*. Bacterial enzymes such as hyaluronidase and lipase are released in the subcutaneous space and destroy the fascia and fatty tissues producing a liquefactive necrosis.
Reference: Pages 594–596

12. C

The principal reason for the performance of a "bowel prep" is to reduce the incidence of postoperative infectious morbidity. The rate of infection associated with intestinal resection in unprepared bowel is as high as 40%, whereas it is 5% to 10% after a preparation. When resection of the colon is a possibility, the intestinal preparation should include mechanical and antibiotic preparation (see Table 19.7).
Reference: Pages 596–597

Table 19.7. Bowel Preparation Regimens to Begin Day Prior to Surgery

Time	Mechanical Prep	Antibiotic Prep
Preoperative day 2 PM	Clear liquid diet	
Preoperative day 1 Noon	Clear liquid diet *Magnesium citrate* (240 cc PO), or *GoLYTELY* (4 L PO over 3 hr)	
1 PM		*Erythromycin* base 500 mg PO, plus *Neomycin* 1 gm PO *Metronidazole* 500 mg PO may be substituted
2 PM		Repeat PO antibiotics
8 PM	Enemas until clear IV D5/0.5 NS + 20 mEq KCl at 125 cc/hr (optional)	
11 PM		Repeat PO antibiotics
Operative day 12 midnight AM	Nothing by mouth Surgery	Prophylactic IV antibiotics

IV, intravenous; D5, 5% dextrose; NS, normal saline; PO, per os.

13. C

Although the mechanism of ileus is somewhat unclear, there is a disruption in normal intestinal motility that is associated with peritoneal infection, various surgical procedures performed in the abdomen, and electrolyte disturbances. The primary therapy is decompression of the bowel, typically with a nasogastric tube, and careful administration of fluids and electrolytes. Pharmacologic and radiologic stimulants are of limited value. Surgery should be performed if the condition does not resolve over several days and a true mechanical obstruction is suspected.
Reference: Pages 597–598

14. C

With complete colonic obstruction (typically by a gynecologic or colonic neoplasm), the colon can rapidly dilate and perforate. A normal cecum may dilate to 4 to 5 cm, but when it reaches 10 to 12 cm, the colon is dangerously dilated. Immediate treatment with colostomy or colectomy is warranted.
Reference: Pages 598–599

15. D

The use of external pneumatic compression results in a reduction of postoperative venous thromboembolic complications by nearly threefold. This reduction is similar to that seen with low-dose *heparin* and has the advantage of not increasing the likelihood of bleeding complications.
Reference: Pages 602–604

16. B

A randomized trial of a 5-day versus a 10-day regimen of *heparin* showed that the 5-day regimen was equally effective and had a lower risk of complications.
Reference: Pages 601–602

17. D

The preoperative variable that most likely predisposes to a postoperative myocardial infarction is the presence of jugular venous distention or an S₃ gallop (indicating congestive heart failure) and the occurrence of a myocardial infarction in the preceding

Table 19.8. Risk Factors for Perioperative Cardiovascular Risk (160)

Major

Unstable or severe angina
Recent myocardial infarction (>7 days but <30 days)
Decompensated congestive heart failure
Symptomatic arrhythmias

Intermediate

Mild angina
Prior myocardial infarction by history or ECG
Compensated or prior congestive heart failure
Diabetes mellitus

Minor

Advanced age
Abnormal ECG (LVH, LBBB, ST-T abnormalities)
Rhythm other than sinus
Low functional capacity
History of stroke
Uncontrolled systemic hypertension

ECG, electrocardiogram; LVH, left ventricular hypertrophy; BBB, bundle branch block.

6 months (see Table 19.8). Therefore, in women who have had a recent myocardial infarction, elective surgery should be postponed at least for 6 months.
Reference: Pages 611–615

18. C

Otherwise known as the "wedge pressure," the measurement of the pulmonary capillary wedge pressure (PCWP) reflects the LVEDP and is most useful in the management of fluid replacement in the perioperative period.
Reference: Page 619

19. A

The American Heart Association recommends this regimen for antibiotic valvular prophylaxis (see Table 19.12). The use of *vancomycin hydrochloride/gentamicin* is for *penicillin*-allergic patients. Oral *amoxicillin* is recommended for low-risk patients for minor procedures only.
Reference: Pages 616–617

Table 19.12. Recommendations for Prophylaxis of Bacterial Endocarditis for Genitourinary and Gastrointestinal Procedures (185)

High-Risk Patients	Agents	Regimen
Standard regimen	*Ampicillin* and	2.0 g IM or IV within 30 min of starting procedure; 1.0 g IM or IV 6 hr later
	Gentamicin	1.5 mg/kg (not to exceed 120 mg) within 30 min of starting procedure
Penicillin-allergic	*Vancomycin* and	1.0 g IV over 1–2 hr completed within 30 min of starting procedure
	Gentamicin	1.5 mg/kg (not to exceed 120 mg) within 30 min of starting procedure
Moderate-Risk Patients	*Agents*	*Regimen*
Standard regimen	*Ampicillin* or *Amoxicillin*	2.0 g IM or IV within 30 min of starting procedure 2.0 g orally 1 hr before procedure
Penicillin-allergic	*Vancomycin*	1.0 g IV over 1–2 hr completed within 30 min of starting procedure

20. D

With extensive blood loss, the most likely requirement for transfusion relates to the consumption of clotting factors and platelets. Therefore, intraoperative determinations of the platelet count and the partial thromboplastin time are useful to help assess whether platelets or fresh-frozen plasma should be transfused.
Reference: Pages 620–622

21. D

Chronic bronchitis and emphysema are diseases that often occur in tandem. Cigarette smoking is involved in the pathogenesis of both. Preoperative treatment with bronchodilators, antibiotics, respiratory therapy, and cessation of smoking are important to decrease the risk of postoperative pulmonary complications.
Reference: Pages 625–627

22. A

Atelectasis accounts for 90% of all pulmonary complications. The most important maneuvers for prevention and therapy are those that promote maximal inspiratory pressure. These include the use of incentive spirometry, deep breathing exercises, coughing, and in some cases, the use of positive end-expiratory pressure with a mask. Oversedation should be avoided and early ambulation should be encouraged.
Reference: Page 627

23. D

Otherwise known as noncardiogenic pulmonary edema, ARDS is a condition requiring aggressive pulmonary resuscitation and treatment of the underlying cause. In gynecologic patients, the underlying cause is usually septicemia, and thus, the broad-spectrum antibiotics in addition to the specific treatment of respiratory failure, which typically involves ventilator support and shock management, are used.
Reference: Pages 628–629

24. D

Immediate treatment of postoperative deep-vein thrombosis is aimed at preventing propagation of deep thrombosis and prevention of pulmonary embolism. Long-term treatment should aim at prevention of rethrombosis while at the same time minimize the risks of bleeding complications. *Streptokinase* is contraindicated in the postoperative surgical patient except under the most life-threatening conditions. The risks of postoperative hemorrhage are extremely high with this therapy. The most widely evaluated and recognized method of deep-vein thrombosis treatment is the use of intravenous *heparin* therapy with the goal of achieving an activated partial thromboplastin time (APTT) of approximately 1.5 to 2.0 times the control value. This is usually accomplished with immediate intravenous bolus of *heparin* followed by continuous infusion.

The duration of *heparin* therapy has been evaluated in randomized prospective studies comparing what had been "traditional" therapy of 10 days of *heparin* versus a shorter infusion of 5 days of *heparin*. Both *heparin* regimens were then followed with 3–6 months of oral *coumadin* administration achieving an international normalized ration (INR) of approximately 2.0 times control value. Five days of *heparin* therapy were found to be equally effective in preventing rethrombosis and, at the same time, shortened the hospital stay by approximately 5 days.
Reference: Pages 605–606

25. D

An elderly patient undergoing surgery for gynecologic cancer is at very high risk of developing postoperative venous thrombolic complications. Prophylactic methods are clearly warranted, and prospective studies have identified that both low-dose *heparin, low molecular weight heparin,* and intermittent pneumatic leg compression are effective in this patient group. However, the intensity of prophylaxis is critical.

Randomized trials have shown that *heparin* given every 12 hours (answer **A**) and short-duration (24 hours) pneumatic compression (answer **C**) are not effective in patients with gynecologic cancers, although they are effective in lower risk groups of patients. Low-dose *heparin* given as an 8-hour regimen or pneumatic compression continued for 5 days postoperatively have both been found to be effective in preventing venous thrombolic complications in this high-risk group of patients. Because of the decreased risks of bleeding complications, intermittent pneumatic leg compression was considered to be the most cost-effective regimen available.
Reference: Pages 601–604

26. D

Necrotizing fasciitis is an uncommon infectious disorder with approximately 1,000 cases occurring annually in the United States. It is characterized by a rapidly progressive bacterial infection that involves the subcutaneous tissues and fascia and characteristically spares underlying muscle. Systemic toxicity is a frequent feature of the disease. The pathogenesis of necrotizing fasciitis involves a polymicrobial infection with common organisms including hemolytic *Streptococcus* as well as other organisms, including gram-positive organisms and anaerobes. Enzymes released by bacteria into the subcutaneous space destroy the fascia, adipose tissue, and induce a liquefactive necrosis. In addition, noninflammatory and intravascular coagulation and thrombosis frequently will occur in the small vessels in the subcutaneous tissues, resulting in ischemia and necrosis of the subcutaneous tissues. Late in the course of infection, destruction of the superficial nerves can produce anesthesia in the involved skin. Release of bacteria and toxins into the systemic circulation can cause septic shock, acid-base abnormalities, and multiorgan impairment.

Predisposing risk factors for necrotizing fasciitis include diabetes mellitus, trauma, alcoholism, an immunocompromised state, hypertension, peripheral vascular disease, intravenous drug abuse, and obesity. The mortality rate of the disease is high. However, early diagnosis and aggressive management has led to improved survival rates. Clinical and laboratory findings can include a disproportionally greater amount of pain than expected from the clinical findings; temperature abnormalities—both hypothermia and hyperthermia; tenderness; erythema and warmth of the involved skin; edema and erythema spread diffusely, invading into normal skin. Most patients have leukocytosis and develop acid-base abnormalities. Successful treatment involves early recognition of the problem and immediate initiation of resuscitative measures, including correction of fluid and acid-base electrolyte and hematologic abnormalities. Aggressive surgical debridement and redebridement need to be performed, and broad-spectrum antibiotic therapy should be initiated. An incision should be made through the infected tissue, down to the fascia. An ability to undermine the skin and subcutaneous tissues with digital palpation often will confirm the diagnosis. Multiple incisions can be made sequentially toward the periphery of the infected tissue until well-vascularized healthy tissue is reached at all margins. Many patients have benefited from central venous monitoring as well as from high-caloric and nutritional support. In addition, in one study, the use of hyperbaric oxygen therapy after surgical debridement was associated with an improvement in overall mortality. Once the infection has resolved and granulation has begun, skin flaps can be mobilized to help cover open wounds.
Reference: Pages 594–596

27. E

Further imaging studies are not likely to change the surgeon's approach to this patient. If she has a solid mass compressing her sigmoid colon, which was present before the chemotherapy, it is probable that this is related to the malignancy and probably represents her ovary. An ultrasound, MRI, and CT scan will not change the treatment or the surgical approach in this patient. A CT scan of the abdomen and pelvis with contrast to identify the anatomy of the pelvic ureter is not only unnecessary but would likely result in acute tubular necrosis in a patient with a history of insulin-dependent diabetes and

Table 19.9. Functional Capacity Assessment from Clinical History (160)

Excellent

Carry 24 lb up eight steps
Carry objects that weigh 80 lb
Outdoor work (shovel snow, spade soil)
Recreation (ski, basketball, squash, handball, jog or walk 5 mph)

Moderate

Have sexual intercourse without stopping
Walk at 4 mph on ground level
Outdoor work (garden, rake, weed)
Recreation (roller skate, dance)

Poor

Shower and dress without stopping
Basic housework
Walk 2.5 mph on level ground
Recreation (golf, bowl)

a prior history of cisplatin. It should be noted that the patient already has a component of nephropathy (creatinine, 1.2 mg/dL), which may be due to the long-standing hypertension, diabetes, and/or the cisplatin treatments. Intravenous contrast agents are associated with approximately a 70% incidence of acute tubular necrosis. Therefore, the right answer would be to proceed with an exploratory laparotomy and then debulk the pelvic mass. Because the patient initially presented with a stage IV lesion, additional debulking should be limited to only those areas in which the colon or small intestine were in jeopardy of obstruction, as it would probably not change her overall survival. Reference: Pages 592–594

28. B

Because of the high mortality and morbidity associated with perioperative myocardial infarction, much effort has been made to predict perioperative cardiac risk. A prospective evaluation of preoperative cardiac risk factors using a multivariate analysis identified independent cardiac risk factors, as presented in Table 19.8. Using these factors, a cardiac risk index has been created that places a patient in one of four risk classes (see Table 19.9). Unstable angina, probably because it is relatively uncommon, does not appear as a risk factor, although many believe that patients with unstable angina should be considered at extremely high risk of perioperative cardiac mortality and should undergo coronary artery revascularization prior to any elective gynecologic surgery. Reference: Pages 611–613

20

Incontinence, Prolapse, and Disorders of the Pelvic Floor

Shawn A. Menefee
L. Lewis Wall

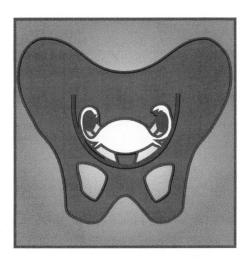

Learning Objectives

1. Describe the functional anatomy of the pelvic floor and its relationship to urinary and fecal continence and incontinence.

2. Understand normal continence mechanisms of the lower urinary tract and colorectal system.

3. Outline the principles of investigation used in the evaluation of patients with incontinence and/or prolapse.

4. Understand clinical urodynamic testing and its application in the evaluation of urinary incontinence.

5. Describe the causes of urinary incontinence and the appropriate means for diagnosing them.

6. Understand the terminology used to describe pelvic relaxation and incontinence.

7. Understand the basic principles involved in nonsurgical management of urinary incontinence.

8. Understand the surgical procedures used for treating urinary incontinence and prolapse, and understand which procedures are useful for which type of incontinence.

9. Describe the evaluation and treatment of patients with colorectal dysfunction.

Questions

1. The main support for the pelvic floor is provided by which structure?

   A. Uterosacral ligaments
   B. Levator ani muscle
   C. Bony pelvis
   D. Round ligament

2. Which treatment option for stress urinary incontinence consistently results in significant improvement?

   A. Anterior colporrhaphy
   B. Electrical stimulation
   C. Retropubic urethropexy
   D. Needle urethropexy

3. In the Pelvic Organ Prolapse Quantification (POPQ) profile, how many points are included in the measurements?

   A. 9
   B. 3
   C. 6
   D. 12

4. When using anticholinergic medications for the treatment of urge incontinence, the most common side effect is which of the following?

   A. Muscle weakness
   B. Urinary retention
   C. Dry mouth
   D. Urinary frequency

5. Which of the following statements about urinary incontinence is true?

   A. Urinary incontinence is a normal part of aging.
   B. Urinary incontinence is normal after vaginal childbirth.
   C. Urinary incontinence does not occur in women who have cesarean deliveries.
   D. Urinary incontinence is almost always treatable.

6. Which of the following assists the provider the most in the evaluation of a patient with primary stress urinary incontinence?

   A. Complex cystometrogram report
   B. Pressure-flow study
   C. Urethral pressure profile
   D. Carefully taken history and thorough physical examination

7. In a patient with a history consistent with an overactive bladder, which of the following urodynamic study is the most useful?

   A. Valsalva leak point pressure
   B. Frequency/volume bladder chart over 48 hours
   C. Pelvic ultrasound
   D. Pressure-flow study

8. To be a useful urodynamics study, which of the following criteria must be met?

   A. It must be performed at a continence center.
   B. The study must be performed on a multichannel urodynamics machine.

C. It must provide objective evidence about lower urinary tract function.
D. It needs to performed with the bladder empty.

9. As a worldwide problem, obstetrical fistulas have a tremendous impact. Which of the following considerations is the most important factor in the management of this condition?

   A. Three-layer closure with delayed absorbable suture
   B. Improved access to adequate obstetrical care
   C. Bladder drainage for 7 days after traumatic delivery or fistula surgery
   D. The encorporation of a vascular flap over the fistula repair

10. Which of the following items is true about anal incontinence?

    A. Disorders of rectal function are uncommon in women.
    B. Anal incontinence is referred to as passage of stool from the vagina.
    C. Anal incontinence is referred to as involuntary passage of flatus or feces through the anal canal.
    D. Patients affected by anal incontinence will promptly seek care to correct this condition.

    For each of the questions below, one or more of the responses is correct. Select the best answer based on the following:

    A. If A, B, C are correct
    B. If only A and C are correct
    C. If only B and D are correct
    D. If only D is correct

11. Overactive bladder is also known by which of the following terms?

    A. Detrusor instability
    B. Urgency/frequency syndrome
    C. Urge incontinence
    D. Urinary retention

12. The initial treatment for patients with overactive bladder includes which of the following treatments?

    A. Behavioral modification
    B. Bladder neck suspension
    C. Anticholinergic medications
    D. α-Agonist medications

13. Nonobstructive voiding dysfunction in females can be treated by the following:

    A. Cholinergic medications
    B. Clean intermittent self-catheterization
    C. Urethrolysis
    D. Sacral neuromodulation

14. In examining a patient with complaints of stress urinary incontinence who does not leak during initial evaluation, which of the following considerations may demonstrate this bothersome problem?

    A. Ensuring that the bladder is not empty
    B. Full cough stress test in the standing position
    C. Replacement of any prolapse beyond the hymenal ring
    D. Running water in the sink

15. Which of the following items are true about pelvic floor exercises?

    A. Handouts are sufficient instruction.
    B. Supervised instruction is beneficial.
    C. Should be taught and performed only when pregnant.
    D. Additional benefit may be obtained using biofeedback devices.

16. Which of the following is associated with the syndrome of interstitial cystitis?

    A. Frequency
    B. Urgency
    C. Bladder pain
    D. Painful voiding

For each numbered item, select the one heading most closely associated with it. Each lettered heading may be used once, more than once, or not at all. Match the procedure with the technique.

    A. Polypropylene mesh attached to a trocar placed under the midurethra with minimal tension and no fixed attachment point
    B. The plication of the vaginal muscularis layer or endopelvic fascia in the midline through a vaginal incision
    C. The attachment of endopelvic fascia at the level of the bladder neck to the iliopectineal ligament
    D. The lateral endopelvic fascia along the urethra and bladder is reattached to the arcus tendinous fascia pelvis

17. Paravaginal repair

18. Anterior colporrhaphy

19. Tension-free vaginal tape (TVT)

20. Retropubic urethropexy (Burch)

Answers

  1. B

The striated muscles of the pelvic floor, in combination with their fascial attachments, work together across the entire pelvis to prevent pelvic organ prolapse, to maintain continence, and to control expulsive activities. The pelvic organs are supported primarily by the muscular activity of the pelvic floor, aided by ligamentous attachments. Rather than functioning as a rigid structure, the pelvic floor muscles provide dynamic support through constant activity, functioning more like a self-regulating trampoline that continually adjusts its tension in response to changing circumstances. The pelvic floor muscles consist of a diaphragmatic portion (iliococcygeus) and the pubovisceral (pubococcygeus) portion. This unit of muscle is commonly referred to as the levator ani muscle. When the pubovisceral muscle contracts, it pulls the rectum, vagina, and urethra anteriorly toward the pubic bone and constricts the lumina of these pelvic organs. It is this constant contractile property that is so important in maintaining pelvic support and continence. The pelvic ligaments are often erroneously believed to be the most important factors in pelvic support. Ligaments are poorly suited to maintain support over time because fibrous tissue elongates when subjected to constant tension. The pelvic ligaments serve mainly to keep structure in positions where they can be supported by muscular activity rather than as weight-bearing structures themselves. The loss of normal muscular support lead to sagging and widening of the urogenital hiatus and predisposes patients to the development of pelvic organ prolapse. The importance

of these ligaments is derived from the amount of attention given to these structures in performing gynecologic surgery. The pelvic ligaments (round, infundibulopelvic, and cardinal) are loose condensations of areolar tissue, blood vessels, and muscle fibers. By themselves, they have little supportive strength but function as "moorings" to hold the uterus and vagina in place.
Reference: Pages 645–650

2. **C**

The treatment of stress urinary incontinence consists of conservative therapy and surgical correction. The mainstay of conservative therapy involves active and/or passive pelvic floor muscle rehabilitation. This conservative therapy may include basic instruction and clinical feedback in the form of Kegel exercise or formal biofeedback therapy. In women with moderate-to-severe weakness of their pelvic floor muscles who have difficulty performing pelvic floor muscles exercises themselves, a form of passive pelvic floor muscle rehabilitation may be considered as a treatment option. Electrical stimulation of the pelvic floor involves passage of an electrical current through the muscles of the pelvic floor causing them to contract. However, when compared to sham devices and pelvic floor exercises, electrostimulation has produced mixed results in the treatment of stress incontinence. The surgical treatment of stress incontinence resulting from anatomic hypermobility of the urethra has traditionally been classified into the following areas: anterior colporrhaphy, vaginal needle urethropexies, retropubic urethropexies, and suburethral sling procedures. Most surgical series that have evaluated techniques of anterior colporrhaphy for stress incontinence have shown long-term success rates of only 35% to 65%, a figure that most would regard as unacceptably low. The initial cure rates with numerous different needle urethropexies were between 70% to 90%, but these rates seem to decrease significantly over time in many series, with 5-year success rates of 50% or less. The long-term success rates for needle urethropexy are poor, thus this operation is falling out of favor. Retropubic urethropexy (i.e. Marshall, Marchetti, and Kratz urethropexy and Burch urethropexy) has demonstrated high long-term success rates for patients undergoing these operations as a primary procedure for stress incontinence in the range of 70% to 90%.
Reference: Pages 668–677

3. **A**

As the result of the deficiencies in the traditional classifications, the International Continence Society standardization of terminology of female pelvic organ prolapse was developed and published in 1996. This descriptive system contains a series of nine site-specific measurements. The classification uses six points along the vagina (two points on the anterior, middle, and posterior compartments) measured in relation to the hymen. Three other measurements include the genital hiatus, the perineal body, and the total vaginal length. All measurements except the total vaginal length are measured at maximal straining. This new classification appears confusing in initial review; however, it is easily learned when instructed by an experienced person or by viewing the instructional videotape. The POPQ examination provides a standardized measurement system to allow for more accurate postoperative outcome assessments and to ensure uniform, reliable, and site-specific descriptions of pelvic organ prolapse.
Reference: Pages 686–688

4. **C**

The drugs used to treat overactive bladder symptoms can be grouped into different categories according to their pharmacologic characteristics; however, for all practical purposes, these drugs are anticholinergic agents that exert their effects on the bladder by blocking the activity of acetylcholine at muscarinic receptor sites. These medications work well for the treatment of overactive bladder. These drugs have side effects, the most common of which are dry mouth resulting from decrease saliva production, increased heart rate because of vagal blockade, feelings of constipation resulting from decreased gastrointestinal motility, and occasional blurred vision. In most patients, dry mouth

is the most common and bothersome symptom. Because of the short half-life and common occurrence of side effects with traditional medications, two new medications have recently been developed and appear to decrease the incidence of dry mouth with similar efficacy in those taking these new agents.
Reference: Pages 679–680

5. D

Urinary incontinence is defined as involuntary loss of urine that is a social or hygienic problem and that is objectively demonstrable. Urinary incontinence is a symptom, not a diagnosis. It is not a normal part of aging, although the prevalence of the problem increases with age. Urinary incontinence affects 13 million Americans with an estimated 1 million new cases diagnosed each year. The condition cost billions of dollars annually in the United States. Stress urinary incontinence does not occur in every woman following a vaginal childbirth, although this condition is more common in parous women. However, the lack of pelvic floor trauma related to vaginal birth does not protect all women from developing stress incontinence. Urinary incontinence usually can be improved and frequently can be cured, often by using relatively simple, nonsurgical interventions.
Reference: Page 654

6. D

The initial evaluation of most patients with incontinence is not difficult, but it requires a systematic approach to consider all possible causes. Multichannel urodynamic studies produce a biophysical profile of a patient's bladder and urethral function. A wide variety of sophisticated studies of bladder and urethral function has been developed to measure various aspects of bladder storage and emptying. These studies include uroflowmetry, filling cystometry, pressure-flow voiding studies, urethral pressure profilometry, and determination of leak point pressure. Clinicians who recommend complex studies without taking a careful history and without performing a thorough physical examination are likely to obtain useless or irrelevant information from these expensive investigations. When combined with some simple urodynamic tests, a detailed history and physical examination often can reliably predict the type of incontinence.
Reference: Pages 654–658

7. B

A frequency/volume bladder chart is an invaluable aid in the evaluation of patients with urinary incontinence, but use of this tool is often neglected. A frequency/volume chart is a voiding record kept by the patient for several days. Patients should be instructed to measure and record each voided amount. The time of any incontinence episodes should be recorded; it is also helpful to maintain an annotated record of symptoms or activities associated with urine loss. A frequency/volume bladder chart gives an accurate record of 24-hour urinary output, the total number of daily voids, the average voided volume, and the functional bladder capacity. This information allows the clinician to confirm complaints with objective data. The bladder diary is the foundation for conservative management of urinary incontinence based on fluid manipulation and behavioral management of voiding habits. Subtracted-filling cystometrography for patients with an overactive bladder should show phasic pressure waves that produce urgency and urge incontinence. False-negative and false-positive results can occur. The measurement of Valsalva leak point pressure is meant to confirm stress urinary incontinence. The pressure-flow study is used to evaluate the voiding mechanism of a patient. Ultrasound is usually used in the assessment of the patient with incontinence to perform estimation of the postvoid residual without requiring catheterization.
Reference: Pages 658–663

8. C

A urodynamics study is anything that provides objective evidence about lower urinary tract function. The use of bladder chart, measurement of postvoid residual and

bladder neck angle, and simple bladder filling with cough stress test are all simple, inexpensive tests that provide a great deal of useful clinical information and can be performed in any office setting. In certain individuals, even after complete history and physical examination, complex urodynamic testing is required for complete evaluation and diagnosis. When diagnosis or treatment is uncertain, the patient may benefit from multichannel urodynamic studies, which are often performed in a continence or pelvic floor center. These studies evaluate both bladder and urethral function and, depending on the specific study, may be performed with the bladder empty, partially full, or near capacity.
Reference: Pages 658–663

9. B

A traumatic opening between the urinary tract and the surface of the body is called a fistula. Worldwide, the most common cause of fistulas is obstructed labor. This was also true in the Western world 150 years ago, but advances in the provision of basic obstetric services and advanced obstetric interventions have virtually eliminated this problem in developed countries. The development of an obstetric fistula is related to social, economic, and medical factors. Obstructed labor often occurs in rural areas where girls marry at a young age and where transportation is poor and access to medical services is limited. The key to decreasing the incidence of this significant worldwide problem is prevention. The development of adequately trained obstetric providers and facilitating access to this care in underdeveloped countries are paramount. The surgical correction of these fistulas is extremely important to the many unfortunate women afflicted with this condition, with many becoming social outcasts if not corrected. The keys to closure of a vesicovaginal fistula include wide mobilization of the tissue plans so that the fistula edges can be approximated without any tension, close approximation of tissue edges, closure of the fistula in several layers, and meticulous attention to postoperative bladder drainage. The closure of large, recurrent, or complex fistulas is enhanced by tissue flaps.
Reference: Pages 664–665

10. C

Pelvic floor disorders span all three anatomic compartments of the pelvis: urinary, genital, and colorectal. No approach to the pelvic floor dysfunction that ignores colonic and rectal problems will meet the needs of female patients. Disorders of colonic and rectal function are disproportionally prevalent among women and represent a major area of continuing clinical neglect in women's health care. Because gynecologists are often the first physicians that women see for pelvic floor disorders, we have an obligation to become knowledgeable about common colorectal complaints. Gynecologists should be familiar with common disorders of the posterior pelvis including anal incontinence, rectal prolapse, constipation, fecal impaction, and irritable bowel syndrome. Anal incontinence refers to the involuntary passage of flatus or feces (either liquid or formed stool) through the anal canal. The passage of stool from the vagina represents a rectovaginal or colovaginal fistula. Although it is becoming more socially acceptable to talk about urinary incontinence, discussion of fecal loss remains a taboo subject. Physicians must ask patients directly (but sensitively) about loss of bowel control in order to elicit this complaint. The problem is more prevalent than most people realize: In one survey, 7.1% of the general population reported some degree of anal incontinence. As we learn more information about the function of the pelvic floor, the posterior compartment must be included in our understanding to best serve our patients.
Reference: Pages 685–690

11. A

The term *overactive bladder* refers detrusor overactivity in patients who have symptoms of urgency, frequency, and urge incontinence. Urge incontinence caused by detrusor overactivity is the most common form of incontinence in older women, and the second-most-common form of incontinence overall. These patients typically experience sudden, unexpected loss of large volumes of urine that cannot be controlled. For

patients who have frequency and urgency without incontinence, detrusor overactivity rarely is the cause of their problem. The cause of these symptoms may represent a disorder of bladder sensation. Urinary retention may be obstructive, related to surgery, or neurologic in nature. In some cases, bladder overdistention may provoke an uninhibited contraction of the detrusor muscle leading to urinary incontinence, but urinary retention should not be termed an overactive bladder. Unlike stress urinary incontinence, the medical terminology associated with an overactive bladder is broad and includes detrusor spasm, detrusor hyperreflexia, urge incontinence, and even urinary urgency/frequency.
Reference: Pages 677–678

12. B

Overactive bladder can be treated using medications or behavioral modification. The best initial choice is probably a combination of the two therapies. The cure rates with behavioral modification are comparable to drug therapy, and any drug therapy for this condition will be enhanced by modifying the behaviors that contribute to detrusor overactivity. Bladder neck suspensions are used to treat stress urinary incontinence related to anatomic hypermobility. This therapy should not be used to treat urge incontinence but may be considered in patients with mixed incontinence, especially if stress incontinence is the major complaint. The tone of the urethra and bladder neck is maintained in large part by α-adrenergic activity from the sympathetic nervous system. These agents may be considered in a select group of women with stress urinary incontinence, but they should not be used in patients with overactive bladder symptoms.
Reference: Pages 679–680

13. C

In patients with voiding dysfunction, elevated postvoid residuals are discovered on evaluation after a spontaneous void. These patients may also present with recurrent urinary tract infections or overflow incontinence. These patients should begin a regime of clean, intermittent self-catheterization to improve bladder emptying. In many cases, this technique may be the only therapy needed to correct the incontinence. However, many women are bothered with daily repetitive catheterization and often desire other therapy. The recent development of sacral nerve root neuromodulation offers an additional treatment option. Voiding dysfunction in females can be related to a prior antiincontinence procedure; thus, it may be obstructive in nature. In these patients, urethrolysis is often beneficial in relieving their symptoms. Cholinergic therapy is not effective in the treatment of voiding dysfunction.
Reference: Pages 682–684

14. A

The physical examination of the patient with incontinence should include detection of general medical conditions that may affect the lower urinary tract. Such conditions include cardiovascular insufficiency, pulmonary disease, occult neurologic processes, as well as abnormalities of genitourinary development. The pelvic examination, including an evaluation of urethral and vaginal support, is of crucial importance. The patient should be examined with a full (not empty) bladder, especially if stress incontinence is a complaint. A cough stress test should be performed to confirm the condition. If negative in a supine position, it is beneficial to have the patient stand with her feet separated to shoulder width and cough several times prior to emptying her bladder. The patient with pelvic relaxation beyond the hymen will often not leak on cough stress test unless the prolapse is reduced in the normal anatomic position. Urinary leakage with replacement of the prolapse is often quite marked and may represent intrinsic sphincter deficiency, which requires preoperative evaluation prior to correction of symptomatic pelvic relaxation. The use of running water during the physical examination may result in an uninhibited detrusor contraction but typically does not assist with demonstrating stress urinary incontinence.
Reference: Page 657

15. C

Kegel was the first person to investigate pelvic muscle strengthening. He developed the patient's awareness of the pubococcygeus muscle and instructed her in exercises to strengthen this muscle with a crude pneumatic biofeedback device called a perineometer. Nearly all gynecologists are familiar with these exercises; however, discussions on this therapy have often degenerated into a few brief words of oral instruction or a copied handout. Programs based on this approach are not only disappointing but can train women to become dysfunctional voiders. Efficient pelvic floor exercises must include supervised instruction by an interested provider (physician, physical therapist, or clinical nurse). The use of vaginal cones or biofeedback units can augment learning in patients having difficulty with a supervised exercise program.
Reference: Pages 669–670

16. A

The classic syndrome associated with interstitial cystitis (sometimes also called "painful bladder syndrome") includes urgency, frequency, and bladder pain in the presence of a small-capacity bladder. Bladder pain tends to increase with bladder filling and is relieved with voiding. The etiology of interstitial cystitis is unknown; most probably, a variety of disorders with a common clinical presentation is lumped together because the underlying pathophysiology is unknown. The diagnosis is often made by the exclusion of other etiologies in patients with painful bladder symptoms.
Reference: Pages 684–685

17. D

18. B

19. A

20. C

The basic understanding of the anatomic defects responsible for anterior vaginal wall prolapse and stress urinary incontinence and the surgical correction should be understood by all gynecologists. Anterior vaginal colporrhaphy is the oldest operation for stress incontinence. In most surgeons' hands, *anterior colporrhaphy* has resulted in suboptimal outcomes for the treatment of stress incontinence. This procedure should be reserved primarily for patients requiring cystocele repair who do not have significant stress incontinence. The procedure is performed by the plication of the vaginal fascia (muscularis) in the midline often including the area under the bladder neck. The use of retropubic urethropexy for stress urinary incontinence has proven to be an effective therapy, which has been discussed in prior sections. The *retropubic urethropexy* or *Burch colposuspension* involves the attachment of the vaginal fascia at the level of the bladder neck to the iliopectineal ligament (Cooper's ligament) with suture. The Burch colposuspension is commonly performed through an abdominal incision; however, it has also been reported by a laparoscopic route. Anterior vaginal prolapse may occur secondary to lateral detachment of the vagina from the pelvic sidewall. This defect is often found associated with hypermobile bladder neck. The *paravaginal repair* can be performed by an abdominal, laparoscopic, or vaginal route and consists of reattachment of the endopelvic fascia to the arcus tendinous. The poor success rates of needle urethropexy operations have led many surgeons to search for a similarly attractive, low-morbidity surgical procedure with better long-term success. Short-term results on studies of the TVT procedure are encouraging, but long-term data must be evaluated before the place of this operation in the treatment of stress incontinence can be determined. This procedure involves the use of polypropylene mesh placed under the midurethra with minimal tension. To perform this operation, a small midurethral incision is made in the vaginal epithelium and trocars are passed lateral to the urethra and through the endopelvic fascia into the retropubic space. Surgical correction remains an important treatment option for women with stress urinary incontinence.
Reference: Pages 671–677

21

Gynecologic Endoscopy

Andrew I. Brill
Malcolm G. Munro

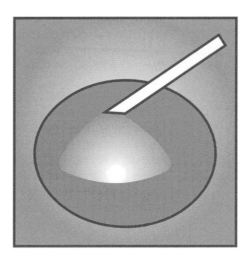

Learning Objectives

1. Understand the role of endoscopy in the diagnosis and treatment of gynecologic conditions.

2. Acquire a technical understanding of the equipment and supplies necessary for performing gynecologic endoscopic procedures.

3. Be able to effectively counsel patients who may be candidates for gynecologic endoscopic procedures.

4. Understand the complications associated with gynecologic endoscopic procedures.

Questions

1. Avoiding injury to the inferior epigastric vessels is facilitated by a thorough understanding of their locations. These vessels are best identified by

   A. Transillumination of the anterior abdominal wall using the laparoscope as a light source
   B. Laparoscopically identifying their origin from the external iliac arteries and tracing their course cephalad and lateral to the medial umbilical ligament
   C. Positioning any lower quadrant trocars within 3 cm of the medial umbilical ligaments, thereby avoiding injury to the inferior epigastric vessels, which invariably course cephalad and more laterally

2. The risk of capacitive coupling associated with monopolar laparoscopic surgery may be minimized by all of the following **except**

   A. Use of all-metal cannula systems
   B. Use of all-plastic cannula systems
   C. Using "cutting" current
   D. Use of coagulation current
   E. All of the above
   F. None of the above

3. Which of the following circumstances are most likely to result in electrosurgical bowel injuries secondary to direct coupling?

   A. Using a monopolar grasping forceps to desiccate a vessel that is being held by a noninsulated laparoscopic needle driver
   B. The use of monopolar "coagulation" to fulgurate oozing vessels through a metal laparoscopic cannula held by a plastic sleeve anchor
   C. The use of bipolar electrosurgical forceps passed through the instrument channel of an operating laparoscope to desiccate the oviducts for purposes of sterilization

4. Which of the following best describes the type of electrical current used for performing electrosurgery?

   A. Low-voltage, direct current
   B. High-wattage, low-frequency, alternating current
   C. Variable-voltage, radiofrequency current

5. Which of the following is considered an acceptable site for placement of an insufflation needle in a woman undergoing laparoscopy with a history of two previous laparotomies for pelvic disease?

   A. Suprapubic
   B. Left upper quadrant
   C. Right upper quadrant
   D. McBurney's point
   E. None of the above

6. Which of the following findings is suggestive of extraperitoneal positioning of the insufflation needle?

   A. An early insufflation pressure of 12 mm Hg
   B. Persistence of dullness to percussion under the right costal margin after insufflation of 500 mL carbon dioxide (CO_2)
   C. The absence of measured negative pressure following elevation of the anterior abdominal wall, prior to insufflation

D. All of the above
E. None of the above

7. Which of the following would *not* be considered an appropriate method for securing the infundibulopelvic ligament when performing laparoscopic oophorectomy?

   A. Suture ligature with extracorporeal tie
   B. Endoscopic stapling device
   C. Bipolar technique using "cutting" current
   D. Monopolar technique using coagulation current
   E. All are equally appropriate

8. Which of the following may be a complication associated with the performance of laparoscopy for prolonged periods of time with the intraperitoneal pressure exceeding 20 mm Hg?

   A. CO_2 embolus
   B. Hypercarbia
   C. Hypotension
   D. All of the above

9. Injury to the great vessels secondary to insertion of a laparoscopic trocar in the umbilicus can be reduced by

   A. Ensuring that the angle of incidences is always between 45° and 90° to horizontal
   B. Utilizing disposable shielded trocars
   C. Maintaining the trocar in the sagittal plane
   D. All of the above

10. Which of the following is true regarding diagnostic hysteroscopy?

    A. It should be part of the workup for all infertile patients.
    B. It is generally difficult to perform in an office setting because of patient discomfort.
    C. Comparative studies have demonstrated it superior to dilatation and curettage (D & C) and hysterosalpingography for the identification of structural anomalies of the uterus.
    D. All of the above
    E. None of the above

11. Which of the following is untrue regarding 1.5% glycine when used as a uterine distention medium for operative hysteroscopy?

    A. Patients may experience hyperglycemia with high infused volumes.
    B. Significant and, occasionally, rapid systemic absorption may result in hypoosmolar encephalopathy.
    C. Hypernatremia is an occasional complication.
    D. None of the above

12. Which of the following causes loss of uterine distention at the time of hysteroscopy?

    A. Uterine perforation
    B. An overdilated cervix
    C. An open outflow valve
    D. All of the above
    E. None of the above

13. Which of the following steps may reduce the incidence and severity of systemic absorption of uterine distention media?

    A. Frequent, accurate measurement of total inflow and outflow in the uterine cavity
    B. Maintain intrauterine pressure above mean arterial pressure

C. Use of an in-line pump

D. Add suction to the outflow collecting system

14. Which of the following is true regarding laparoscopic hysterectomy?

A. It is a procedure that involves complete laparoscopically directed dissection of the bladder and fixation of all vascular and ligament pedicles.

B. It has been demonstrated to be a more cost-effective procedure in both vaginal and abdominal hysterectomies.

C. Postoperative morbidity has been demonstrated to be less than that of a vaginal hysterectomy.

D. All of the above

E. None of the above

15. Which of the following steps may reduce the risk of clinically significant gas embolism during an operative hysteroscopy?

A. Trendelenburg position

B. Keeping the outflow port of the resectoscope closed

C. Utilizing the least amount of pressure for uterine distention

D. Flushing air bubbles from the inflow tubing

E. None of the above

Answers

1. **B (see Fig. 21.3)**

   The inferior epigastric vessels can rarely, if ever, be seen by transillumination because they lie deep to the anterior rectus sheath and usually inferior to the rectus muscle

Figure 21.3   Vascular anatomy of the anterior abdominal wall. Location of the vessels that can be traumatized when inserting trocars into the anterior abdominal wall.

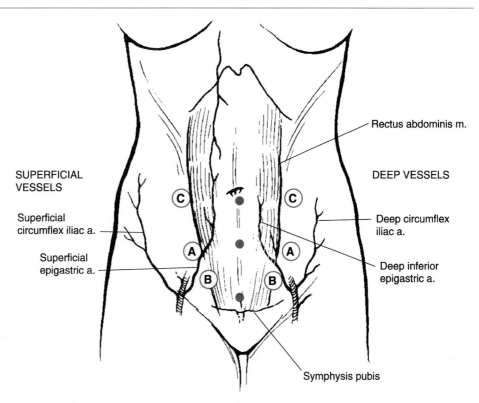

itself. Whereas the *superficial* epigastric vessels may frequently be identified using transillumination, these vessels do not align with the deeper inferior epigastric vessels.

Lower quadrant trocars should be passed *lateral* to, not within, 3 cm of the medial umbilical fold (ligaments) because the inferior epigastric vessels generally course in this area.

The inferior epigastric vessels can usually be identified shortly distal to their origin from the external iliac arteries after they wrap around the inguinal ligament to begin their intraperitoneal course between the internal inguinal ring (marked by the round ligament) and the most distal visible attachment of the medial umbilical ligament in the perivesical space.
Reference: Pages 718–721

2. D (see Fig. 21.16)

All-metal cannula systems generally prevent capacitance by allowing current to be widely dispersed via the relatively large area of the abdominal wall in contact with the conductive surface. All-plastic systems reduce the chance of capacitance to adjacent bowel because of the nonconductive nature of all of the system's materials.

High-voltage currents predispose to the formation of a capacitor. "Cutting" current is of relatively low voltage and is appropriately used for desiccation, vaporization, and the creation of incisions. It is far less likely to result in clinically significant capacitive coupling than "coagulation" current, which has much higher voltage.
Reference: Pages 733–737

3. A (see Fig. 21.15)

Monopolar grasping forceps are invariably insulated while laparoscopy needle drivers are not. If a noninsulated hand instrument is utilized to grasp tissue undergoing monopolar desiccation, the entire shaft becomes a conductor and, therefore, has the potential to directly couple to the bowel. Monopolar fulguration through a metal laparoscopic cannula held by a plastic sleeve anchor is more likely to result in capacitive, not direct, coupling (see Fig. 21.16C). Bipolar forceps may safely be passed through the instrument channel of an "operating" laparoscope without concern. However, when monopolar instruments are inserted through the instrument channel, it causes an increased risk of capacitive coupling to the metal jacket of the laparoscope.
Reference: Pages 733–736

4. C

The electrosurgical generators convert low-frequency alternating wall current (60 Hz in North America) to a frequency similar to that used in AM radio broadcasts (around 500 Hz and higher).
Reference: Pages 732–736

5. B (see Fig. 21.6)

In the presence of known or suspected adhesions under the umbilicus, the left upper quadrant is an ideal site for primary peritoneal entry, provided there is no marked hepatosplenomegaly and no history of exposure to previous potentially adhesiogenic procedures such as splenectomy, gastrectomy, or upper abdominal radiation therapy. Prior to such an entry, the stomach is routinely decompressed with an orogastric or nasogastric tube. Use of a small caliber (<3 mm) "scout" laparoscope via an insufflation needle will minimize postoperative pain and cosmetic concerns, and is usually adequate to allow assessment of the underside of the umbilicus and, if necessary, to direct required adhesiolysis.

The suprapubic area is inappropriate because of risks of adhesions, at least in this patient. Blind insertion at McBurney's point, which is immediately above the right

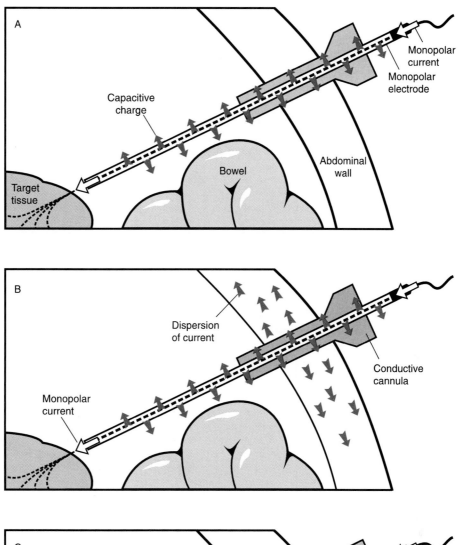

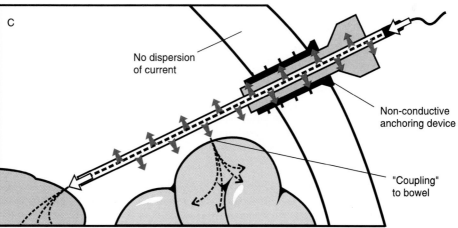

Figure 21.16   Capacitative coupling. All activated monopolar electrodes emit a surrounding charge, proportional to the voltage of the current **(A).** This makes the electrode a potential capacitor. Generally, as long as the charge is allowed to disperse through the abdominal wall **(B),** no sequelae result. However, if the "return" to the dispersive electrode is blocked by insulation, such as a plastic anchor **(C),** the current can couple to a conductive cannula or directly to bowel.

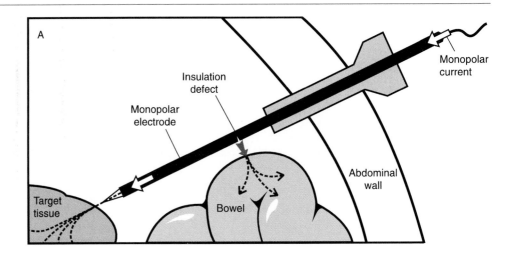

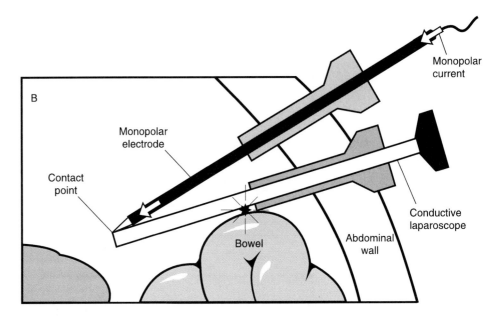

Figure 21.15 Direct coupling. Direct coupling is a potential complication of monopolar electrosurgery and may occur secondary to defects in the insulation **(A)** or, classically, to contract with a conductive instrument that in turn touches other intraperitoneal structures. In the example depicted **(B),** the active electrode is touching the laparoscope, and current is transferred to bowel via a small enough contact point that thermal injury results. Another common target of such coupling is to noninsulated hand instruments.

iliac vessels, should not be performed. Right upper quadrant insertion places the patient at risk for injury to the liver, gallbladder, great hepatic vessels, and biliary collecting system. Some have suggested that open laparoscopy reduces the risk of bowel injury, but there are no data supporting such a contention.
Reference: Pages 721–724

6. D

Insufflation pressure that exceeds 10 mm Hg early in the insufflation process is suggestive of extraperitoneal positioning or of the needle tip being located within the posterior abdominal wall, the lumen of a vessel, or abdominal viscera. Gas dispersing to the left upper quadrant separates the costal margin from the liver resulting in a tympana to percussion—a distinct change from the preexisting dullness to percussion

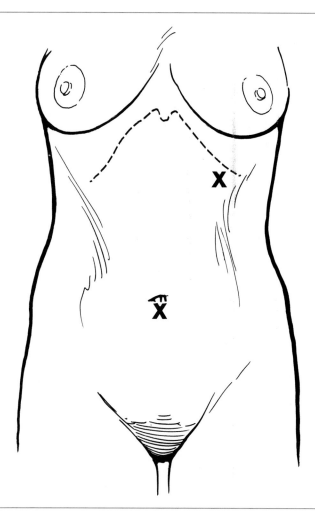

Figure 21.6   Insufflation needle and cannula insertion sites. In most instances, the insufflation needle, if used, and the primary cannula are inserted through the umbilicus. When subumbilical adhesions are known or suspected, the insufflation needle may be placed through the pouch of Douglas or in the left upper quadrant following evacuation of the gastric contents with an orogastric tube.

prior to insufflation. Failure of this tympanitic change by 500 mL of insufflation gas may be an early sign of inappropriate needle placement.

If the insufflation needle is in the peritoneal cavity, the negative intraperitoneal pressure created by lifting the abdominal wall may be demonstrated with the aspiration of a drop of fluid placed at the proximal opening of the needle. This negative pressure gradient is perhaps more accurately demonstrated by attaching the needle to the insufflator using insufflation tubing and reading the pressure gauge as the abdominal wall is abruptly lifted. Reference: Pages 718–721

7. **D**

"Cutting current" of appropriate output results in even desiccation of the tissue interposed between the jaws of the monopolar or bipolar grasping instrument. "Coagulation current" is interrupted and of much higher voltage, resulting in uneven areas of desiccation. These focally desiccated areas of tissue can impede conduction of current throughout the rest of the tissue, potentially leaving parts of the lumen intact. In the case of a fallopian tube, the result could be pregnancy; for blood vessels, the result could be hemorrhage. Reference: Pages 728–730

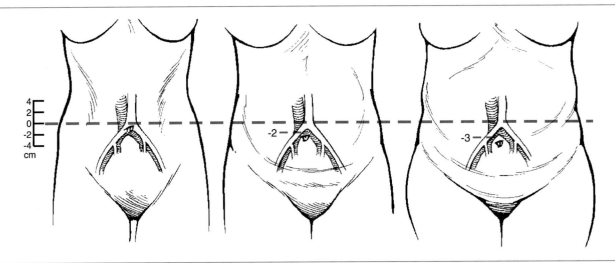

Figure 21.4   Vascular anatomy. Location of the great vessels and their changing relationship to the umbilicus with increasing patient weight (*from left to right*).

8. D

CO$_2$ embolus may be caused by a number of aspects of laparoscopic surgery, including extensive dissection under high intraperitoneal pressures (>25 mm Hg). The risk of hypercarbia has been demonstrated to increase gradually with time, even between 12 and 15 mm Hg.

High intraperitoneal pressure may compress the great veins of the pelvis as well as the vena cava, thereby reducing end diastolic flow to the right atrium, causing reduced cardiac output.
Reference: Pages 731–732

9. C (see Fig. 21.4)

For most patients of normal weight, the incision angle should be approximately 45° to the plane of the operating table. With increasing body habitus, the location of the umbilicus tends to fall below the bifurcation of the great vessels, thereby allowing for a more vertical insertion of the trocar. The plastic shields integrated into the design of many disposable laparoscopy cannulas have never been demonstrated to reduce the rate of injury to the retroperitoneal vessels.

The surgeon should *always* maintain the trocar–cannula in the sagittal plane when inserting at the umbilicus to prevent injury to the common and external iliac vessels. This alone does not necessarily preclude injury to vessels along the sacral promontory.
Reference: Pages 718–720

10. C

Many infertile patients receive adequate primary evaluation of the endometrial cavity with the hysterosalpingogram because it is able to provide information regarding patency of the fallopian tubes. Hysteroscopy is generally performed with ease in an office setting using a small-diameter hysteroscope or one, or a combination, of conscious sedation and an effective intracervical block with local anesthetic. Diagnostic hysteroscopy is clearly superior to both D & C and hysterosalpingogram in detecting structural abnormalities of the uterus.
Reference: Pages 743–746

11. D

Sorbitol is a sugar solution, which, if absorbed in sufficient amounts, can contribute to hyperglycemia, a problem not experienced with glycine. Large amounts of absorbed

electrolyte-free distention media of any type may result in a hypoosmolar state and can potentially result in encephalopathy. Hyponatremia is a complication associated with glycine and other electrolyte-free distention media. Of the "low-viscosity" electrolyte free media, only 5% *mannitol* is essentially isoosmolar.
Reference: Pages 749–750

12. D

Uterine perforation will invariably result in loss of distention of the endometrial cavity. Overdilation of the cervix may also prevent generation of adequate intracavitary pressure. In such instances, the problem usually can be overcome by using an additional tenaculum or other clamp to more tightly secure the cervix around the hysteroscope. If a gravity-flow system is used, the surgeon should always check to ensure that the outflow valve is set appropriately to maintain some degree of intrauterine pressure.
Reference: Page 753

13. A

The incidence and severity of absorption of uterine distention media is decreased when the surgeon operates at pressures that are *below* mean arterial pressure. An in-line pump can result in increasing intracavitary pressure and systemic absorption unless there is a pressure threshold above which the pump shuts off. A constant-pressure, variable-flow infusion pump is more likely to maintain intrauterine pressure at a preset limit. Regardless, frequent and accurate measurement of total inflow and outflow of uterine distention medium must take place at least every 15 minutes during a case or continuously using an automated collection device.
Reference: Pages 754–755

14. E

The term laparoscopic hysterectomy refers to a spectrum of procedures that vary depending upon the relative amount of dissection performed vaginally and laparoscopically. A number of classification systems exist that allow for various types of laparoscopic hysterectomy to be defined.

While laparoscopic hysterectomy *may* be more cost-effective for many women who would otherwise undergo abdominal hysterectomy, neither morbidity nor cost is saved when compared to vaginal hysterectomy.
Reference: Page 714

15. C and D

Because venous gas embolism may occur whenever there is open venous access and a significant pressure differential with the right atrium, Trendelenburg position may increase this risk during hysteroscopic uterine surgery. Keeping the outflow port of the resectoscope open to suction reduces this risk by continuously flushing bubbles out of the uterine cavity. Higher intrauterine distention pressures are more likely to drive air or gas bubbles into the venous circulation. Flushing the inflow line is a *sine qua non* for reducing the incidence for air embolism.
Reference: Pages 753–755

22 Hysterectomy

Jonathan S. Berek
Thomas G. Stovall

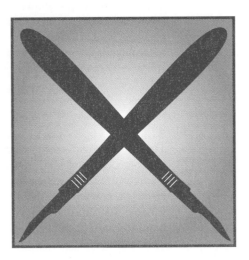

Learning Objectives

1. Know the indications for hysterectomy.

2. Understand the different methods for performing hysterectomy, their advantages, and their disadvantages.

3. Know concurrent surgical procedures that are performed with hysterectomy.

4. Be able to articulate the perioperative complications of hysterectomy.

5. Understand the psychosomatic effects of hysterectomy.

Questions

1. The most common indication for hysterectomy in North America is

   A. Malignancy
   B. Uterine leiomyomata
   C. Abnormal/dysfunctional uterine bleeding
   D. Pelvic pain
   E. Pelvic relaxation

2. A 46-year-old woman who has had two prior full-term pregnancies needs to undergo a hysterectomy because of severe menorrhagia unresponsive to medical therapy. She wishes to preserve her ovaries. In counseling the patient regarding the pros and cons of a vaginal versus an abdominal hysterectomy, an important issue for the discussion is the difference of the two procedures on outcome for which of the following variables?

   A. Sexual function
   B. Ovarian function
   C. Rate of complications
   D. Cancer prophylaxis

3. A 40-year-old woman is to undergo a hysterectomy for symptomatic uterine leiomyomata. She has no personal or family history of ovarian or breast disease. She asks you whether she should undergo bilateral oophorectomy. The principal reason for ovarian preservation is

   A. The risk of malignancy is low and compliance with estrogen replacement therapy is low.
   B. The risk of malignancy is unknown and the morbidity of prophylactic oophorectomy is significant.
   C. The psychological effects of oophorectomy are unknown.
   D. The pelvic support structures are more likely to be retained.

4. During the performance of an abdominal hysterectomy, the best way to identify the ureter is

   A. Observe the course of the ureter transperitoneally.
   B. Palpate the ureter at the pelvic brim.
   C. Enter the retroperitoneum and visualize the ureter.
   D. The ureter need not be identified if proper clamping techniques are used.

5. During the performance of an abdominal hysterectomy for uterine leiomyomata, an inadvertent cystotomy is created in the dome of the bladder. The management of the cystotomy is

   A. Postoperative bladder drainage with an indwelling Foley catheter for 14 days
   B. Resection of the bladder dome with three-layered closure
   C. One- or two-layered closure with absorbable suture
   D. No repair is necessary

6. An inadvertent enterotomy is created in the ileum during the performance of a lysis of adhesions prior to a planned abdominal hysterectomy. The defect is 1 cm. The repair should be

   A. Closed in two layers in a direction perpendicular to the intestinal lumen
   B. Closed in two layers in a direction parallel to the intestinal lumen
   C. A small-bowel resection 2 cm proximal and distal to the defect with an end-to-end reanastomosis
   D. A small-bowel resection and diverting colostomy

7. After the performance of a hysterectomy for benign disease, the best predictor of postoperative sexual functioning is

A. The results of psychological testing
B. The patient's preoperative sexual satisfaction
C. Whether the cervix has been preserved
D. Whether the ovaries have been preserved
E. Vaginal length

8. Indications for the removal of the uterus in patients with uterine leiomyomata include which of the following?

A. Uterine size of 12 weeks' gestation or greater
B. Growth following menopause
C. Impingent on other pelvic structures
D. Infertility/fetal wastage

Answers

1. B
The most common indication listed for the performance of a hysterectomy is uterine leiomyomata. However, available data strongly suggest that hysterectomy for leiomyomata should only be considered in symptomatic patients who do not desire future fertility.
Reference: Pages 761–763

2. C
The risk of one or more complications after abdominal hysterectomy is 1.7 times the risk after vaginal hysterectomy. The two major categories of complications are febrile morbidity and hemorrhage requiring transfusion. The risk of febrile morbidity is 2.1 times higher for abdominal hysterectomy than vaginal hysterectomy, and the risk of transfusion is 1.9 times higher.
Reference: Page 765

3. A
The risk of developing ovarian cancer after a hysterectomy performed in women for benign conditions is low. If there is no significant family history of ovarian cancer or a history of ovarian pathology, the risk of subsequent malignancy may be as low as 0.14%. A 40-year-old woman is more than 10 years younger than her anticipated menopause. Long-term compliance with posthysterectomy estrogen replacement therapy is about 20% to 40% at 5 years. The optimal duration of replacement therapy is unknown.
Reference: Page 767

4. C (see Fig. 22.4)
The most consistent means of identification of the ureter is by entering the retroperitoneal space. This is accomplished by extending the incision made into the broad ligament in a cephalad direction on the medial leaf of the broad ligament. The ureter is identified crossing the common iliac artery.
Reference: Pages 770–771, 775–776

5. C
Uncomplicated cystotomy should be repaired in the manner described. Postoperative drainage for 2 to 3 days should be sufficient. Defects near the trigone are more involved and often require passage of retrograde ureteral catheters and, occasionally, ureteral reimplantation.
Reference: Page 777

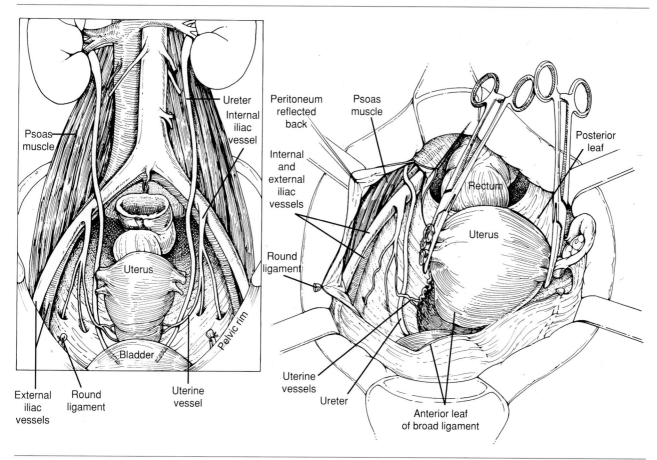

Figure 22.4   Identification of the ureter in the retroperitoneal space on the medial leaf of the broad ligament.
(From **Mann WA, Stovall TG.** *Gynecologic surgery.* New York: Churchill Livingstone, 1996, with permission.)

6. **A**

When a small inadvertent enterotomy occurs, it should be repaired in this manner to minimize the risk of lumenal stenosis, Resection or diversion of the intestine is unnecessary.
Reference: Pages 777–778

7. **B**

Reports in the literature support the belief that hysterectomy does not cause psychiatric sequelae or diminished sexual functioning in most patients.
Reference: Pages 796–797

8. **B, C, and D**

It has been previously taught that the uterus should be removed when it reached a size of 12 weeks' gestation or greater. This recommendation was based on the fact that the ovaries could not be palpated (ovarian cancer detection) and that hysterectomy would be more difficult if the uterus were larger. It has been demonstrated that these factors are not true and therefore it is no longer recommended that the uterus be removed on the basis of size alone.
Reference: Pages 762–763

REPRODUCTIVE ENDOCRINOLOGY

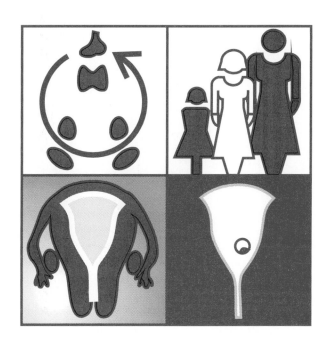

23 Puberty

Robert W. Rebar

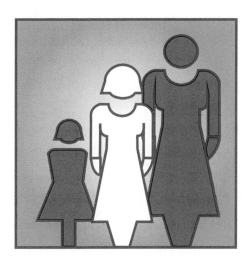

Learning Objectives

1. Describe the physical and hormonal changes that occur during normal pubertal development.

2. Classify the possible disorders of pubertal development.

3. Evaluate delayed and precocious puberty.

4. Evaluate the newborn infant with genital ambiguity.

Questions

1. The usual events in normal pubertal development from first to last are:

    A. Peak growth velocity, appearance of pubic hair, breast budding, menarche
    B. Breast budding, appearance of pubic hair, peak growth velocity, menarche
    C. Appearance of pubic hair, peak growth velocity, breast budding, menarche
    D. Breast budding, menarche, appearance of pubic hair, peak growth velocity
    E. Appearance of pubic hair, breast budding, menarche, peak growth velocity

2. Each of the following hormonal changes occurs early in normal pubertal development in girls **except**

    A. Increased circulating estradiol
    B. Sleep-entrained increases in luteinizing hormone (LH) and follicle-stimulating hormone (FSH)
    C. Increased circulating dehydroepiandrosterone sulfate (DHEAS)
    D. Decreased circulating estrone
    E. Increased circulating dehydroepiandrosterone (DHEA)

3. Each of the following statements about Turner's syndrome is true **except**

    A. Affected individuals may have a variety of karyotypes, including 45,X; 45,X/46,XY; and 45,X/46,XX.
    B. 45,X is the most common chromosomal disorder in humans.
    C. Associated abnormalities include multiple pigmented nevi, lymphedema at birth, hyperconvex nails, coarctation of the aorta, and abnormalities of the kidneys.
    D. Most individuals have below average intelligence.
    E. Diabetes mellitus and thyroid disorders are common.

4. Genital ambiguity at birth may be caused by maternal ingestion of which of the following steroids?

    A. *Ethinyl estradiol*
    B. *Prednisolone*
    C. *Danazol*
    D. *Medroxyprogesterone acetate*
    E. *17α-hydroxyprogesterone*

5. Causes of precocious puberty may include each of the following **except**

    A. McCune-Albright syndrome
    B. Langerhans cell–type histiocytosis
    C. Prader-Labhardt-Willi syndrome
    D. Granulosa–theca cell tumors
    E. Hypothalamic hamartomas

6. The initial change in the hypothalamic–pituitary–gonadal axis with puberty in girls is

    A. Decreased sensitivity to inhibitory effects of the low levels of sex steroids
    B. Maturation of the positive feedback response to estrogen
    C. Reversal of the estrogen/estradiol ratio with concomitant follicular development
    D. Reversal of the LH/FSH ratio in response to changing gonadotropin-releasing hormone (GnRH) pulse frequency

7. Treatment of Turner's syndrome can begin with

    A. *Conjugated estrogen* 0.625 mg daily plus *medroxyprogesterone acetate* 5 mg daily
    B. *Conjugated estrogen* 1.25 mg daily plus *medroxyprogesterone acetate* 10 mg for 14 days each month

C. *Conjugated estrogen* 0.3 mg daily
D. *Medroxyprogesterone acetate* 10 mg daily

8. The most common cause of delayed puberty is

   A. Isolated gonadotropin deficiency
   B. Craniopharyngioma
   C. Constitutional delay
   D. Anorexia nervosa
   E. Primary hypothyroidism

9. A 6-year-old girl is brought to your office with Tanner III breast and pubic hair development. Gonadotropin levels are low, but serum estradiol is 60 pg/mL. Which of the following diagnoses is consistent with these findings?

   A. Constitutional precocious puberty
   B. McCune-Albright syndrome
   C. Hypothalamic hamartoma
   D. Hydrocephalus
   E. Septooptic dysplasia

10. A young girl presents with what you believe is heterosexual precocious puberty and hyperandrogenism. Investigation reveals elevated levels of 17-hydroxypregnenolone and DHEA; 17α-hydroxyprogesterone is low. The most likely diagnosis is

    A. 21-hydroxylase deficiency
    B. 11β-hydroxylase deficiency
    C. 17α-hydroxylase deficiency
    D. 3β-hydroxysteroid dehydrogenase (3β-HSD) deficiency
    E. 17,20-desmolase deficiency

Answers

1. B

In girls, pubertal development typically requires 4.5 years in all (see Fig. 23.2). Although the first sign of puberty is generally accelerated growth, breast budding is usually the first recognized pubertal change, followed by the appearance of pubic hair, peak growth velocity, and, later, menarche. The stages initially described by Marshall and Tanner are commonly used to describe breast and pubic hair development.
Reference: Pages 807–810

2. D

Several of the hormonal changes associated with pubertal development begin even before any of the physical changes are obvious. Early in puberty, there is increased sensitivity of LH to GnRH. Sleep-entrained increases in both LH and FSH can be documented early in puberty. In boys, the nocturnal increases in gonadotropins are accompanied by simultaneous increases in circulating testosterone levels. In girls, in contrast, the nighttime increases in circulating gonadotropin levels are followed by increased secretion of estradiol the next day. This delay in estradiol secretion is believed to be due to the additional synthetic steps required in the aromatization of estrogens from androgens. Basal levels of both FSH and LH increase through puberty, with the patterns differing in boys and girls and with LH levels, in terms of milli-International Units per milliliter, eventually becoming greater than FSH. Although it now appears that gonadotropins are always secreted in an episodic or pulsatile fashion, even before puberty, the pulsatile secretion of gonadotropins is more easily documented as puberty progresses and basal levels increase.

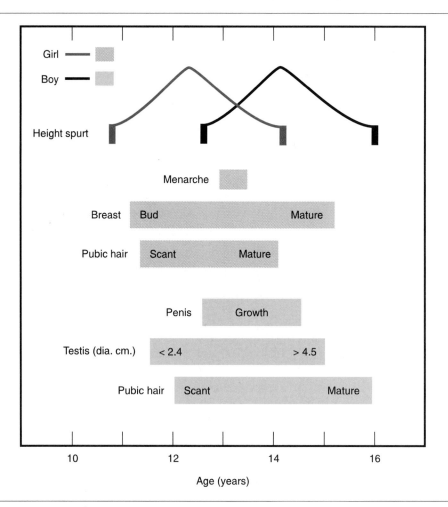

Figure 23.2   Schematic sequence of events at puberty. An idealized average girl (*upper panel*) and an idealized average boy (*lower panel*) are represented. (From **Rebar RW.** Practical evaluation of hormonal status. In: **Yen SSC, Jaffe RB,** eds. *Reproductive endocrinology: physiology, pathophysiology and clinical management.* 3rd ed. Philadelphia: WB Saunders, 1991:830, with permission. Based on data from **Marshall WA, Tanner JM.** Variations in patterns of pubertal changes in girls. *Arch Dis Child* 1969;44:291; and **Marshall WA, Tanner JM.** Variation in the pattern of pubertal changes in boys. *Arch Dis Child* 1970;45:13.)

Increased adrenal androgen secretion is important in stimulating adrenarche—the appearance of pubic and axillary hair—in both boys and girls. (Pubarche specifically refers to the appearance of pubic hair.) Progressive increases in circulating levels of the major adrenal androgens, DHEA and its sulfate (DHEAS), begin as early as 2 years of age, accelerate at 7 to 8 years of age, and continue until 13 to 15 years of age. The accelerated increases in adrenal androgens begin about 2 years before the increases in gonadotropin and gonadal sex steroid secretion when the hypothalamic–pituitary–gonadal axis is still functioning at a low prepubertal level.

In girls, estradiol, secreted predominantly by the ovaries, increases during puberty. Although, increases in estradiol first appear during the daytime hours, basal levels increase during both the day and night. Estrone, which is secreted in part by the ovaries and arises in part from extraglandular conversion of estradiol and androstenedione, also increases early in puberty but plateaus by midpuberty. Thus, the ratio of estrone to estradiol decreases throughout puberty, indicating that ovarian production of estradiol

becomes increasingly important and peripheral conversion of androgens to estrone less important during maturation.
Reference: Pages 810–813

3. D

Most affected individuals have a 45X karyotype and Turner's syndrome; still others have mosaic karyotypes (45,X/46,XX; 45,X/46,XY; etc.) and may present with the Turner's phenotype as well. These patients generally grow slowly beginning in the second or third year of life. They typically have many of the associated stigmata, including lymphedema at birth; a webbed neck; multiple pigmented nevi; disorders of the heart, kidneys (horseshoe), and great vessels (most commonly coarctation of the aorta); and small hyperconvex fingernails. Diabetes mellitus, thyroid disorders, essential hypertension, and other autoimmune disorders are often present in individuals with 45,X karyotypes. Most patients with 45,X have normal intelligence, but many affected individuals have an unusual cognitive defect characterized by an inability to appreciate the shapes and relations of objects with respect to one another (i.e., space-form blindness). Affected children typically become shorter compared to their peers as they get older. Although they do not develop breasts at puberty, some pubic or axillary hair may develop because of appropriate adrenarche with failure of thelarche (i.e., breast development). Although less severe short stature and some adolescent development may occur with chromosomal mosaicism, the tenet that any short, slowly growing, sexually infantile girl has Turner's syndrome until proved otherwise is reasonable because this disorder is so prevalent (approximately 1 in 2,500 newborn phenotypic females). In fact, the 45,X karyotype is the single most frequent chromosomal disorder in humans, but most affected fetuses are aborted spontaneously early in pregnancy.
Reference: Pages 813–815

4. C

It is important to recognize that ambiguous genitalia can result from the maternal ingestion of various teratogens, most of which are synthetic steroids (Table 23.3). Exposure to the teratogen must occur early in pregnancy during genital organogenesis. Moreover, not all exposed fetuses manifest the same anomalies or even the presence of any anomalies.

In principle, most synthetic steroids with androgenic properties, including weakly androgenic progestins, can affect female genital differentiation. However, the doses required to produce genital ambiguity are generally so great that the concern is only

Table 23.3. Androgens and Progestogens Potentially Capable of Producing Genital Ambiguity[a]

Proved	No Effect	Insufficient Data
Testosterone enanthate	Progesterone	Ethynodiol diacetate
Testosterone propionate	17α-Hydroxyprogesterone	Dimethisterone
Methylandrostenediol	Medroxyprogesterone acetate	Norgestrel
6α-Methyltestosterone	Norethynodrel	Desogestrel
Ethisterone		Gestodene
Norethindrone		Norgestimate
Danazol		

[a] Those agents proved to cause genital ambiguity do so only when administered in relatively high doses. Insufficient data exist regarding effects of dimethisterone and norgestrel. In low doses (e.g., as in oral contraceptives), progestins, even including norethindrone, seem unlikely to virilize a female fetus.

theoretical. The one agent that clearly can lead to genital ambiguity when ingested in clinically used quantities is danazol. There is no evidence that inadvertent ingestion of oral contraceptives, which contain relatively low doses of *ethinyl estradiol* and a 19-nor-steroid, results in virilization.
Reference: Pages 837–838

5. C (see Table 23.1)

Precocious puberty may be defined by some as pubertal development beginning before the age of 7 years in white girls and before the age of 6 years in African-American girls. Others claim that evaluation for breast or pubic hair development before the age of 8 or 9 years, respectively, is still warranted despite the fact that younger girls are much more likely to have a pathologic basis for their early development. Precocious pubertal development is characterized in several ways. In isosexual precocious puberty, the early changes are common to the phenotypic sex of the individual. In heterosexual precocious puberty, the development is characteristic of the opposite sex. Precocious puberty is sometimes termed "true" when it is of central origin with activation of the hypothalamic–pituitary unit. In precocious pseudopuberty, also known as precocious puberty of peripheral origin, secretion of hormones in the periphery (commonly by neoplasms) stimulates pubertal development.
Reference: Pages 814–815

6. A

The mechanisms responsible for the numerous hormonal changes occurring during puberty are poorly understood, although it is recognized that a "central nervous system (CNS) program" must be responsible for initiating puberty. It appears that the hypothalamic–pituitary–gonadal axis in girls develops in two distinct stages during puberty. First, sensitivity to the negative or inhibitory effects of the low levels of circulating sex steroids present in childhood decreases early in puberty. Second, late in puberty, there is maturation of the positive or stimulatory feedback response to estrogen, which is responsible for the ovulatory midcycle surge of LH.

Current evidence suggests that the CNS inhibits the onset of puberty until the appropriate time. Based on this theory, the neuroendocrine control of puberty is mediated by GnRH-secreting neurons in the medial basal hypothalamus, which act together as an endogenous pulse generator. At puberty, the GnRH pulse generator is reactivated (i.e., disinhibited), leading to increased amplitude and frequency of GnRH pulses. In turn, the increased GnRH secretion results in increased gonadotropin and then gonadal steroid secretion. What causes this "distinhibition" of GnRH release is unknown.
Reference: Pages 812–813

7. C

To increase final adult height, treatment strategies utilizing exogenous growth hormone (GH) are commonly accepted. It is not yet known what dose of GH is optimal or if an anabolic steroid such as oxandrolone will provide additional growth. However, GH in doses 25% greater than those recommended for GH deficiency are proving safe and effective, with a net increase in height of 8.1 cm over the average height of approximately 146 cm in untreated individuals.

The treatment of patients with Turner's syndrome is as follows:

1. To promote sexual maturation, therapy with exogenous estrogen should be initiated when the patient is psychologically ready, at approximately 12 to 13 years of age, and after GH therapy is completed.
2. Because the intent is to mimic normal pubertal development, low-dose estrogen alone (such as 0.3 mg *conjugated estrogens* orally each day) should be initiated.
3. Progestins (5–10 mg *medroxyprogesterone acetate* given orally for 12–14 days every 1–2 months) can be added to prevent endometrial hyperplasia after the patient

Table 23.1. Aberrations of Pubertal Development

I. Delayed or interrupted puberty
   A. *Anatomic abnormalities of the genital outflow tract*
      1. Müllerian dysgenesis (Rokitansky–Küster–Hauser syndrome)
      2. Distal genital tract obstruction
         a. Imperforate hymen
         b. Transverse vaginal septum
   B. *Hypergonadotropic (follicle-stimulating hormone >30 mIU/mL) hypogonadism (gonadal "failure")*
      1. Gonadal dysgenesis with stigmata of *Turner's syndrome*
      2. Pure gonadal dysgenesis
         a. 46,XX
         b. 46,XY
      3. Early gonadal "failure" with apparent normal ovarian development
   C. *Hypogonadotropic (luteinizing hormone and follicle-stimulating hormone <10 mIU/mL) hypogonadism*
      1. Constitutional delay
      2. Isolated gonadotropin deficiency
         a. Associated with midline defects (*Kallmann's syndrome*)
         b. Independent of associated disorders
         c. Prader-Labhardt-Willi syndrome
         d. Laurence-Moon-Bardet-Biedl syndrome
         e. Many other rare syndromes
      3. Associated with multiple hormone deficiencies
      4. Neoplasms of the hypothalamic–pituitary area
         a. Craniopharyngiomas
         b. Pituitary adenomas
         c. Other
      5. Infiltrative processes (Langerhans cell–type histiocytosis)
      6. After irradiation of the central nervous system
      7. Severe chronic illnesses with malnutrition
      8. Anorexia nervosa and related disorders
      9. Severe hypothalamic amenorrhea (rare)
    10. Antidopaminergic and gonadotropin-releasing hormone–inhibiting drugs (especially psychotropic agents, opiates)
    11. Primary hypothyroidism
    12. Cushing's syndrome

II. Asynchronous pubertal development
   A. Complete androgen insensitivity syndrome (testicular feminization)
   B. Incomplete androgen insensitivity syndrome

III. Precocious puberty
   A. *Central (true) precocious puberty*
      1. Constitutional (idiopathic) precocious puberty
      2. Hypothalamic neoplasms (most commonly hamartomas)
      3. Congenital malformations
      4. Infiltrative processes (Langerhans cell–type histiocytosis)
      5. After irradiation
      6. Trauma
      7. Infection
   B. *Precocious puberty of peripheral origin (precocious pseudopuberty)*
      1. Gonadotropin-secreting neoplasms
         a. Human chorionic gonadotropin secreting
            i. Ectopic germinomas (pinealomas)
            ii. Choriocarcinomas
            iii. Teratomas
            iv. Hepatoblastomas
         b. Luteinizing hormone–secreting (pituitary adenomas)
      2. Gonadal neoplasms
         a. Estrogen secreting
            i. Granulosa–theca cell tumors
            ii. Gonadal sex-cord tumors
         b. Androgen-secreting
            i. Arrhenoblastomas
            ii. Teratomas

Table 23.1.—continued

III. Precocious puberty
    3. Congenital adrenal hyperplasia
        a. 21-Hydroxylase (P450c21) deficiency
        b. 11 β-Hydroxylase (P450c11) deficiency
        c. 3 β-Hydroxysteroid dehydrogenase deficiency
    4. Adrenal neoplasms
        b. Adenomas
        b. Carcinomas
    5. Autonomous gonadal hypersecretion
        a. Cysts
        b. McCune-Albright syndrome
    6. Iatrogenic ingestion/absorption of estrogens or androgens

IV. Heterosexual puberty
    A. Polycystic ovarian syndrome
    B. Nonclassic forms of congenital adrenal hyperplasia
    C. Idiopathic hirsutism
    D. Mixed gonadal dysgenesis
    E. Rare forms of male pseudohermaphroditism (*Reifenstein's syndrome*, 5α-reductase deficiency)
    F. Cushing's syndrome (rare)
    G. Androgen-secreting neoplasms (rare)

first experiences vaginal bleeding or after 6 months of unopposed estrogen use if the patient has not yet had any bleeding.

4. The dose of estrogen is increased slowly over 1 to 2 years until the patient is taking about twice as much estrogen as is administered to postmenopausal women.

5. Girls with gonadal dysgenesis must be monitored carefully for the development of hypertension with estrogen therapy.

6. The patients and their parents should be counseled regarding the emotional and physical changes that will occur with therapy.

Reference: Pages 819–821

8. C

Hypothalamic–pituitary disturbances are usually associated with low levels of circulating gonadotropins (with both LH and FSH < 10 mIU/mL). There are both sporadic and familial causes of hypogonadotropic hypogonadism, and the differential diagnosis is extensive. It is important to remember, however, that low levels of LH and FSH are normally present in the prepubertal years; thus, girls with constitutionally delayed puberty may be mistakenly presumed to have hypogonadotropic hypogonadism. In fact, constitutional delay is the most common cause of delayed puberty. Constitutional delayed growth and adolescence can be diagnosed only after careful evaluation excludes other causes of delayed puberty and longitudinal follow-up documents normal sexual development. The farther below the third percentile for height that the young girl is, the less likely it is that constitutional explanations are correct.
Reference: Pages 821–822

9. B

In central precocious puberty, GnRH prematurely stimulates increased gonadotropin secretion. Central precocious puberty may occur in children in whom no structural abnormality exists, in which case it is termed *constitutional* or *idiopathic*. Alternatively, central precocious puberty may result from a tumor, infection, congenital abnormality, or traumatic injury affecting the hypothalamus. Tumors of the hypothalamus include hamartomas and, less frequently, neurogliomas and pinealomas. It appears that hamartomas produce GnRH in a pulsatile manner and thus stimulate gonadotropin secretion. A number of congenital malformations, including hydrocephalus, craniostenosis,

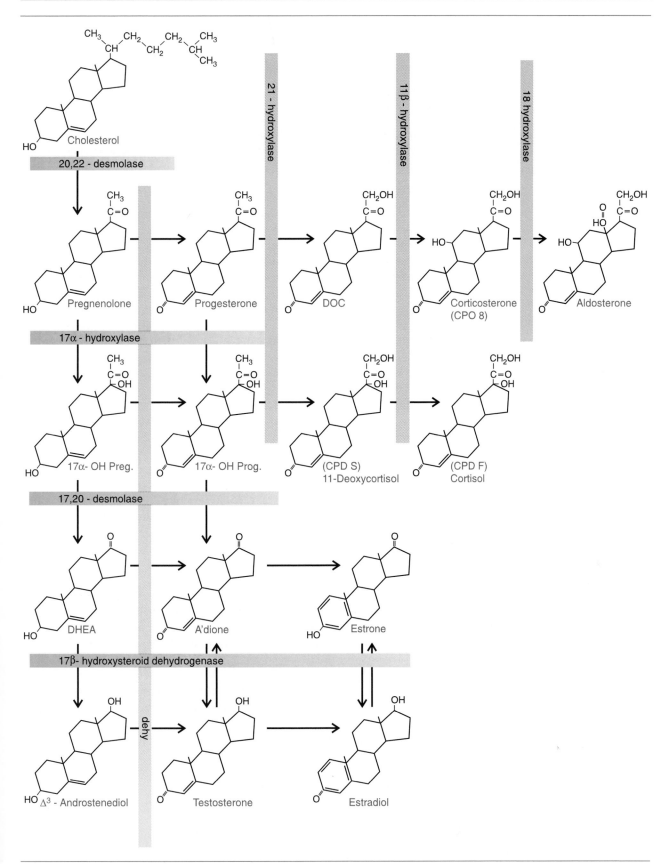

Figure 23.19   Gonadal and adrenal steroid pathways and the enzymes required for steroid conversion. (From **Rebar RW, Kenigsberg D, Hodgen GD.** The normal menstrual cycle and the control of ovulation. In: **Becker KL,** ed. *Principles and practice of endocrinology and metabolism.* 2nd ed. Philadelphia: JB Lippincott, 1995:868, with permission.)

arachnoid cysts, and septooptic dysplasia, can also be associated with precocious puberty (as well as with sexual infantilism).

In gonadotropin-independent precocious puberty, production of estrogens or androgens from the ovaries, adrenals, or rare steroid-secreting neoplasms leads to early pubertal development. Small functional ovarian cysts, typically asymptomatic, are common in children and may cause transient sexual precocity. Simple cysts (with a benign ultrasonographic appearance) can be observed and usually resolve over time. Of the various ovarian neoplasms that can secrete estrogens, granulosa–theca cell tumors occur most frequently but are still rare. Although such tumors may grow rapidly, more than two thirds are benign.

McCune-Albright syndrome is associated with estrogen secretion in the absence of increased gonadotropin and is one possibility for the clinical scenario described. The syndrome is characterized by polyostotic fibrous dysplasia of bone, irregular *café au lait* spots on the skin, and hyperfunctioning endocrinopathies. Girls develop sexual precocity as a result of functioning ovarian cysts. Other endocrinopathies may include hyperthyroidism, hypercortisolism, hyperprolactinemia, and acromegaly. It is now known that mutations of the $G_{s\alpha}$ subunit of the G protein, which couples extracellular hormonal signals to the activation of adenylate cyclase, are responsible for the autonomous hyperfunction of the endocrine glands and, presumably, for the other defects present in this disorder. Exposure to exogenous estrogens can mimic gonadotropin-independent precocious puberty. Ingestion of oral contraceptives, other estrogen-containing pharmaceutical agents, and estrogen-contaminated foods and the topical use of estrogens have been implicated in cases of precocious development in infants and children. Severe primary hypothyroidism has also been associated with sexual precocity; associated hyperprolactinemia may result in galactorrhea in affected individuals.
Reference: Pages 829–830

10. D

Heterosexual precocious puberty is always of peripheral origin and is most often caused by congenital adrenal hyperplasia (CAH). Three adrenal enzyme defects—21-hydroxylase deficiency, 11β-hydroxylase deficiency, and 3β-HSD deficiency—can lead not only to heterosexual precocity but also to virilization of the external genitalia because of increased androgen production beginning in utero.

Deficiency of 3β-HSD affects the synthesis of glucocorticoids, mineralocorticoids, and sex steroids. Typically, levels of 17-hydroxypregnenolone and DHEA are elevated (see Fig. 23.19). The classic form of the disorder, detectable at birth, is quite rare, and affected girls may be masculinized only slightly. In severe cases, salt-wasting may also be present.

A nonclassic form of this disorder may be associated with heterosexual precocious pubertal development (as in the classic form if untreated), but postpubertal hyperandrogenism occurs more often. The androgen excess in individuals with nonclassic 3β-HSD deficiency appears to result from androgens derived from the peripheral conversion of increased serum concentrations of DHEA. This disorder is inherited in autosomal recessive fashion, with allelism at the 3β-HSD gene on chromosome believed to be responsible for the varying degrees of enzyme deficiency.
Reference: Pages 830–833

24 Amenorrhea

Wendy J. Schillings
Howard D. McClamrock

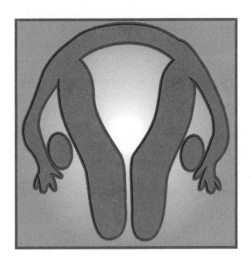

Learning Objectives

1. Understand organ system abnormalities that may cause amenorrhea.

2. Understand the relationship of amenorrhea to anovulation and luteal phase defect.

3. Be able to present a strategy for the workup of the patient with amenorrhea.

4. Be able to determine the appropriate treatment for the patient with amenorrhea according to medical needs and personal desires.

Questions

1. The underlying etiology of premature ovarian failure may be any of the following **except**

   A. Turner's syndrome
   B. Autoimmune dysfunction
   C. Hyperandrogenism
   D. Galactosemia
   E. Radiation exposure

2. The following are all associated with Kallmann's syndrome, **except**

   A. XX karyotype
   B. Insufficient pulsatile secretion of gonadotropin-releasing hormone (GnRH)
   C. Blind vaginal pouch
   D. Anosmia
   E. Normal height for age

3. The following are associated with congenital androgen insensitivity, **except**

   A. Blind vaginal pouch
   B. Absence of uterus and fallopian tubes
   C. Serum total testosterone concentrations in the normal male range
   D. Anosmia
   E. Breast development at puberty

4. Asherman's syndrome is most commonly seen with which one of the following:

   A. Curettage, especially postpartum
   B. Imperforate hymen
   C. Transverse vaginal septum
   D. Congenitally absent endometrium
   E. Use of intrauterine device

5. A luteal phase defect is caused by

   A. Abnormal pulsatility of GnRH
   B. Absence of oocytes in the ovary
   C. Absence of nerve cells that secrete GnRH
   D. Uterine scarring
   E. Chromosomal abnormalities

6. Patients with the following conditions may present initially with amenorrhea, anovulation, or luteal phase defects, **except**

   A. Hyperprolactinemia
   B. Hypothyroidism
   C. Anorexia nervosa
   D. Polycystic ovarian syndrome
   E. Müllerian agenesis

7. The following conditions may be associated with ovulation in the presence of amenorrhea, **except**

   A. Asherman's syndrome
   B. Mayer-Rokitansky-Küster-Hauser syndrome
   C. Imperforate hymen
   D. Congenitally absent endometrium
   E. Androgen insensitivity

8. The following conditions may be associated with anovulation and amenorrhea, because of abnormalities of GnRH production or release, **except**

   A. Asherman's syndrome
   B. Exercise-induced amenorrhea
   C. Kallmann's syndrome
   D. Stress-induced amenorrhea
   E. Physiologic delay of puberty

9. The initial workup for a patient with secondary sexual characteristics and amenorrhea usually includes all of the following **except**

   A. Pregnancy test
   B. Pelvic ultrasound
   C. Prolactin level
   D. Thyrotropin level
   E. Assessment of estrogen status

10. The following disorder is associated with absent secondary sexual characteristics, lack of an anatomic cause for amenorrhea demonstrable on physical examination, and an elevation of follicle-stimulating hormone (FSH) level:

    A. Physiologic delay of puberty
    B. Kallmann's syndrome
    C. Pure gonadal dysgenesis
    D. Disorders of low-estrogen status occurring before puberty
    E. Central nervous system tumors

11. The following condition has an anatomic defect demonstrable on physical examination that is associated with amenorrhea:

    A. Pure gonadal genesis
    B. Savage syndrome
    C. Congenital adrenal hyperplasia
    D. Androgen insensitivity
    E. Hypothalamic dysfunction

12. All of the following conditions are treated surgically **except**

    A. Asherman's syndrome
    B. Imperforate hymen
    C. Transverse septum of the vagina
    D. Absent endometrium
    E. Androgen insensitivity

13. Estrogen replacement therapy is generally needed in the following conditions, **except**

    A. Turner's syndrome (45X)
    B. Eugonadotropic chronic anovulation
    C. Hypothalamic hypogonadism
    D. Savage syndrome
    E. Premature ovarian failure

14. Clomiphene citrate is generally ineffective in inducing ovulation in the following conditions, **except**

    A. Hypogonadotropic hypogonadism
    B. Hypergonadotropic hypogonadism
    C. Anorexia nervosa
    D. Savage syndrome
    E. Eugonadotropic chronic anovulation

15. All of the following statements regarding treatment options are correct, **except**

   A. *Clomiphene citrate* is one of the first agents used when attempting to induce ovulation in a patient with polycystic ovarian syndrome.
   B. Injectable human menopausal gonadotropins or pulsatile GnRH therapy may be used to induce ovulation in patients with hypogonadotropic hypogonadism.
   C. Oral contraceptives may be effective in treating hirsutism by decreasing ovarian androgen production and by decreasing circulating levels of sex-hormone binding globulin (SHBL).
   D. *Spironolactone* may be effective in treating hirsutism by decreasing androgen production and by competing with androgens for the androgen receptor.
   E. Patients with Turner's syndrome may become pregnant using donated oocytes through *in vitro* fertilization.

Answers

1. C (see Table 24.3)

Premature ovarian failure occurs due to decreased follicular endowment or accelerated follicular atresia. It occurs in approximately 1% of the population. Once this condition has been diagnosed, the underlying etiology should be explored. Genetic abnormalities such as Turner's syndrome, iatrogenic causes such as radiation exposure, metabolic dysfunction such as galactosemia, and autoimmune disorders all cause accelerated follicular atresia. Hyperandrogenism causes abnormalities in gonadotropic secretions and the local environment that a follicle is exposed to but it does not cause accelerated atresia of the follicles.
Reference: Pages 845–848

2. C

Kallmann's syndrome was originally described as a triad of hypogonadism, anosmia, and color blindness in men. Although it is more common in men, women also may be affected. It is also known as isolated gonadotropin deficiency and occurs as a result of an absence of GnRH neurons in the hypothalamus and olfactory bulbs and, consequently, hypogonadotropic hypogonadism and anosmia. Cleft lip and palate may also be associated with the syndrome. Patients with Kallmann's syndrome traditionally have normal height for age, in contrast to patients with physiologic delay of puberty, who generally are short for their chronologic age but are of normal height for their bone age. Kallmann's syndrome is not associated with reproductive organ defects, therefore, it is not associated with a blind vaginal pouch.
Reference: Page 848

Table 24.3. Causes of Ovarian Failure After Development of Secondary Sexual Characteristics

Chromosomal etiology
Iatrogenic causes
   Radiation
   Chemotherapy
   Surgical alteration of ovarian blood supply

Infections

Autoimmune disorders

Galactosemia (mild form or heterozygote)

Savage syndrome

Cigarette smoking

Idiopathic

3. D

Androgen insensitivity (previously known as testicular feminization) occurs in individuals with an XY karyotype, but a defect in androgen receptor function that leads to development of the female phenotype. Antimüllerian hormone is present and functions normally in these patients, therefore, internal female (müllerian) structures such as a uterus, vagina, and fallopian tubes are absent. The gonads are testes rather than ovaries and occur in the abdomen or inguinal hernias where they secrete testosterone leading to circulating testosterone concentrations in the normal male range. Testosterone does not function during development to suppress formation of breast tissues, and at puberty, the conversion of androgens to estrogens stimulates breast growth, often leading to well-developed breasts. Due to the defect in androgen receptor function, external genitalia are phenotypically female and a blind vaginal pouch is characteristic of the disorder. There is no association with anosmia or midline facial defects.
Reference: Pages 852–853

4. A (see Fig. 24.1 and Table 24.2)

Imperforate hymen, transverse vaginal septum, and congenitally absent endometrium are all causes of amenorrhea associated with normal secondary sexual characteristics. Asherman's syndrome is not associated with imperforate hymen or transverse vaginal septum because there is no history of uterine instrumentation in those individuals. Congenitally absent endometrium is a very rare condition and is a diagnosis of exclusion. Asherman's syndrome may be seen in patients after infections related to the use of an intrauterine device, however, it is much more common after a pregnancy-related uterine curettage. It has been reported to occur in 39% of patients undergoing hysterosalpingography who have previously undergone postpartum curettage.
Reference: Pages 845, 852

5. A

In the luteal phase of the cycle, progesterone is secreted from the corpus luteum. This promotes development of the endometrial lining to support implantation of an embryo. Abnormalities in the luteal phase are caused by abnormal stimulation of the follicle development in the follicular phase leading to inadequate development of the corpus luteum. GnRH secreted in a pulsatile manner stimulates FSH to be secreted from the pituitary, which in turn stimulates estrogen production by granulosa cells in the ovarian follicle. Both FSH and estrogen stimulate the granulosa cells to multiply and differentiate. Estrogen through positive feedback causes the midcycle surge of luteinizing hormone (LH), which leads to ovulation and luteinization of follicular cells (formation of the corpus luteum). Luteinized cells secrete progesterone. If the frequency of the GnRH pulses is altered, ovulation may occur but the corpus luteum formation may not be adequate. Patients with uterine scarring are not considered to have luteal phase defects because the defect is not related to hormonal abnormalities. Patients with absent oocytes cannot ovulate and, therefore, do not have any luteal phase. Likewise, patients who have no cells that secrete GnRH cannot stimulate follicles to ovulate and, therefore, cannot have a luteal phase defect. Chromosomal abnormalities cause rapid loss of oocytes.
Reference: Pages 848–850

6. E

Any condition that effects gonadotropin pulsatility leads to disruption of the hormonal signals that control the normal reproductive cycle. Gonadotropins need to be released in pulses in order to stimulate follicular growth and estrogen production in the ovary, which leads to ovulation and adequate corpus luteum development. Gonadotropin secretion is directly stimulated by the pulsatile release of GnRH from the hypothalamus. GnRH release is influenced by a variety of neurotransmitters and hormones. Prolactin, thyroid hormone, and androgens all can cause abnormal secretion of GnRH.

Anorexia nervosa, malnutrition, and chronic diseases can also disrupt the normal secretion of GnRH. If the normal GnRH pulsatile secretion is severely disrupted, amenorrhea

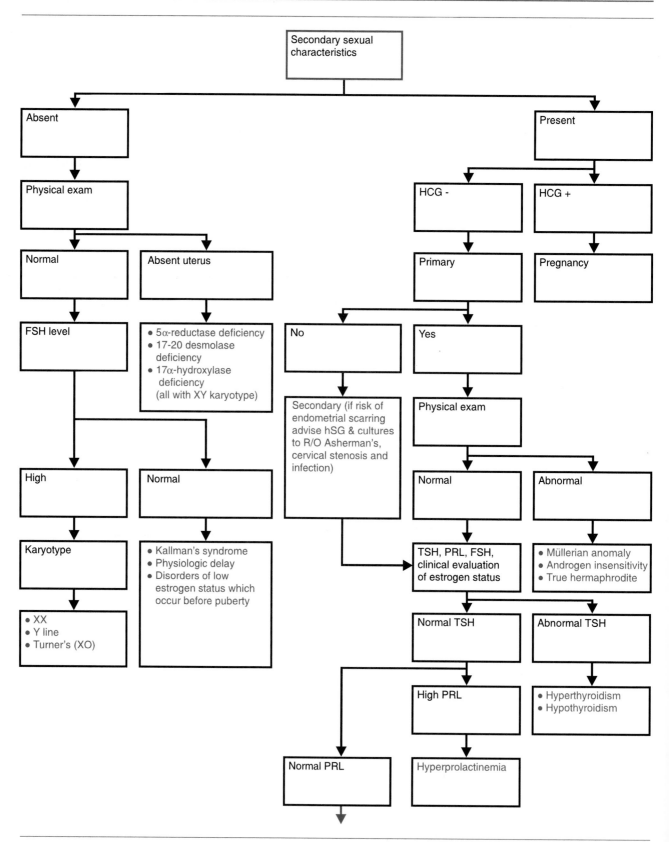

Figure 24.1   Decision tree for evaluation of amenorrhea.

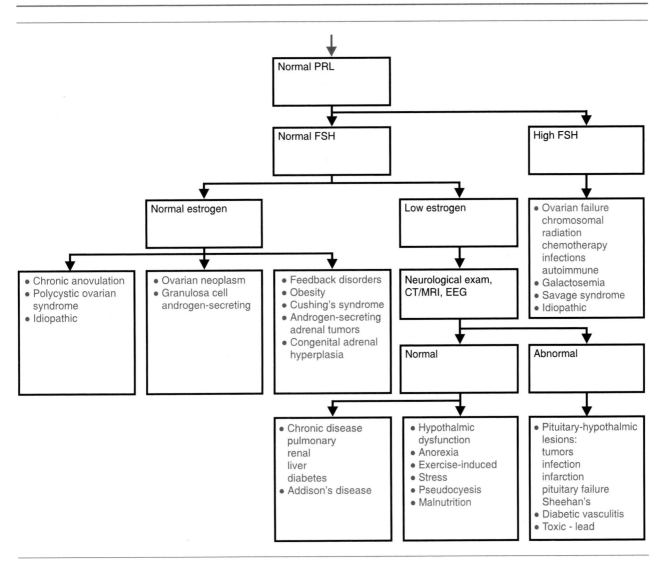

Figure 24.1—*continued*

Table 24.2. Anatomic Causes of Amenorrhea

Secondary sexual characteristics present

Müllerian anomalies
   Imperforate hymen
   Transverse vaginal septum
   Mayer-Rokitansky-Küster-Hauser syndrome
Androgen insensitivity
True hermaphrodites
Absent endometrium
Asherman's syndrome
   Secondary to prior uterine or cervical surgery
     Currettage, especially postpartum
     Cone biopsy
     Loop electroexcision procedure
   Secondary to infections
     Pelvic inflammatory disease
     IUD-related
     Tuberculosis
     Schistosomiasis

IUD, intrauterine device.

Table 24.4. Pituitary and Hypothalamic Lesions

Pituitary and hypothalamic

Craniopharyngioma
Germinoma
Tubercular granuloma
Sarcoid granuloma
Dermoid cyst

Pituitary

Nonfunctioning adenomas
Hormone-secreting adenomas
  Prolactinoma
  Cushing's disease
  Acromegaly
  Primary hyperthyroidism
Infarction
Lymphocytic hypophysitis
Surgical or radiologic ablations
Sheehan's syndrome
Diabetic vasculitis

---

will result. Less severe abnormalities in GnRH secretion cause the patient to develop oligomenorrhea. Minor disruptions in the secretion of GnRH lead to luteal phase defect where ovulation occurs, but the corpus luteum is not able to secrete enough progesterone to allow for normal development of the endometrial lining to support implantation. Müllerian agenesis is an anatomic defect that presents as amenorrhea and is frequently associated with cyclic pain.
Reference: Pages 858–859

7. E (see Tables 24.4 and 24.5)

Asherman's syndrome results in amenorrhea due to intrauterine scarring, often because of pregnancy-related uterine curettage. Ovulation is not affected. Mayer-Rokitansky-Küster-Hauser syndrome is a congenital absence of the uterus, cervix, and/or vagina, with the ovaries intact, which leads to normal ovulation. Imperforate hymen results in amenorrhea because of outflow obstruction but, again, ovulation is not affected. Amenorrhea in patients with a congenitally absent endometrium is a result of the inability of the endometrium to develop despite normal circulating hormone levels in association with ovulation. Ovulation does not occur in androgen insensitivity, because the gonads are testes rather than ovaries and the individuals are genotypically male.
Reference: Pages 852–853

8. A

Kallmann's syndrome is also known as isolated gonadotropin deficiency due to an absence GnRH neurons in the hypothalamus and olfactory bulbs. Amenorrhea induced by exercise or stress occurs as a result of hypogonadotropic hypogonadism and the resulting abnormalities of GnRH production. Physiologic delay of puberty results in amenorrhea because of a delayed reactivation of the hypothalamic pulse generator. Asherman's syndrome occurs as a result of intrauterine scarring and is not associated with any abnormalities of GnRH production.
Reference: Pages 822–823, 848

9. B

Any patient of reproductive age with amenorrhea should be tested for pregnancy. History and physical, including a pelvic examination, are always necessary when evaluating a patient with secondary sexual characteristics and amenorrhea. Unless the diagnosis is made by the physical examination, one needs to determine if thyroid hormone, prolactin, and estrogen are normally secreted. Serum levels for prolactin and thyrotropin

---

Table 24.5. Abnormalities Affecting Release of Gonadotropin-Releasing Hormone

---

Variable estrogen status[a]

Anorexia nervosa
Exercise-induced
Stress-induced
Pseudocyesis
Malnutrition
Chronic diseases
    Diabetes mellitus
    Renal disorders
    Pulmonary disorders
    Liver disease
    Chronic infections
    Addison's disease
Hyperprolactinemia
Thyroid dysfunction

Euestrogenic states

Obesity
Hyperandrogenism
    Polycystic ovary syndrome
    Cushing's syndrome
    Congenital adrenal hyperplasia
    Androgen-secreting adrenal tumors
    Androgen-secreting ovarian tumors
Granulosa cell tumor
Idiopathic

---

[a]Severity of the condition determines estrogen status—the more severe, the more likely to manifest as hypoestrogenism.

hormone should be obtained. For secondary sexual characteristics to develop, estrogen secretion had to be adequate at some point in development. However, evaluation of estrogen status needs to be obtained, usually by a progesterone withdrawal test but physical examination and estradiol level may also be helpful. A pelvic ultrasound is not usually part of the initial workup but could be considered if an anatomic defect is found on physical examination.
Reference: Pages 843–844

10. C

Physiologic delay of puberty and Kallmann's syndrome are both associated with an absence of secondary sexual characteristics and the lack of an anatomic cause for amenorrhea demonstrable on physical exam. Physiologic delay of puberty is due to a delayed reactivation of the hypothalamic pulse generator; therefore, FSH levels remain low. Kallmann's syndrome is associated with extremely low FSH levels due to absence of GnRH neurons in the hypothalamus. Disorders of low estrogen status occurring before puberty and central nervous system tumors may also be associated with lack of sexual characteristics if these occur prior to the development of sexual characteristics. Again, patients lack demonstrable anatomic causes for amenorrhea on physical examination, and FSH levels remain low to normal because the ovaries remain normal and these patients have a normal complement of oocytes. FSH elevation implies gonadal failure and the resultant lack of oocytes. In the selections given for this question, only gonadal dysgenesis is associated with ovarian failure.
Reference: Pages 848–849

11. D (see Table 24.1)

Pure gonadal dysgenesis is a genetic disorder resulting in ovarian failure. In Savage syndrome, amenorrhea again results from anovulation due to ovarian resistance. Because oocytes are present in the ovary, they do not respond with follicular development and ovulation in response to gonadotropin stimulation. There is no anatomic defect

Table 24.1. Amenorrhea Associated with a Lack of Secondary Sexual Characteristics

Abnormal physical examination

5α-reductase deficiency in XY individual
17, 20-desmolase deficiency in XY individual
17α-hydroxylase deficiency in XY individual

Hypergonadotropic hypogonadism

Gonadal dysgenesis
Pure gonadal dysgenesis
Partial deletion of X chromosome
Sex chromosome mosaicism
Environmental and therapeutic ovarian toxins
17α-hydroxylase deficiency in XX individual
Galactosemia
Other

Hypogonadotropic hypogonadism

Physiologic delay
Kallmann's syndrome
Central nervous system tumors
Hypothalamic/pituitary dysfunction

associated with Savage syndrome. Congenital adrenal hyperplasia results in increased circulating androgen levels, which in turn interferes with feedback mechanisms leading to amenorrhea in some individuals. Patients with congenital adrenal hyperplasia are anatomically normal. Any of the many conditions associated with hypothalamic dysfunction result in amenorrhea due to abnormalities in the pulsatile release of GnRH. These individuals are generally anatomically normal. Androgen insensitivity is associated with a blind vaginal pouch that is demonstrable on physical exam. Despite circulating testosterone levels in the normal male range, external genitalia remain female in phenotype due to receptor defects. The uterus, cervix, fallopian tubes, and upper vagina are absent, however, due to normal function of antimüllerian hormone. Reference: Page 847

12. D

There is no surgical treatment for an absent endometrium. An imperforate hymen and a transverse septum need to be removed surgically to allow for the release of menstrual flow. Asherman's syndrome (uterine scarring) can be treated surgically to improve menstrual flow and pregnancy outcome. A patient with androgen sensitivity has intrabdominal testes that can develop malignancies. Therefore, the testes should be removed surgically after puberty to prevent tumor development. Reference: Pages 854–855

13. B

Estrogen replacement therapy is needed in conditions where circulating estrogen levels are low (hypoestrogenism). Hypoestrogenism may be a result of ovarian failure or a result of hypothalamic dysfunction leading to insufficient ovarian stimulation and estrogen production. Tumer's syndrome and premature ovarian failure are both associated with hypoestrogenism as a result of ovarian failure and the associated lack of oocytes. Savage syndrome is associated with oocytes in the ovary, but these oocytes do not respond to gonadotropin stimulation resulting in hypoestrogenism. Hypoestrogenism also results in hypothalamic hypogonadism because of inappropriate GnRH production. This leads to insufficient gonadotropin levels for ovarian stimulation of folliculogenesis and a resulting hypoestrogenism. Eugonadotropic chronic anovulation is not associated with hypoestrogenism. In some cases, the patient may be in a state of chronic unopposed estrogen. Androgen levels may be elevated, which in turn may be converted to estrogens. These patients do not need estrogen replacement, but

may need cyclic progestin therapy to combat the unopposed estrogen state and to lead to withdrawal bleeding.
Reference: Pages 863–864

14. E

Clomiphene citrate is primarily indicated in patients with adequate levels of estrogen and normal levels of FSH and prolactin. It is generally ineffective in patients with a poor estrogen supply. This includes patients with hypogonadotropic hypogonadism and patients with hypergonadotropic hypogonadism resulting from a decreased supply of oocytes. It may be ineffective in anorexia nervosa because these patients are also hypoestrogenic. Patients with Savage syndrome may have oocytes demonstrable by biopsy, but these oocytes do not respond to stimulation with either clomiphene citrate or human menopausal gonadotropins. *Clomiphene citrate* is generally effective in eugonadotropic chronic anovulation and up to 80% of well-selected patients can be expected to ovulate after therapy with clomiphene citrate.
Reference: Pages 864–866

15. C

Clomiphene citrate is generally the first agent used for ovulation induction as long as the patient is not hypoestrogenic. Patients with polycystic ovarian syndrome are not hypoestrogenic and may respond to *clomiphene citrate,* however, rates of ovulation in patients with polycystic ovarian syndrome are lower than in patients with other forms of chronic anovulation. In patients with hypogonadotropic hypogonadism, *clomiphene citrate* is generally ineffective. These patients will respond to either injectable human menopausal gonadotropins or pulsatology GnRH therapy. *Spironolactone* is one of several agents that may be used in treating hirsutism. This mechanism acts by decreasing the androgen production and by competing with androgens for the androgen receptor.

Patients with Turner's syndrome or other forms of ovarian failure may become pregnant using donated oocytes through *in vitro* fertilization. Oocytes obtained from donors may be fertilized with sperm from the recipient's husband and transferred into the recipient's uterus after the endometrium has been appropriately prepared with hormonal regimens. Estrogen and progestins are used to prepare the endometrium for implantation of the transferred embryos. Patients with Turner's syndrome, other forms of ovarian failure, or natural menopause may all carry pregnancies derived from oocyte donation. Pregnancy rates from anonymous oocyte donation are very high and average over 50% per transfer in better programs.

Oral contraceptives may be effective in treating hirsutism in some patients. The mechanism acts by decreasing ovarian androgen production and by increasing circulating levels of sex-hormone binding globulin (SHBG). Oral contraceptives have a net estrogenic effect leading to increases in SHBG. The increases in SHBG are associated with the increased androgen binding, which therefore leaves less free androgen available.
Reference: Pages 864–866

25

Endocrine Disorders

Avner Hershlag
C. Matthew Peterson

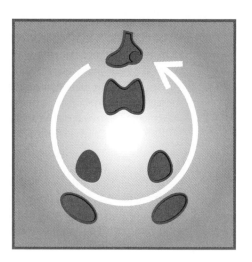

Learning Objectives

1. Understand the evaluation and treatment of the hirsute patient.

2. Be able to explain the pathophysiology and treatment of polycystic ovarian disease.

3. Be aware of the causes of Cushing's syndrome.

4. Understand the different types of congenital adrenal hyperplasia (CAH), including the genetics, time of onset, manifestations, and diagnosis.

5. Recognize the many causes of hyperprolactinemia, including their diagnoses and treatment.

6. Realize the prevalence increase of thyroid disease in women.

Questions

1. Arrange the following androgens: (a) dehydroepiandrosterone sulfate (DHEAS), (b) dihydrotestosterone (DHT), (c) androstenedione, and (d) testosterone in order of increasing androgenicity:

   A. c, a, b, d
   B. a, c, b, d
   C. a, d, c, b
   D. a, c, d, b

2. Decrease in sex-hormone binding globulin (SHBG) may be caused by all of the following **except**

   A. Hyperinsulinemia
   B. Obesity
   C. Pregnancy
   D. Cushing's Disease

3. All of the following statements regarding androgens in menopause are true **except**

   A. Overweight women may be less at risk of osteoporosis because of extragonadal aromatization of androgens.
   B. The ovary makes more estrone (E_2).
   C. Ovarian contribution to elevations in testosterone and androstenedione increases.
   D. The adrenals produce less dehydroepiandrosterone (DHEA) and DHEAS.

4. Of the following criteria for polycystic ovary syndrome (PCOS) mark (a) for major and (b) for minor.

   A. Elevated luteinizing hormone (LH)/follicle-stimulating hormone (FSH) ratio
   B. Hyperandrogenism
   C. Hyperinsulinism
   D. Chronic anovulation

5. All of the following are true statements regarding PCOS, **except**

   A. The ovaries of patients with PCOS are more sensitive to gonadotropins than patients who do not have PCOS.
   B. Androgen levels in patients with PCOS drop more rapidly than estrogen levels in response to gonadotropin-releasing hormone (GnRH) agonists.
   C. Total and free testosterone correlate directly with LH levels.
   D. LH is not always elevated in PCOS.

6. Of the following statements, which are false and which are true?

   A. Glucose intolerance or frank diabetes are detected in 20% of patients with PCOS.
   B. GnRH analogs reduce elevated insulin levels in PCOS.
   C. Elevated LH and FSH levels in PCOS are the result of increased GnRH pulse frequency.
   D. Elevated prolactin levels seen in 25% of patients with PCOS are frequently the result of a coexisting pituitary microadenoma.

7. Oral contraceptives (OCs) in PCOS offer all of the following benefits **except**

   A. LH suppression, therefore reduced androgens
   B. Reduced free T resulting from increased SHGB stimulated by estrogen
   C. 5α-reductase is inhibited by estrogen
   D. All reduction in androgens are the results of OC's effects on LH and SHBG

8. *Spironolactone* works to reduce hirsutism in all of the following mechanisms **except**

    A. Inhibition of 5α-reductase activity
    B. Competitive inhibition of DHT
    C. Increase in cytochrome P450 (CYP) enzymes
    D. Increase in androgen catabolism

9. Compared to *spironolactone,* the following drugs should be expected to be

    a. More effective
    b. Less effective
    c. About the same in reducing hirsutism

    A. *Cyproterone acetate*
    B. *Cimetidine*
    C. *Flutamide*
    D. *Finasteride*

10. Of the following statements about ovarian electrocautery, which are true?

    A. Reportedly, about 70% of patients ovulate, and 70% of those conceive.
    B. Even with careful technique, most patients will develop significant pelvic adhesions.
    C. Unilateral diathermy leads to bilateral ovarian activity.
    D. Androgens and LH and FSH levels are increased postoperatively.

11. True statements about the action of insulin sensitizers in PCOS include all of the following **except**

    A. Enhance insulin sensitivity at the postreceptor level
    B. Stimulate insulin-mediated glucose disposal
    C. Enhance peripheral glucose uptake
    D. Have no effect on hepatic glucose production

12. The following are true statements regarding insulin sensitizers in PCOS:

    A. Should not be given to patients with renal dysfunction.
    B. Should always be tried as single agent before clomiphene citrate.
    C. There are no known teratogenic effects.
    D. Only works exclusively in patients with elevated fasting insulin levels

13. True statements about corticotropin-dependent Cushing's syndrome include all of the following, **except**

    A. Small cell carcinoma of the lung is the most common cause.
    B. Diurnal cortisol secretion is lost
    C. The most common pituitary lesions are microadenoma
    D. Bronchial carcinoids may cause Cushing's through corticotropin-releasing hormone (CRH) secretion.

14. Of the following statements regarding CAH, which are true?

    A. Simple virilizing is the most common type.
    B. Easier to diagnose in newborn males.
    C. Associated with elevated 17-hydroxyprogesterone (17-OHP).
    D. Cortisol production is decreased.

15. Match the following enzymatic defects

    a. 21-hydroxylase deficiency

b. 11β-hydroxylase

c. 3β-hydroxysteroid dehydrogenase

With the following genetic findings or clinical manifestations

A. Short arm of chromosome 6
B. Hypertension
C. Human leukocyte antigen (HLA) linkage
D. Enzyme is found in both the adrenals and the ovaries

16. Which of the following statements is true regarding androgenizing ovarian tumors?

A. Testosterone levels over 2.5 times the norm are typical.
B. Computed tomography (CT) scan is highly diagnostic
C. Duplex Doppler ultrasound is first step.
D. DHEAS levels are usually elevated.

17. In the patient with hyperprolactinemia who desires future fertility, the imaging technique of choice is

A. None
B. Coned down x-ray of the sella turcica
C. CT scan
D. Tomograms
E. Magnetic resonance imaging (MRI)

18. Which of the following statements is true regarding pituitary adenomas in pregnancy?

A. *Bromocriptine mesylate* does not work to reduce symptoms.
B. Prolactin levels are followed to determine clinical course.
C. Breastfeeding is contraindicated.
D. These tumors rarely create complications during pregnancy.

19. The laboratory test that represents the best single screen for thyroid function is

A. Free T_4 index
B. Total serum T_4
C. T_3 resin uptake
D. Free T_3 index
E. Thyrotropin

20. The most common clinical state associated with autoimmune thyroid disease is

A. Hypothyroidism
B. Hyperthyroidism
C. Euthyroidism

Answers

1. D

For testosterone to exert its biologic effects on many target tissues, it must be converted into its active metabolite, DHT, by 5α-reductase (a cytosolic enzyme that reduces testosterone and androstenedione levels). Two isozymes of 5α-reductase exist: type 1, which predominates in the skin, and type 2, or acidic 5α-reductase, which is found in the liver, prostate, seminal vesicle and genital skin. The type 2 isozyme has a 20-fold higher affinity for testosterone than type 1. Both type 1 and 2 deficiencies in males result in ambiguous genitalia, and both isozymes may play a role in androgen effects on hair growth.

DHT is more potent than testosterone, primarily because of its higher affinity and slower dissociation from the androgen receptor. The relative androgenicity of androgens is as follows: DHT = 300, testosterone = 100, androstenedione = 10, and DHEAS = 5.
Reference: Page 874

2. C

The concentration of free testosterone has an inverse relationship with the SHBG concentration. Increased SHBG levels are noted in conditions associated with high estrogen levels. Thus, pregnancy and the luteal phase, use of estrogen (including OCs), and conditions causing elevated thyroid hormone levels and cirrhosis of the liver are associated with reduced free testosterone levels caused by elevated SHBG levels. Conversely, levels of SHBG decrease and result in elevated free testosterone levels in response to androgens, androgenic medications (progestational agents with androgenic biologic activities, danazol), androgenic disorders (PCOS, CAH, Cushing's syndrome), glucocorticoids, growth hormone, prolactin, insulin, and obesity.
Reference: Page 874

3. B

With age, the adrenal glands produce less DHEA and DHEAS. Once the ovaries cease production of estrogen during menopause, the production of testosterone and androstenedione increases. The diurnal variation is maintained by the adrenal contribution. These androgens are ultimately converted to estrone (E_1) and estradiol (E_2) via extragonadal aromatization.
Reference: Pages 874–875

4. A (b), B (a), C (b), and D (a)

The most common cause of hyperandrogenism and hirsutism is PCOS. The association of amenorrhea with bilateral polycystic ovaries was first described in 1935 by Stein and Leventhal and was known for decades as the Stein–Leventhal syndrome. In the past, the clinical diagnosis rested on the triad of hirsutism, amenorrhea, and obesity. Subsequently it has been recognized that PCOS has an extremely heterogeneous presentation and is multifactorial in etiology. Following are diagnostic criteria based on the "modified" consensus of the National Institutes of Health and Child Health and Human Development.

Major

Chronic anovulation

Hyperandrogenemia

Clinical signs of hyperandrogenism

Other etiologies excluded

Minor

Insulin resistance

Perimenarchal onset of hirsutism and obesity

Elevated LH/FSH ratio

Intermittent anovulation associated with hyperandrogenemia (free testosterone, DHEAS)

In this schema, there are only two major criteria for PCOS: anovulation and the presence of laboratory or clinical evidence or both of hyperandrogenism in the absence of other pathologies such as ovarian and adrenal neoplasms, pituitary disease, or CAH.

All other frequently encountered manifestations are less consistent findings and therefore qualify only as minor criteria. They include: insulin resistance, perimenarchal onset of hirsutism and obesity, elevated LH-to-FSH ratio, ultrasonographic evidence of PCOS, and oligoovulation.
Reference: Page 876

5. B

In patients with PCOS, the ovarian compartment is the most consistent contributor of androgens. Dysregulation of CYP17, the androgen-forming enzyme in both the adrenals and the ovaries, may be one of the central pathogenetic mechanisms underlying hyperandrogenism in PCOS. The ovarian stroma, theca, and granulosa contribute to ovarian hyperandrogenism and are stimulated by LH. This hormone relates to ovarian androgenic activity in PCOS in a number of ways:

1. Total and free testosterone levels correlate directly with LH levels.
2. The ovaries are more sensitive to gonadotropic stimulation, possibly as a result of CYP17 dysregulation.
3. Treatment with a GnRH agonist effectively suppresses serum testosterone and androstenedione levels.
4. Larger doses of a GnRH agonist are required for androgen suppression than for estrogen suppression.

Reference: Page 877

6. A (T), B (F), C (F), and D (F)

The increased testosterone levels in patients with PCOS are considered ovarian in origin. The serum total testosterone levels are usually no more than twice the upper normal range (20–80 ng/dL). However, in ovarian hyperthecosis, values may reach 200 ng/dL or more. High intraovarian androgen concentrations inhibit follicular maturation. Although ovarian theca cells are hyperactive, the retarded follicular maturation results in inactive granulosa cells with minimal aromatase activity for conversion to estrogens.

The adrenal compartment also plays a role in the development of PCOS. Although the hyperfunctioning CYP17 androgen-forming enzyme coexists in both the ovaries and the adrenal glands, DHEAS is increased in only about 50% of PCOS patients. The hyperresponsiveness of DHEAS to stimulation with corticotropin, the onset of symptoms around puberty, and the observation that 17,20-lyase activation (one of the two CYP17 enzymes) is a key event in adrenarche have led to the concept of PCOS as an exaggerated adrenarche.

The peripheral compartment, defined as the skin and the adipose tissue, manifests its contribution to the development of PCOS in several ways:

1. The presence and activity of 5α-reductase in the skin largely determines the presence or absence of hirsutism.
2. Aromatase and 17β-hydroxysteroid dehydrogenase activities are increased in fat cells, and peripheral aromatization is increased with body weight.
3. The metabolism of estrogens, by way of reduced 2-hydroxylation and 17α-oxidation, is decreased.
4. Whereas E_2 is at a follicular phase level in patients with PCOS, E_1 levels are increased as a result of peripheral aromatization of androstenedione.
5. A chronic hyperestrogenic state results with reversal of the E_1:E_2 ratio.

The hypothalamic–pituitary compartment also participates in aspects critical to the development of PCOS:

1. An increase in LH pulse frequency is the result of increased GnRH pulse frequency.
2. This increase in LH pulse frequency typically results in elevated LH and LH: FSH ratio.
3. FSH is not increased with LH, probably because of the synergistic negative feedback of chronically elevated estrogen levels and normal follicular inhibin.
4. About 25% of patients with PCOS exhibit elevated prolactin levels. The hyperprolactinemia may result from abnormal estrogen feedback to the pituitary gland. In some patients with PCOS, bromocriptine mesylate has reduced LH levels and restored ovulatory function.

Genetic association and linkage analysis studies presently under way suggest an oligogenic origin for PCOS. Patients with PCOS are at risk for hyperinsulinemia and insulin resistance. The most common cause of insulin resistance and compensatory hyperinsulinemia is obesity. The insulin resistance seen in PCOS seems to be independent of the expected insulin resistance that occurs with obesity alone. The following observations provide evidence that the insulin resistance associated with PCOS is not the result of hyperandrogenism:

1. Hyperinsulinemia is not a characteristic of hyperandrogenism in general but is uniquely associated with PCOS.
2. In obese women with PCOS, 30% to 45% have glucose intolerance or frank diabetes mellitus, whereas ovulatory hyperandrogenic women have normal insulin levels and glucose tolerance. It seems that the negative effects of PCOS and obesity on the action of insulin are synergistic.
3. Treatment with long-acting GnRH analogs does not change insulin levels or insulin resistance.
4. Oophorectomy in patients with hyperthecosis accompanied by hyperinsulinemia and hyperandrogenemia does not change insulin resistance, despite a decrease in androgen levels.

Reference: Pages 878–879

7. D

Combination OCs decrease adrenal and ovarian steroid production and reduce hair growth in nearly two thirds of hirsute patients. Treatment with OCs offers the following benefits:

1. The progestin component suppresses LH, resulting in diminished ovarian androgen production.
2. The estrogen increases hepatic production of SHBG, resulting in decreased free testosterone concentration.
3. Circulating androgen levels are reduced, which to some extent is independent of the effects of both LH and SHBG.
4. Estrogens decrease conversion of testosterone to dihydrotestosterone in the skin by inhibition of 5α-reductase.
5. Adrenal androgen secretion is reduced.

When an OC is used to treat hirsutism, a balance must be maintained between the decrease in free testosterone levels and the intrinsic androgenicity of the progestin. Three progestin compounds that are present in OCs (*norgestrel, norethindrone,* and *norethindrone acetate*) are believed to be androgen dominant. The androgenic bioactivity of these steroids may be a factor of their shared structural similarity with 19-nortestosterone steroids. OCs containing the "new progestins"(*desogestrel, gestodene, norgestimate,* and *drospirenone*) have minimized androgenic activity.

The use of OCs alone may be relatively ineffective ($>10\%$ success rate) in the treatment of hirsutism in women with PCOS. Insulin resistance may also be enhanced by OCs in these patients.
Reference: Page 880

8. C

Spironolactone is a specific antagonist of aldosterone, which competitively binds to the aldosterone receptors in the distal tubular region of the kidney. It is, therefore, an effective potassium-sparing diuretic, which was originally used for treatment of hypertension. The effectiveness of spironolactone in the treatment of hirsutism is based on the following mechanisms:

1. Competitive inhibition at the intracellular receptor level for DHT.
2. Suppression of testosterone biosynthesis by a decrease in the CYP enzymes.

3. Increase in androgen catabolism (with increased peripheral conversion of testosterone to E_2).

4. Inhibition of skin 5α-reductase activity.

Although total and free testosterone levels are significantly reduced in patients with both PCOS and idiopathic hirsutism (hyperandrogenism with regular menses) after treatment with spironolactone, total and free testosterone levels in patients with PCOS remain higher than those with idiopathic hirsutism (hyperandrogenism with regular menses). In both groups, SHBG levels are unaltered. The reduction in circulating androgen levels observed within a few days of *spironolactone* treatment partially accounts for the progressive regression of hirsutism.

At least a modest improvement in hirsutism can be anticipated in 70% to 80% of women using at least 100 mg of *spironolactone* per day for 6 months. *Spironolactone* reduces the daily linear growth rate of sexual hair, hair shaft diameters, and daily hair volume production. The most common doses are 25 to 100 mg twice daily. Women treated with 200 mg/d show a greater reduction in hair shaft diameter than women receiving 100 mg/d. Maximal effect on hair growth is noted between 3 and 6 months but continues for 12 months. Electrolysis can be recommended 9 to 12 months after the initiation of *spironolactone* for permanent hair removal.

The most common side effect of *spironolactone* is menstrual irregularity (usually metrorrhagia), which may occur in over 50% of patients with a dose of 200 mg/d.. Normal menses may resume with reduction of the dosage. Infrequently, other side effects such as urticaria, mastodynia, or scalp hair loss occur. Nausea and fatigue can occur with high doses. Because *spironolactone* can increase serum potassium levels, its use is not recommended in patients with renal insufficiency or hyperkalemia. Periodic monitoring of potassium and creatinine levels is required.

Return of normal menses in amenorrheic patients is reported in up to 60% of cases. Patients must be counseled to use contraception while taking *spironolactone* because it theoretically can feminize a male fetus.
Reference: Pages 881–882

9. A (c), B (b), C (b), and D (c)
Cyproterone acetate is a synthetic progestin derived from 17-OHP that has potent antiandrogenic properties. The primary mechanism of *cyproterone acetate* is competitive inhibition of testosterone and DHT at the level of androgen receptors. This agent also induces hepatic enzymes and may increase the metabolic clearance rate of plasma androgens.

The combination of ethinyl estradiol with *cyproterone acetate,* which was commonly used in Europe for many years, significantly reduces plasma testosterone and androstenedione levels, suppresses gonadotropins, and increases SHBG levels. *Cyproterone acetate* also shows mild glucocorticoid activity and may reduce DHEAS levels. Administered in a reverse sequential regimen (*cyproterone acetate,* 100 mg/d on days 5–15, and ethinyl estradiol, 30–50 mg/d on cycle days 5–26), this cyclic schedule allows regular menstrual bleeding, provides excellent contraception, and is effective in the treatment of even severe hirsutism and acne. When a desired clinical response is achieved, the dose of *cyproterone acetate* may be tapered gradually at 3- to 6-month intervals.

Side effects of *cyproterone acetate* include fatigue, weight gain, decreased libido, irregular bleeding, nausea, and headaches. These symptoms occur less often when ethinyl estradiol is added. *Cyproterone acetate* administration has been associated with liver tumors in beagles and is not approved by the U.S. Food and Drug Administration for use in the country.

Flutamide, a pure nonsteroidal antiandrogen, is approved for treatment of advanced prostate cancer. Its mechanism of action is inhibition of nuclear binding of androgens in target tissues. Although it has a weaker affinity to the androgen receptor than *spironolactone* or *cyproterone acetate,* larger doses (250 mg two or three times daily) may compensate for the reduced potency. *Flutamide* is also a weak inhibitor of testosterone biosynthesis.

In a single, 3-month study of *flutamide* alone, most patients demonstrated significant improvement in hirsutism with no change in androgen levels. Significant improvement in hirsutism with a significant drop in androstenedione, DHT, LH, and FSH levels was observed in an 8-month follow-up of *flutamide* and low-dose OC in women who did not respond to OC alone. The side effects of *flutamide* treatment combined with low-dose OC included dry skin, hot flashes, increased appetite, headaches, fatigue, nausea, dizziness, decreased libido, liver toxicity, and breast tenderness. Many patients taking *flutamide* (50%–75%) report of dry skin or a blue-green discoloration of urine. The risk of liver toxicity precludes *flutamide* as a routine option for the treatment of hirsutism.

Cimetidine is a histamine (H$_2$) receptor antagonist that has demonstrated a weak antiandrogenic effect as a result of its ability to occupy androgen receptors and inhibit DHT binding at the level of the hair follicles. Although *cimetidine* has been reported to reduce hair growth in women with hirsutism, two later studies show no beneficial effect.

Finasteride is a specific inhibitor of type 2, 5α-reductase enzyme activity that has been approved in the United States at a 5-mg dose for the treatment of benign prostate hyperplasia and at a 1-mg dose to treat male-pattern baldness. In a study in which *finasteride* (5 mg daily) was compared with *spironolactone* (100 mg daily), both drugs resulted in similar significant improvement in hirsutism despite differing effects on androgen levels. Most of the improvement in hirsutism occurred at 6 months of therapy with 7.5 mg of *finasteride* daily. The improvement in hirsutism in the presence of rising testosterone levels serves as convincing evidence that it is the binding of DHT and not testosterone to the androgen receptor that is responsible for hair growth. *Finasteride* does not prevent ovulation or cause menstrual irregularity. The increase in SHBG caused by OC further decreases free testosterone levels; thus and in combination with *finasteride* is more effective in reducing hirsutism than *finasteride* alone. As with *spironolactone, finasteride* could theoretically feminize a female fetus; therefore, both of these agents are used only with additional contraception.
Reference: Pages 882–883

10. **A (T), B (F), C (T), and D (F)**
Bilateral ovarian wedge resection is associated with only transient reduction in androstenedione levels and a prolonged minimal decrease in plasma testosterone. In patients with hirsutism and PCOS who have had wedge resection, hair growth was reduced by approximately 16%. Although Stein's original report cited a pregnancy rate of 85% following wedge resection and maintenance of ovulatory cycles, subsequent reports show lower pregnancy rates and a concerning incidence of periovarian adhesions.

Laparoscopic ovarian electrocautery is used as an alternative to wedge resection in patients with severe PCOS whose condition is resistant to *clomiphene citrate.* In a recent series, ovarian drilling was achieved laparoscopically with an insulated electrocautery needle, using 100 W cutting current to aid in entry and 40 W coagulating current to treat each microcyst over 2 seconds (8-mm needle in ovary). In each ovary, 10 to 15 punctures were created. This led to spontaneous ovulation in 73% of patients, with 72% conceiving within 2 years. Of those who had undergone a follow-up laparoscopy, 11 of 15 were adhesion-free. To reduce adhesion formation, a technique that cauterized the ovary only in four points led to a similar pregnancy rate with a miscarriage rate of

14% (much lower than the usual miscarriage rate of 30%–40% for patients with PCOS). Most series report a decrease in both androgen and LH concentrations and an increase in FSH concentrations. Unilateral diathermy has been shown to result in bilateral ovarian activity. Further studies are anticipated to define candidates who may benefit most from such a procedure. The risk of adhesion formation should be discussed with the patient.
Reference: Pages 883–884

11. D

Since hyperinsulinemia appears to play a role in PCOS-associated anovulation, treatment with insulin sensitizers may shift the endocrine balance toward ovulation and pregnancy, either alone or in combination with other treatment modalities.

Metformin hydrochloride (Glucophage) is an oral biguanide antihyperglycemic drug used extensively in Europe for non–insulin-dependent diabetes. Given its category-B status, there has been limited use of the drug in pregnant women with diabetes. Preliminary studies evaluating *Metformin hydrochloride* use in pregnancy suggest no teratogenicity and a reduced miscarriage rate but a potential increased risk of preeclampsia and perinatal mortality.

Metformin hydrochloride lowers blood glucose mainly by inhibiting hepatic glucose production and by enhancing peripheral glucose uptake. *Metformin hydrochloride* enhances insulin sensitivity at the postreceptor level and stimulates insulin-mediated glucose disposal.

The hyperandrogenism of PCOS is substantially relieved with *metformin hydrochloride* therapy, which leads to a drop in insulin levels and improved reproductive function. *Metformin hydrochloride* (500 mg three times daily) increases ovulation rates both spontaneously when used in combination with *clomiphene citrate* in obese patients with PCOS. In the latter group, a 90% ovulation rates has been achieved.

The most common side effects are gastrointestinal, including nausea, vomiting, diarrhea, bloating, and flatulence. Because the drug has caused fatal lactic acidosis in men with diabetes who have renal insufficiency, baseline renal function testing is suggested. The drug should not be given to women with elevated serum creatinine levels.

A prevailing concern over the increased incidence of spontaneous abortions in women with PCOS and the potential reduction afforded by insulin sensitizers suggest that insulin sensitizers may be beneficial in combination with gonadotropin therapy for ovulation induction or in-vitro fertilization.
Reference: Pages 884–885

12. A (T), B (F), C (T), and D (F)
See comments for Question 11.
Reference: Page 885

13. A
The six recognized noniatrogenic causes of Cushing's syndrome can be either corticotropin-dependent or corticotropin-independent (see Table 25.3). The corticotropin-dependent causes can result from corticotropin secreted by pituitary adenomas or from an ectopic source. The hallmark of corticotropin-dependent forms of Cushing's syndrome is the presence of normal or high plasma corticotropin concentrations with increased cortisol levels. The adrenal glands are hyperplastic bilaterally. Pituitary corticotropin-secreting adenoma, or Cushing's disease, is the most common cause of Cushing's syndrome. These pituitary adenomas are usually microadenomas (>10 mm in diameter) that may be as small as 1 mm. They behave as if they are resistant, to a variable degree, to the "feedback" effect of cortisol. Like the normal gland, these tumors secrete corticotropin in a pulsatile fashion; unlike the

Table 25.3. Causes of Cushing's Syndrome

Category	Cause	Relative Incidence
ACTH-dependent	Cushing's syndrome	60%[a]
	Ectopic ACTH-secreting tumors	15%
	Ectopic CRH-secreting tumors	Rare
ACTH-independent	Adrenal cancer	15%
	Adrenal adenoma	10%
	Micronodular adrenal hyperplasia	Rare
	Iatrogenic/factitious	Common

ACTH, adrenocorticotropic hormone; CRH, corticotropin-releasing hormone.
[a] ACTH-dependent Cushing's syndrome may be caused by pituitary adenoma, basophil hyperplasia, nodular adrenal hyperplasia, or cyclic Cushing's syndrome.

normal gland, the diurnal pattern of cortisol secretion is lost. Ectopic corticotropin syndrome most often is caused by malignant tumors. About one half of these tumors are small cell carcinomas of the lung. Other tumors include bronchial and thymic carcinomas, carcinoid tumors of the pancreas, and medullary carcinoma of the thyroid.

Ectopic CRH tumors are rare and include such tumors as bronchial carcinoids, medullary thyroid carcinoma, and metastatic prostate carcinoma. The presence of an ectopic CRH-secreting tumor should be suspected in patients who react biochemically similar to those with pituitary corticotropin-dependent disease but who have rapid disease progression and very high plasma corticotropin levels.

The most common cause of corticotropin-independent Cushing's syndrome is exogenous or iatrogenic (i.e., superphysiologic therapy with corticosteroids) or factitious (self-induced). Glucocorticoids are used in pharmacologic quantities to treat a variety of diseases with an inflammatory component. Over time, this practice will result in Cushing's syndrome. When glucocorticoids are taken by the patient but not prescribed by a physician, the diagnosis may be especially challenging. The diagnostic workup for Cushing's syndrome is summarized in Figure 25.2, Table 25.4, and Table 25.5
Reference: Page 886

14. A (F), B (F), C (T), and D (T)
Deficiency of 21-hydroxylase is responsible for over 90% of all cases of CAH. The disorder produces a spectrum of conditions. Salt-wasting CAH, which is the most severe form, affects 75% of patients in whom, during the first 2 weeks of life, a hypovolemic salt-wasting crisis is manifest, accompanied by hyponatremia, hyperkalemia, and acidosis. The salt-wasting crisis results from ineffective aldosterone synthesis. The condition is usually diagnosed earlier in affected women than in men because it causes genital virilization (e.g., clitoromegaly, labioscrotal fusion, and abnormal urethral course).

In simple virilizing CAH, affected patients are diagnosed as virilized newborn females or as rapidly growing masculinized boys at 3 to 7 years.

1. Basal follicular phase 17-OHP less than 200 ng/dL virtually excludes the disorder; no further testing is required.
2. Basal 17-OHP more than 500 ng/dL establishes the diagnosis; there is no need for further testing.
3. Basal 17-OHP higher than 200 ng/dL and less than 500 ng/dL requires corticotropin stimulation testing.
4. In the corticotropin stimulation test, plasma levels of 17-OHP are checked 1 hour following intravenous administration of a bolus of 0.25 mg corticotropin

Figure 25.2   The workup of Cushing's syndrome.

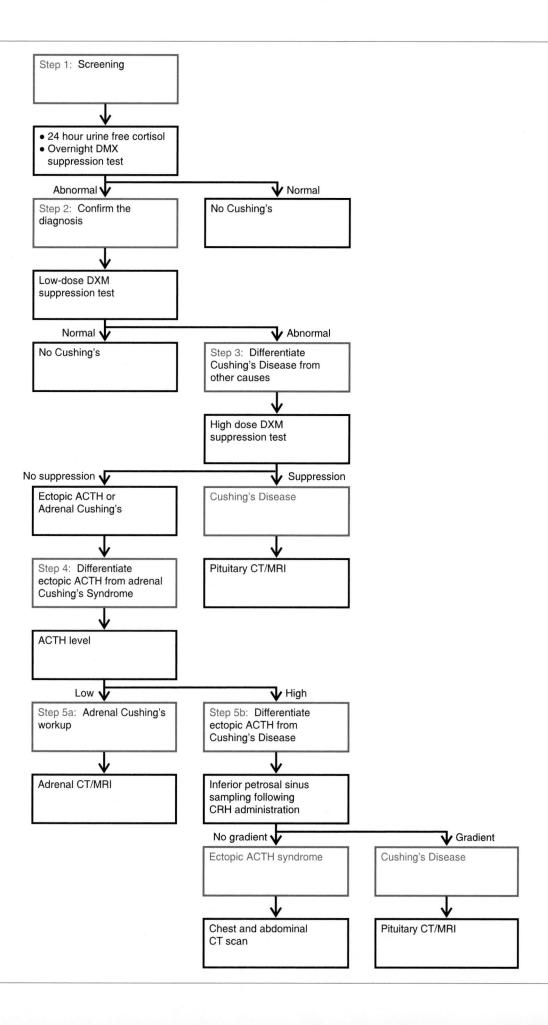

Table 25.4. Diagnostic Workup for Cushing's Syndrome

Screening	**Women with hirsutism who are suspected of having Cushing's syndrome should be tested for urinary free cortisol in a 24-hour collection and should undergo an overnight *dexamethasone* suppression test.** Two consecutive collections are recommended with creatinine determination. Normal urinary free cortisol should range from 30 to 80 μg/day. The overnight *dexamethasone* suppression test is an 8:00 AM cortisol determination after the patient is given 1 mg of *dexamethasone* at 11:00 PM the previous night.
Confirmation of diagnosis	**Confirmation of diagnosis at this stage can be performed by the 2-day, low-dose *dexamethasone* suppression test of Liddle (117).** The patient is given 0.5 mg of *dexamethasone* every 6 hours for 2 days. A 24-hour urine specimen is collected during the second day. Cushing's syndrome is ruled out if there is suppression of urinary 17-hydroxycorticosteroids to <3 mg/24 hr (or to 0% of baseline), suppression of plasma cortisol to <4 μg/day, or suppression of urinary free cortisol to <25 μg/24 hr.
Differentiation of Cushing's syndrome	**The high-dose *dexamethasone* suppression test is used to differentiate Cushing's syndrome from other causes (2 mg every 6 hours).** Normally, urinary 17-hydroxycorticoids should be 40% of baseline after 2 days. This test partially suppresses adrenocorticotropic hormone (ACTH) section with a resulting decrease in cortisol production in most patients with Cushing's syndrome; however, it has no effect on the majority of patients with ectopic or adrenal Cushing's syndrome.
Differentiation of ectopic ACTH syndrome	**High plasma ACTH (>4.5 pmol/L or >20 pg/ml) is consistent with ectopic ACTH production from adrenal glands.** A low ACTH level (<1.1 pmol/L or <5 pg/ml) identifies a patient who most likely has adrenal Cushing's syndrome.
ACTH-independent and -dependent	**A patient with ACTH-independent Cushing's syndrome should undergo an adrenal scan by MRI and should be prepared for adrenal surgery.** A patient with ACTH-dependent Cushing's syndrome should initially receive an administration of cortical-releasing hormone (1 ug/kg IV over 1 minute), which is followed 3–5 minutes later by simultaneous sampling of both the inferior petrosal sinuses and of the peripheral vein. The ratio of ACTH levels from the inferior petrosal sinuses to peripheral plasma is then calculated. An inferior petrosal sinus is virtually diagnostic of a pituitary tumor. Moreover, 95% of patients with Cushing's syndrome are found to have ratios over 2. If the test indicates a patient has Cushing's syndrome, a pituitary MRI with gadolinium enhancement should be obtained in preparation for transsphenoidal surgery. If the results indicate ectopic ACTH secretion, a computed tomography scan of the chest and possibly the abdomen should be performed (118, 119).

IV, intravenous; MRI, magnetic resonance imaging.

1-24 (Cortrosyn) (see Fig. 25.3). 17-OHP levels after corticotropin stimulation in adult-onset adrenal hyperplasia are generally higher than 1,000 ng/dL (Fig. 25.3).

5. Individuals who are heterozygous (carriers) for both adult-onset adrenal hyperplasia and CAH reveal stimulated 17-OHP values less than 1,000 ng/dL. In many cases, an overlap with the normal population is observed (Fig. 25.3).

The nonclassic type 21-hydroxylase deficiency represents partial deficiency in 21-hydroxylation, which produces a late-onset, milder hyperandrogenemia. Some

Table 25.5. Laboratory Diagnosis of Cushing's Syndrome

Diagnosis	24-Hour Urinary Cortisol	DEX Low Dose	DEX High Dose	ACTH
ACTH-dependent				

Cushing's syndrome (60%)
  Pituitary adenoma
  Basophil hyperplasia
  Nodular adrenal hyperplasia
  Cyclic Cushing's syndrome
	Increased	Increased	Decreased	Normal

Ectopic ACTH (15%)	Increased	Increased	Increased	Increased
Ectopic CRH (rare)	Increased	Increased	Increased or decreased	Increased
ACTH-independent				

Adrenal neoplasia
  Adenoma (10%)
  Carcinoma (15%)
  Primary adrenocorticoid
    nodular dysplasia (<1%)
	Increased	Increased	Increased	Decreased

Pseudo-Cushing's syndrome (alcohol-related, <1%)	Increased	Increased	Decreased	Normal

Exogenous
  glucocorticoids/factitious
  (not cortisol)
	Increased or decreased	Decreased	Decreased	Decreased

DEX, dexamethasone; ACTH, adrenocorticotropic hormone; CRH, corticotropin-releasing hormone.

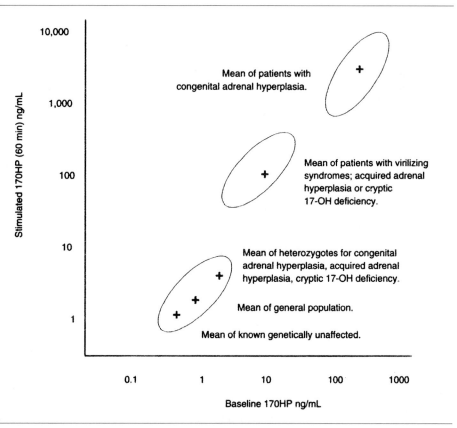

Figure 25.3   Basal and stimulated 17-hydroxyprogesterone concentration.

women with a mild gene defect demonstrate elevated circulating 17-OHP concentrations but no clinical symptoms or signs.

The hyperandrogenic symptoms of adult-onset CAH are mild and typically present at or after puberty. There are three phenotypic varieties:

1. PCOS (39%)
2. Hirsutism alone without oligomenorrhea (39%)
3. Cryptic (22%) (hyperandrogenism but no hyperandrogenic symptoms)

The need for screening patients with hirsutism for adult-onset adrenal hyperplasia depends on the patient population. The disease frequency is estimated to occur in 0.1% of the general population, 1% to 2% of Hispanics and Yugoslavs, and 3% to 4% of Ashkenazi Jews.
Reference: Pages 890–892

15. A (a), B (b), C (a), and D (c)
Genetics of 21-Hydroxylase Deficiency

1. The 21-hydroxylase gene is located on the short arm of chromosome 6, in the midst of the HLA region.
2. The 21-hydroxylase gene is now termed *CYP21*. Its homologue is the pseudogene CYP21P.
3. Because CYP21P is a pseudogene, the lack of transcription renders it nonfunctional. The *CYP21* is the active gene.
4. The *CYP21* gene and the CYP21P pseudogene alternate with two genes called *C4B* and *C4A*, both of which encode for the fourth component (C4) of serum complement.
5. The close linkage between the 21-hydroxylase genes and HLA alleles has allowed the study of 21-hydroxylase inheritance patterns in families through blood HLA-typing (e.g., linkage of HLA-B14 was found in Ashkenazi Jews, Hispanics, and Italians).

In families at risk for CAH, first-trimester prenatal screening is advocated. Currently, the fetal DNA is used for specific amplication of the *CYP21* gene using PCR (polymerase chain reaction) amplification. An aggressive and controversial approach involves the use of dexamethasone treatment for all pregnant women at risk of having a child with CAH. The dosage is 20 mg/kg in three divided doses administered as soon as pregnancy is recognized and no later than 9 weeks of gestation. This is done before performing chorionic villus sampling or amniocentesis in the second trimester. *Dexamethasone* crosses the placenta and suppresses corticotropin in the fetus. If the fetus is determined to be an unaffected female or a male, treatment is discontinued. If the fetus is an affected female, dexamethasone therapy is continued. When *dexamethasone* is administered before 9 weeks of gestation and is continued to term, it effectively reduces genital ambiguity in genetic females. However, at least two thirds of treated females still require surgical repair of the genitalia. Although prenatal treatment reduces virilization in females, the efficacy and safety to both mother and baby have not been verified. The unnecessary treatment of 7 of 8 pregnancies poses a serious ethical dilemma.

In a small percentage of patients with CAH, hypertension rather than mineralocorticoid deficiency develops. The hypertension responds to glucocorticoid replacement. Most of these patients have a deficiency in 11β-hydroxylase. In most populations, 11β-hydroxylase deficiency accounts for 5% to 8% of the cases of CAH, or 1 in 100,000 births. A much higher incidence, 1 in 5,000 to 7,000, has been described in Moroccan Jewish immigrants.

Two 11β-hydroxylase isoenzymes are responsible for cortisol and aldosterone synthesis, respectively, CYP11 B1 and CYP11 B2. They are encoded by two genes on the middle of the long arm of chromosome 8. No HLA linkage has been identified.

Inability to synthesize a fully functional 11β-hydroxylase enzyme causes a decrease in cortisol production, a compensatory increase in corticotropin secretion, and increased production of 11-deoxycortisol, 11-deoxycorticosterone, DHEA, and androstenedione. The diagnosis of 11β-hydroxylase-deficient late-onset adrenal hyperplasia is determined when 11-deoxycortisol levels are higher than 25 ng/mL 60 minutes after corticotropin 1-24 stimulation.

Patients with 11β-hydroxylase deficiency may present with either a classic pattern of the disorder or symptoms of a mild deficiency. The severe, classic form occurs in about two thirds of the patients with mild-to-moderate hypertension during the first years of life. In about one third of the patients it is associated with left ventricular hypertrophy, with or without retinopathy, and death is occasionally reported from cerebrovascular accident. Signs of androgen excess are common in the severe form and are similar to those seen in the 21-hydroxylase deficiency.

In the mild, nonclassic form, children are found to have virilization or precocious puberty but not hypertension. Adult women will present with postpubertal onset of hirsutism, acne, and amenorrhea.

Deficiency of 3β-hydroxysteroid dehydrogenase occurs with varying frequency in hirsute patients. The enzyme is found in both the adrenal glands and ovaries (unlike 21- and 11-hydroxylase) and is responsible for transforming Δ-5 steroids into the corresponding Δ-4 compounds. The diagnosis of this disorder relies on the relationship of Δ-5 and Δ-4 steroids. A marked elevation of DHEA and DHEAS in the presence of normal or mildly elevated testosterone or androstenedione may be a signal to initiate a screening protocol for 3β-hydroxysteroid dehydrogenase deficiency using exogenous corticotropin stimulation. Following intravenous administration of 0.25 mg corticotropin 1-24 bolus, 17-hydroxypregnenolone levels rise significantly within 60 minutes in women with 3β-hydroxysteroid dehydrogenase deficiency compared with normal women (2,276 ng/dL compound with normal of 1,050 ng/dL). The mean poststimulation ratio between 17-hydroxypregnenolone and 17-OHP was markedly elevated (mean ratio of 11 compared with 3.4 in normal controls and 0.4 in 21-hydroxylase deficiency). Because of the rarity of this disorder, routine screening of hyperandrogenic patients is not justified.
Reference: Pages 892–893

16. **A (T), B (F), C (F), and D (F)**
Patients with severe hirsutism, virilization, or recent and rapidly progressing signs of androgen excess require careful investigation for the presence of an androgen-secreting neoplasm. In prepubertal girls, virilizing tumors may cause signs of heterosexual precocious puberty in addition to hirsutism, acne, and virilization. A markedly elevated total testosterone level (2.5 times the upper normal range or over 200 ng/dL) is typical of an ovarian androgen-secreting tumor, and a DHEAS level greater than 800 μg/dL is typical of an adrenal tumor. An adrenal tumor is unlikely when serum DHEAS and urinary 17-ketosteroid excretion measurements are in the normal basal range and the serum cortisol concentration is greater than 3.3 μg/dL after dexamethasone administration. The results of other dynamic tests, especially testosterone suppression and stimulation, are unreliable.

A vaginal and abdominal ultrasound is the first step in the evaluation of an ovarian neoplasm. Duplex Doppler scanning may increase the accuracy of tumor localization. CT scanning is capable of detecting tumors greater than 10 mm (1 cm) in the adrenal gland but may not distinguish between different types of solid tumors. In the ovaries, CT scanning cannot differentiate hormonally active from functional tumors.

MRI is comparable, if not superior, to CT scanning in detecting ovarian neoplasm. When CT and selective venous catheterization fail, nuclear medicine scanning of the abdomen and pelvis after injection with NP-59 (iodomethylnorcholesterol), preceded by adrenal and thyroid suppression, may facilitate tumor localization.

If all four vessels are catheterized transfemorally, selective venous catheterization allows direct localization of the tumor. Samples are obtained for hormonal analysis, with positive localization defined as a 5:1 testosterone gradient compared with lower vena cava values. Under such circumstances specificity approaches 80% but this rate should be weighed against the 5% rate of significant complications such as adrenal hemorrhage and infarction, venous thrombosis, hematoma, and radiation exposure.

Ovarian neoplasms are the most frequent androgen-producing tumor. *Granulosa cell tumors* constitute 1% to 2% of all ovarian tumors and occur mostly in adult women (in postmenopausal more frequent than in premenopausal) (see Chapter 33). Usually associated with estrogen production, they are the most common functioning tumors in children and lead to isosexual precocious puberty. Total abdominal hysterectomy and bilateral salpingo-oophorectomy are the treatments of choice. If fertility is desired, in the absence of contralateral or pelvic involvement, unilateral salpingo-oophorectomy is justifiable. The 10-year survival rates vary from 60% to 90%, depending on the stage, tumor size, and histologic atypia.

Thecomas are rare and occur in older patients. In one study only 11% were found to be androgenic, even in the presence of steroid-type cells (luteinized thecomas). The tumor is rarely malignant and rarely bilateral, and a simple oophorectomy is sufficient treatment.

Sclerosing stromal tumors are benign neoplasms that usually occur in patients younger than 30 years. A few cases with estrogenic or androgenic manifestations have been reported.

Sertoli-Leydig cell tumors, previously classified as androblastoma or arrhenoblastoma, account for 11% of solid ovarian tumors. They contain various proportions of Sertoli cells, Leydig cells, and fibroblasts. Sertoli-Leydig cell tumors are the most common virilizing tumors in women of reproductive age; however, masculinization occurs in only one third of patients. The tumor is bilateral in 1.5%. In 80% of cases, it is diagnosed at stage Ia. Treatment with unilateral salpingo-oophorectomy is justified in patients with stage Ia disease who desire fertility. Total abdominal hysterectomy, bilateral salpingo-oophorectomy, and adjuvant therapy are recommended for postmenopausal women who have advanced stage disease.

Pure Sertoli cell tumors are usually unilateral. For a premenopausal woman with stage I disease, a unilateral salpingo-oophorectomy is the treatment of choice. Malignant tumors are rapidly fatal.

Gynandroblastomas are benign tumors with well-differentiated ovarian and testicular elements. A unilateral oophorectomy or salpingo-oophorectomy is sufficient treatment.

Sex cord tumors with annular tubules (SCTAT) are frequently associated with Peutz-Jeghers syndrome (gastrointestinal polyposis and mucocutaneous melanin pigmentation). Their morphologic features range between those of the granulosa cell and Sertoli cell tumors.

Whereas SCTAT with Peutz-Jeghers syndrome tends to be bilateral and benign, SCTAT without Peutz-Jeghers syndrome are usually unilateral and are malignant in one fifth of cases.

Steroid cell tumors are composed entirely of steroid-secreting cells subclassified into stromal luteoma, Leydig cell tumors (hilar and nonhilar), and steroid cell tumors that are not otherwise specific. Virilization or hirsutism is encountered with three fourths of Leydig cell tumors, with one-half of steroid cell tumors that are not otherwise specific, and with 12% of stromal luteomas.

Ovarian neoplasms, which are usually nonsteroid-producing, are occasionally associated with androgen excess and include serous and mucinous cystadenomas, Brenner tumors, Krukenberg tumors, benign cystic teratomas, and dysgerminomas. Gonadoblastomas arising in the dysgenetic gonads of patients with a Y chromosome are associated with androgen and estrogen secretion.

Stromal hyperplasia is a nonneoplastic proliferation of ovarian stromal cells. *Stromal hyperthecosis* is defined as the presence of luteinized stromal cells at a distance from the follicles. *Stromal hyperplasia,* which is typically seen in patients between 60 and 80 years old, may be associated with hyperandrogenism, endometrial carcinoma, obesity, hypertension, and glucose intolerance. *Hyperthecosis* also is seen in a mild form in older patients. In patients of reproductive age, hyperthecosis may demonstrate severe clinical manifestations of virilization, obesity, and hypertension. Hyperinsulinemia and glucose intolerance may occur in up to 90% of patients with hyperthecosis and probably play a role in the etiology of stromal luteinization and hyperandrogenism. Hyperthecosis is found in many patients with hyperandrogenemia, insulin resistance, and acanthosis nigricans (HAIR-AN syndrome).

In patients with hyperthecosis, levels of ovarian androgens, including testosterone, DHT, and androstenedione, are increased, usually in the male range. The predominant estrogen, as in PCOS, is E_2, which is derived from peripheral aromatization. The E_1:E_2 ratio is increased. Unlike in PCOS, gonadotropin levels are normal.

Wedge resection for the treatment of mild hyperthecosis has been successful and has resulted in resumption of ovulation and even in a pregnancy. However, in cases of more severe hyperthecosis and high free testosterone levels (1–3 ng/dL), the ovulatory response to wedge resection is only transient. In a study in which bilateral oophorectomy was used to control severe virilization, hypertension and glucose intolerance sometimes disappeared. Moreover, when a GnRH agonist was used to treat patients with severe hyperthecosis, ovarian androgen production was dramatically suppressed.

Luteomas of pregnancy are frequently associated with maternal and fetal masculinization. This is not a true neoplasm but rather a reversible hyperplasia, which usually regresses postpartum. A review of the literature reveals a 30% incidence of maternal virilization and a 65% incidence of virilized females in the presence of a pregnancy luteoma and maternal masculinization.

Other tumors causing virilization in pregnancy include (in descending order of frequency), Krukenberg tumors, mucinous cystic tumors, Brenner tumors, serous cystadenomas, endodermal sinus tumors, and dermoid cysts. Five cases of virilization of a female child have been reported.

High testosterone levels in the tumor range, accompanied by normal or only moderately elevated DHEAS levels, should not divert attention from the adrenal gland to the ovary. In fact, patients with these adenomas manifest increased testosterone production following stimulation with human chorionic gonadotropin (hCG) or LH and decreased testosterone secretion following LH suppression.

Of the fewer than 100 reported cases of pure virilizing adrenal neoplasms, 90% were benign. Although the peak age for the diagnosis of adenomas was 20 to 40 years, most of the pure testosterone-producing tumors occurred in menopausal women. With one exception, all cases of adenomas and carcinomas were unilateral. Fifty percent were abdominally palpable in children; in adults, none was solely detected by physical examination.

Reference: Pages 893–896

17. E

In patients with larger microadenomas and macroadenomas prolactin levels usually are higher than 100 ng/mL. However, levels lower than 100 ng/mL may be associated with smaller microadenomas and other suprasellar tumors that may be easily missed on a "coned-down" view of the sella turcica. In patients with a clearly identifiable drug-induced or physiologic hyperprolactinemia, scanning may not be necessary. MRI imaging of the sella and pituitary gland with *gadolinium* enhancement appears to provide the best anatomic detail (see Fig. 25.7). The cumulative radiation dose from multiple CT scans may cause cataracts, and the coned-down views or tomograms of the sella are very insensitive and likewise expose the patient to radiation. Even modest elevations of prolactin can be associated with microadenomas or macroadenomas, nonlactotroph pituitary tumors, and other central nervous system abnormalities; thus imaging of the

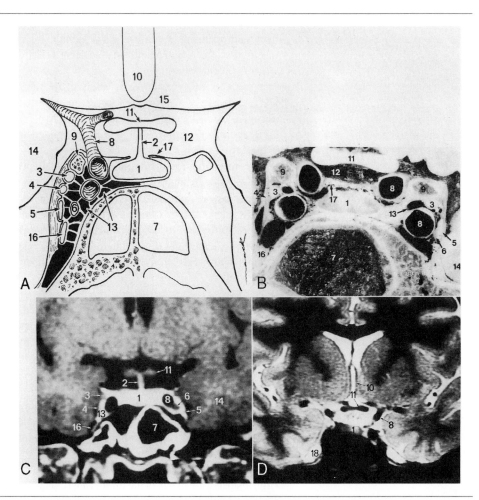

Figure 25.7   Anatomy of the intrasellar region and cavernous sinus by: (A) anatomic diagram, **(B)** coronal cytomicrosome section, **(C)** coronal postcontrast T1-weighted MRI, and **(D)** coronal postcontrast T2-weighted MRI. (1, pituitary gland; 2, infundibular stalk; 3, cranial nerve (CN) III; 4, CN IV; 5, CN VI; 6, CN VI; 7, sphenoid sinus; 8, internal carotid artery; 9, anterior clinoid process; 10, third ventricle; 11, optic chiasm; 12, suprasellar cistern; 13, venous spaces of cavernous sinus; 14, temporal lobe; 15, hypothalamus; 16, CN V$_2$; 17, diaphragma sellae; 18, Meckel's cave.)

Table 25.7. Sellar and Suprasellar Tumors and Conditions That May Result in Hyperprolactinemia

Abscess	Lipoma
Aneurysm	Lymphoma
Arachnoid cyst	Meningioma
Cephalocele	Meningitis (bacterial, fungal,
Chloroma (granulocytic sarcoma)	granulomatous)
Colloid cyst	Metastasis
Craniopharyngioma	Mucocele
Dermoid	Nasopharyngeal carcinoma
Ectopic neurohypophysis	Opticochiasmatic-hypothalamic
"Empty" sella	glioma
Epidermoid tumor	Osteocartilaginous tumor
Germinoma	Paracytic cyst
Hamartoma (tuber cinereum/hypothalmus)	Pars intermedia cysts
Histiocytosis	Pituitary adenoma
Hyperplasia	Rathke's cleft cyst
Hypophysitis	Sarcoidosis

pituitary gland must be considered (see Table 25.7). For patients with hyperprolactinemia who desire future fertility, MRI is indicated to differentiate a pituitary microadenoma from a macroadenoma as well as to identify other potential sellar-suprasellar masses. Although rare, when pregnancy-related complications of a pituitary adenoma occur, they occur more frequently in the presence of macroadenomas (Table 25.7).

In over 90% of untreated women; microprolactinomas do not enlarge over a 4- to 6-year period. For that reason, the argument that medical therapy will prevent a microadenoma from growing is false. Whereas prolactin levels correlate with tumor size, both elevations and reductions in prolactin levels may occur without any change in tumor size. If during follow-up a prolactin level rises significantly or central nervous system symptoms (headache, visual changes) are noted, repeat scanning may be indicated.
Reference: Pages 901–903

18. D

The workup for hyperprolactinemia is outlined in Figure 25.5 and the causes of hyperprolactinemia are listed in Table 25.6. Prolactin-secreting microadenomas rarely create complications during pregnancy. However, monitoring of patients with serial gross visual field examinations and fundoscopic examination is recommended. If persistent headaches, visual field deficits, or visual or fundoscopic changes occur, MRI scanning is advisable. Because serum prolactin levels are elevated throughout pregnancy, prolactin measurements are of no value.

Although not recommended, *Bromocriptine mesylate* use during pregnancy in women with symptomatic (visual field defects, headaches) microadenoma enlargement has resulted in resolution of deficits and symptoms.

Pregnant women with previous transsphenoidal surgery for microadenomas or macroadenomas may be monitored additionally with monthly Goldman perimetry visual field testing. Periodic MRI scanning may be necessary in women with symptoms or visual changes. Bromocriptine has been used on a temporary basis to resolve symptoms and visual field deficits in symptomatic patients with macroadenoma to allow completion of pregnancy before initiation of definitive therapy. Breastfeeding is not contraindicated in the presence of microadenomas or macroadenomas.
Reference: Pages 900–905

19. E

Total serum T4 is measured by radioimmunoassay. Conditions that elevate the levels of thyroid-binding globulin (TBG) (pregnancy, OC use, estrogen replacement,

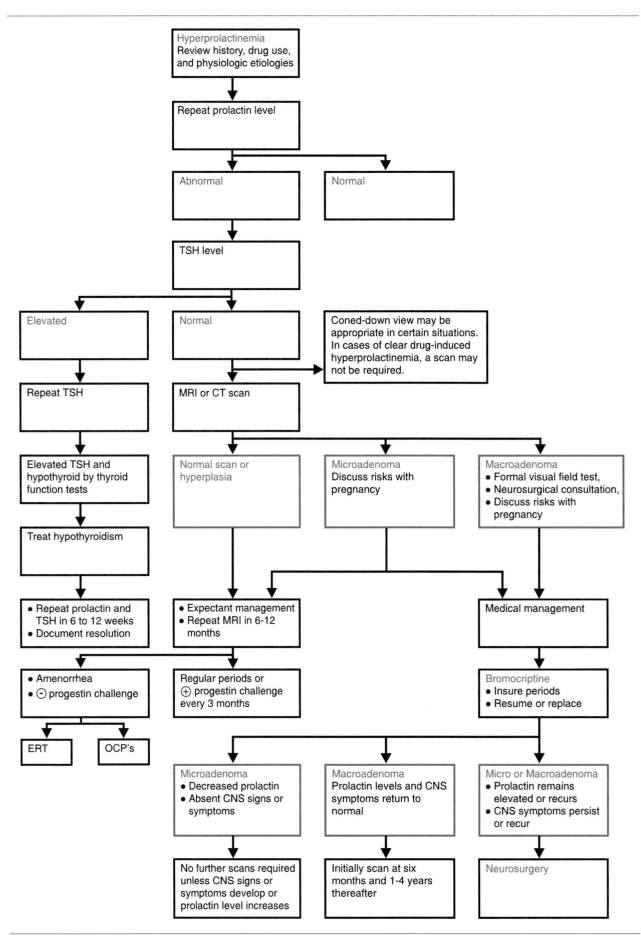

Figure 25.5   Workup for hyperprolactinemia.

Table 25.6. Chemical Factors Modulating Prolactin Release and Conditions That Result in Hyperprolactinemia

Inhibitory factors

Dopamine
γ-Aminobutyric acid
Histidyl-proline diketopiperazine
Pyroglutamic acid
Somatostatin

Stimulatory factors

β-Endorphin
17β-Estradiol
Enkephalins
Gonadotropin-releasing hormone
Histamine
Serotonin
Substance P
Thyrotropin-releasing hormone
Vasoactive intestinal peptide

Physiologic conditions

Anesthesia
Empty sella syndrome
Idiopathic
Intercourse
Major surgery and disorders of chest wall (burns, herpes, chest percussion)
Newborns
Nipple stimulation
Pregnancy
Postpartum (nonnursing: days 1–7; nursing: with suckling)
Sleep
Stress
Postpartum

Hypothalamic conditions

Arachnoid cyst
Craniopharyngioma
Cystic glioma
Cysticercosis
Dermoid cyst
Epidermoid cyst
Histiocytosis
Neurotuberculosis
Pineal tumors
Pseudotumor cerebri
Sarcoidosis
Suprasellar cysts
Tuberculosis

Pituitary conditions

Acromegaly
Addison's disease
Craniopharyngioma
Cushing's syndrome
Hypothyroidism
Histiocytosis
Lymphoid hypophysitis
Metastatic tumors (especially of the lungs and breasts)
Multiple endocrine neoplasia
Nelson's syndrome
Pituitary adenoma (microadenoma or macroadenoma)
Post–oral contraception
Sarcoidosis
Thyrotropin-releasing hormone administration

Table 25.6.—continued

Trauma to stalk
Tuberculosis

Metabolic dysfunction

Ectopic production (hypernephroma, bronchogenic sarcoma)
Hepatic cirrhosis
Renal failure
Starvation refeeding

Drug conditions

α *Methyldopa*
Antidepressants (*amoxapine, imipramine, amitriptyline*)
Cimetidine
Dopamine antagonists (phenothiazines, thioxanthenes, *butyrophenone,
    diphenylbutylpiperidine, dibenzoxazepine, dihydroindolone, procainamide,
    metaclopramide*)
Estrogen therapy
Opiates
Reserpine
Sulpiride
Verapamil

hepatitis, and genetic abnormalities of TBG) necessitate measuring T_3 resin uptake for clarification.

The T_3 resin uptake determines the concentration of radiolabeled T_3 bound to serum TBG and an artificial resin. The number of binding sites available in TBG is inversely proportional to the amount of labeled T_3 bound to the artificial resin. Therefore, high TBG T_3 receptor site availability results in a low T_3 resin uptake.

The free T_4 index (FTI) is obtained by multiplying the serum T_4 concentration by the T_3 resin uptake percentage, yielding an indirect measurement of free T_4:

$$\% \text{ free } T_4 \times T_4 \text{ total} = \text{free } T_4$$

Equilibrium dialysis may be used to determine the percentage of free T_4. Free T_4 and T_3 may also be determined by radioimmunoassay.

The present thyrotropin sandwich immunoassays are extremely sensitive and are capable of differentiating low-normal from pathological or iatrogenically subnormal values and elevations. Thus, thyrotropin measurements provide the best single screen for thyroid dysfunction and accurately predict thyroid hormone dysfunction in about 80% of cases.
Reference: Page 908

20. A

Thyroid disorders are 10 times more common in women than men. Approximately 1% of the female population of the United States will develop overt hypothyroidism. Even before the discovery of the long-acting thyroid stimulator (LATS) in women with Graves' disease in 1956, numerous investigations demonstrated a link between these autoimmune thyroid disorders and reproductive physiology and pathology.
Reference: Page 906

26 Endometriosis

Thomas M. D'Hooghe
Joseph A. Hill

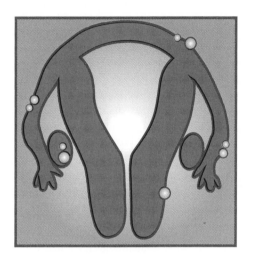

Learning Objectives

1. To understand the spontaneous evolution of endometriosis

2. To understand the rationale and methods for the surgical treatment of endometriosis

3. To understand the rationale and methods for the medical treatment of endometriosis

4. To understand the pathogenesis of endometriosis

Questions

Please answer the following questions as either true (T) or false (F).

1. Endometriosis is

   A. A progressive disease over 6 to 12 months in at least 30% of women.
   B. A disease that always appears the same.
   C. A dynamic condition with a progressive character.
   D. A disease without significant progression over several years.

2. Surgical treatment of endometriosis

   A. Should preferably be performed by laparoscopy in infertile women.
   B. Results in pain relief in all patients with endometriosis.
   C. Is not effective for pain relief in women with moderate-to-severe disease.
   D. Is proven to be effective in restoring infertility in women with minimal endometriosis.

3. Medical treatment of endometriosis

   A. Using oral contraceptives continuously may be an effective treatment.
   B. Using progestins, *gestrinone, danazol,* or gonadotropin-releasing hormone (GnRH) analogues are equally effective for relief of endometriosis-associated pain.
   C. Improves endometriosis-associated infertility.
   D. Results in long-term (at least 2 years) disease suppression and pain relief after cessation of therapy.

4. Pathogenesis:

   A. Endometriosis can be explained in all cases by the Sampson theory of retrograde menstruation with subsequent implantation of endometrial cells in the pelvic cavity.
   B. The Sampson theory and the induction theory are mutually exclusive.
   C. Menstrual endometrial cells can implant on the pelvic peritoneum.
   D. Strong clinical and experimental evidence supports the coelomic metaplasia theory.

5. Pathogenesis/genetics:

   A. Endometriosis is an autosomal recessive disorder.
   B. The endometriosis risk is increased in a patient if her mother or sister has (had) endometriosis.
   C. Genetic screening for aneuploidy should be routine in the investigation of a woman with suspected endometriosis.
   D. Twins are always concordant for the presence of endometriosis.

6. Pathogenesis/environment:

   A. Endometriosis is caused by increased exposure to dioxin.
   B. The Seveso study has demonstrated a link between dioxin exposure and the severity of endometriosis.
   C. Dioxins are not associated with endometriosis in primates.
   D. The link between dioxin exposure and endometriosis is not proven.

7. Diagnosis/clinical presentation:

   A. Women with endometriosis always have dysmenorrhea or chronic pelvic pain.
   B. All women with endometriosis are symptomatic.
   C. The degree of pelvic pain during menses is positively correlated with the degree of endometriosis in some but not in all women.

    D. Gastrointestinal symptoms, including bloating, nausea, and diarrhea, are not often associated with endometriosis.

8. Diagnosis:

    A. Gynecologic examination during menstruation does not add new information in the diagnosis of endometriosis.

    B. Lateral displacement of the cervix can be a sign of significant pelvic endometriosis.

    C. In women with infertility, endometriosis should be suspected if the external diameter of the cervical ostium measures at least 3 mm.

    D. A rectal examination is not needed for the diagnosis of deeply invasive pelvic endometriosis.

9. Diagnosis:

    A. A magnetic resonance imaging (MRI) pelvic evaluation is superior to gynecologic ultrasound in the diagnosis of peritoneal endometriosis.

    B. An MRI pelvic evaluation is superior to gynecologic ultrasound in the diagnosis of ovarian endometriosis.

    C. A combination of pelvic MRI and gynecologic ultrasound is needed for the diagnosis of endometriosis.

    D. Gynecologic ultrasound is equivalent to MRI in the diagnosis of pelvic endometriosis in more than 95% of the cases.

10. Laparoscopic and histologic aspects:

    A. Peritoneal endometriosis is found in all women of reproductive age undergoing a laparoscopy for pain and infertility.

    B. A brown-orange peritoneal patch in the ovarian fossa is unlikely to be endometriosis.

    C. Biopsy and histologic examination for the presence of endometrial glands and stroma are needed for the diagnosis of endometriosis.

    D. Endometriosis is only rarely seen in women undergoing laparascopic sterilization.

11. Surgical treatment:

    A. Minimal or mild endometriosis should be treated surgically in women with infertility only.

    B. Minimal or mild endometriosis should be treated surgically in women with pain only.

    C. Minimal or mild endometriosis should never be treated surgically, only medically.

    D. Minimal or mild endometriosis should always be treated surgically.

12. Medical treatment, GnRH analogues:

    A. GnRH analogues only cause osteoporosis when taken more than 6 months continuously.

    B. All progestogens are equivalent as "add-back" therapy in the medical management of endometriosis.

    C. Add-back therapy is known to significantly reduce the effectiveness of GnRH treatment in the management of endometriosis.

    D. Women with endometriosis should not receive GnRH analogues without add-back estrogens and/or progestins.

13. Recurrent endometriosis:

    A. Recurrence of endometriosis only occurs if all endometriotic foci have not been removed during surgery.

    B. Recurrence of endometriosis is more likely in women with moderate-to-severe endometriosis.

C. Endometriosis is not a recurrent disease, but cannot be completely treated because microscopic endometriosis is present in nearly every woman.

D. Recurrent endometriosis should always be treated surgically in women with chronic pain.

14. Assisted reproduction and endometriosis:

A. The implantation rate per embryo is decreased in women with ovarian endometriosis.

B. The number of oocytes is decreased in women with ovarian endometriosis.

C. The pregnancy rate per insemination cycle is similar in women with endometriosis and those with unexplained infertility.

D. Women without pregnancy within 1 year after endometriosis surgery should undergo a second surgical intervention, rather than assisted reproduction.

Answers

1. A (T), B (F), C (T), and D (F)

Endometriosis has a highly variable appearance, and has been reported to be progressive in 30% to 50% of patients within 2 years of follow-up.
Reference: Pages 936–937, 946–947

2. A (T), B (F), C (F), and D (F)

The multicenter Canadian study and other studies have clearly shown that laparascopic destruction of peritoneal endometriotic lesions and removal of endometriosis-associated adhesions and cysts can improve fertility.
Reference: Pages 947–950

3. A (T), B (T), C (F), and D (F)

Current effective medical treatment of endometriosis-associated pain includes the continuous use of oral contraceptives, progestins, and GnRH agonists with add-back. Danazol and gestrinone are less frequently prescribed due to their side effects. However, during medical treatment, patients cannot conceive. Furthermore, fertility is not increased after medical treatment, and there is a problem of endometriosis recurrence and pain recurrence within 6 to 12 months after cessation of medical treatment.
Reference: Pages 951–957

4. A (F), B (F), C (T), and D (F)

It is hard to explain the occurrence of endometriosis in brain, lungs, or umbilicus by the Sampson theory. On the other hand, the idea of retrograde menstruation allows the application of both the Sampson theory (implantation of endometrial cells in the pelvis) and the induction theory (menstrual fluid contains substances that cause metaplasia from peritoneum to ectopic endometrium). However, the coelomic metaplasia theory is not supported by strong clinical or experimental evidence.
Reference: Pages 931–932

5. A (F), B (T), C (F), and D (F)

There is a well-known increased risk for women to develop endometriosis if their first-degree relatives are known to have endometriosis. However, there is no clear genetic pattern and endometriosis seems to be a genetically complex and multifactorial disease without recessive or dominant inheritance pattern, without specific karyotype abnormality in white blood cells of patients with endometriosis, and without complete concordance in monozygotic twins.
Reference: Pages 932–933

6. A (F), B (F), C (F), and D (T)

Whereas there is a lot of attention from the media, patients, and patient organizations with respect to the link between dioxin and endometriosis, there are no hard data from which to draw any firm conclusions. Several studies suggest a positive correlation between the degree of endometriosis and the degree of dioxin exposure in primates. However, there is no evidence that women with endometriosis have an increased concentration of dioxin in their body.

Reference: Page 934

7. A (F), B (F), C (T), and D (F)

Many women with endometriosis, even advanced stages of endometriosis, are completely asymptomatic. Gastrointestinal problems occur together with endometriosis, although few clinicians are aware of this link.

Reference: Page 937

8. A (F), B (T), C (F), and D (F)

Clinical examination is very important in the diagnosis of endometriosis. In **speculo,** a very narrow cervix (ostium < 3 mm) and lateral displacement of the cervix can be signs of intrapelvic endometriosis. At the time of menstruation, it is easier to detect deeply infiltrative endometriosis during a bimanual pelvic exam than at other phases of the cycle. When deep infiltrative endometriosis of the rectovaginal septum is suspected, it is advisable to do a rectal examination or a combined rectovaginal examination.

Reference: Page 938

9. A (F), B (F), C (F), and D (T)

Gynecologic ultrasound, carried out by an experienced clinician using state-of-the-art equipment, can detect most of the ovarian endometriotic cysts and deeply infiltrating endometriotic nodules with a size of 1 cm or more. MRI is also very accurate, but not significantly more accurate than ultrasound, and is much more expensive.

Reference: Pages 938–939

10. A (F), B (F), C (T), and D (F)

Endometriosis is commonly found in women of reproductive age, but not in all. Endometriosis can be found in about 5% to 10% of women at the time of sterilization. Because the visual diagnosis of endometriotic lesions is often false-positive, systematic histologic confirmation is needed. Practically, it can be suggested that at least one endometriotic lesion per patient should be positive for endometrial glands and stroma to make the diagnosis of endometriosis.

Reference: Pages 939–941

11. A (F), B (F), C (F), and D (T)

Surgery for endometriosis-associated pain and infertility is effective and can be recommended as first line therapy. The Canadian multicenter study has shown that the monthly pregnancy rate is significantly higher (5%) after surgical removal of minimal-to-mild endometriosis than after expectant management (2.5%). As such, it can be recommended that minimal-to-mild endometriosis should be treated when diagnosed at laparoscopy.

Reference: Pages 949–951

12. A (F), B (F), C (F), and D (T)

The use of GnRH analogues is an effective treatment of endometriosis, but can cause osteoporosis, even if taken for less than 6 months. Therefore, effective add-back with estrogens and/or progestins should be combined with GnRH analogues, because this combination is known to largely prevent the osteoporosis side effects without reducing the efficacy of endometriosis treatment.

Reference: Pages 955–956

13. A (F), B (T), C (F), and D (F)

Endometriosis is a recurrent disease, and the recurrence rate is positively correlated with the stage of endometriosis. Complete surgery is an illusion, because it is clinically impossible to be sure that the last microscopic areas of visual endometriosis have been removed. If endometriosis has recurred several times after surgery, it is advisable to treat the patient medically with continuous oral contraceptives, progestagens, or with a *levonorgestrel*-containing intrauterine device (IUD). If the patient wants to become pregnant, *in vitro* fertilization (IVF) can be considered immediately following GnRH medical suppression of endometriosis. The goal should be to limit the number of menstruations, preferable by medically creating a continuous state of amenorrhea that is only interrupted by IVF treatment.

Reference: Pages 957–958

14. A (F), B (T), C (F), and D (F)

This is a controversial topic. In general, it can be stated that patients who have not become spontaneously pregnant within 1 year after fertility surgery for endometriosis are unlikely to conceive afterwards and should be offered assisted reproduction (controlled ovarian hyperstimulation with intrauterine insemination [IUI], or IVF). However, the pregnancy rate per IUI cycle is lower in patients with endometriosis than in controls, whereas there is not sufficient evidence that the pregnancy rate per embryo transfer or the implantation rate per embryo is decreased in women with endometriosis when compared to controls. On the other hand, there is sufficient evidence to state that the number of oocytes is decreased in women with ovarian endometriosis, and that these patients need higher doses of gonadotropins for their ovarian stimulation in an IVF program.

Reference: Pages 958–959

27

Infertility

Mylene W. M. Yao
Daniel J. Schust

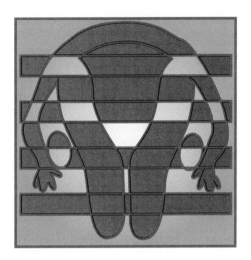

Learning Objectives

1. Understand the epidemiology of infertility.

2. Know the initial evaluation of the infertile couple.

3. Be able to articulate the different causes of infertility in the male and female.

4. Understand the indications for various diagnostic tests and procedures in an infertility investigation.

5. Understand treatments available to treat the infertile couple, their relative efficacies, and possible complications.

6. Know the different types of treatment available in assisted reproduction.

Questions

For each of the following questions, choose:

A. If only 1, 2, and 3 are correct
B. If only 1 and 3 are correct
C. If only 2 and 4 are correct
D. If only 4 is correct
E. If all are correct

1. Which of the following is/are true?

   1. The fecundity of a normal fertile couple is 20% to 25%.
   2. Fecundability is the probability of achieving a live birth within a single menstrual cycle.
   3. Fecundity is the probability of achieving a pregnancy within a single menstrual cycle.
   4. Fecundability is typically greater than fecundity.

2. It is estimated that the incidence of tubal infertility associated with a history of pelvic inflammatory disease (PID) is

   1. Approximately 12% after a single documented episode of PID
   2. Greater than 50% after three documented episodes of PID
   3. Greater than 20% after two documented episodes of PID
   4. Independent of the number of episodes of PID

3. Which of the following statements concerning artificial insemination is/are true?

   1. Pregnancy rates using intracervical insemination (ICI) are higher than those with intrauterine insemination (IUI).
   2. Pregnancy rates are higher with the use of fresh semen than with use of frozen donor specimens.
   3. When using IUI to treat male infertility, it is recommended that the female partner be treated with clomiphene citrate or gonadotropins to maximize the pregnancy rate even if she has no known fertility defects.
   4. It is recommended that frozen semen samples be used for all donor inseminations.

4. Which of the following is/are accepted indication(s) for use of intracytoplasmic sperm injection?

   1. Severe male factor infertility (<0.5 million total motile sperm)
   2. Previous fertilization failure in standard *in vitro* fertilization (IVF) cycles
   3. Use of surgically recovered epididymal and testicular sperm
   4. Preimplantation genetic diagnosis

5. Which of the following statements is/are true regarding the use of ovarian reserve screening?

   1. The clomiphene citrate challenge test (CCCT) should be used because it is more sensitive and specific than day-3 FSH.
   2. A normal CCCT is a reliable indicator of normal ovarian function.
   3. Serum inhibin B has recently been established to be the best method for ovarian reserve testing.
   4. Age over 40 years and an abnormal CCCT are poor prognostic factors in IVF treatment.

6. Which of the following causes contribute to the increase in spontaneous abortion rate seen in older women?

   1. There is an increase in polypoidy with age.
   2. There is an increase in trisomies 16, 18, 20, 21 and 22 with age.
   3. There is an increase in monosomy X with age.
   4. There is an increase in abnormal fetal karyotype with age.

7. Which of the following is/are false regarding the use of urine luteinizing hormone (LH) detection kits to document ovulation?

   1. A positive test is usually followed by ovulation.
   2. Up to 5% to 10% of women may have urine LH tests that fail to document an LH surge.
   3. Enzyme-linked immunosorbent assays (ELISA) using 40 mIU/mL as the threshold for detection is the basis of these urine LH kits.
   4. For women whose LH surge cannot be detected by these urine LH kits, the only alternative methods are basal body temperature, midluteal serum progesterone assessment, and transvaginal ultrasound.

8. Which of the following statements is/are true regarding ovulation induction in patients with polycystic ovary syndrome (PCOS)?

   1. Because weight reduction in overweight patients with PCOS significantly increases the spontaneous ovulation and pregnancy rates, other medical interventions should be withheld until a trial of weight reduction has been attempted.
   2. Clomiphene citrate has a lower success rate in patients with PCOS with obesity and insulin resistance.
   3. *Troglitazone* is an insulin sensitizer that is effective in inducing ovulation and is the first line treatment for patients with PCOS and insulin resistance.
   4. Clomiphene citrate can be added to the *metformin hydrochloride* regimen to increase the chance of ovulation in patients with PCOS with increased body mass index (BMI), significant hyperandrogenism, and hyperinsulinemia.

9. In addition to the surgical risks associated with laparoscopic surgery, which of the following should be included in the informed consent for a patient who is considering undergoing laparoscopic ovarian drilling for ovulation induction?

   1. Risk of premature ovarian failure
   2. Risk of failure to induce ovulation
   3. Anovulation can recur
   4. Potential adhesion formation, which may interfere with fertility

10. Which of the following is/are contraindications to hysterosalpingography?

   1. Previous tubal reversal surgery (or tubal reanastamosis)
   2. Known hydrosalpinx
   3. Normal hysterosalpingography examination within 5 years
   4. Undiagnosed adnexal mass

11. Which of the following is/are good prognostic factors for surgical sterilization reversal?

   1. The length of each tube is 7 cm.
   2. There is no significant difference in the tubal diameters at the sites of reanastamosis.
   3. Tubal ligation was performed with Fallope rings.
   4. Tubal ligation was performed using the Pomeroy technique.

12. Which of the following statements is/are true regarding diagnostic imaging in infertility?

   1. Hysterosalpingography has a high sensitivity in detecting uterine anomalies such as uterine septum but can only detect 50% to 65% of tubal obstructions.
   2. Sonohysterography increases the sensitivity and specificity in the diagnosis of intrauterine abnormalities and is superior to regular transvaginal ultrasonography.
   3. Diagnostic hysteroscopy and laparoscopic chromotubation are considered the best method for detecting uterine anomalies and tubal blockage, respectively, and should be performed routinely as part of initial infertility investigations.
   4. The use of contrast media in sonohysterography may increase its sensitivity in detecting tubal blockage compared with that of laparoscopic chromotubation.

13. Which of the following is/are true regarding the treatment of unexplained infertility?

   1. *Clomiphene citrate* administration should always be combined with intrauterine insemination in unexplained infertility.
   2. *Clomiphene citrate* alone is a reasonable first-line superovulation treatment without the risks of intrauterine insemination.
   3. Endometriosis that is seen at the time of diagnostic laparoscopy should be surgically ablated.
   4. Expectant management for 1 year is reasonable if no cause is identified, especially if there is no evidence of endometriosis on diagnostic laparoscopy.

14. Which of the following is/are benefit(s) of IVF as a treatment for unexplained infertility?

   1. The pregnancy rate per IVF cycle is higher than that of combined controlled ovarian hyperstimulation (COH) and IUI.
   2. IVF is a diagnostic and therapeutic procedure because fertilization defects can be detected.
   3. The risk of higher-order multiple gestation (HOMG) is lower in IVF than COH/IUI if the number of embryos transferred is dictated by a stringent protocol.
   4. The routine use of intracytoplasmic sperm injection (ICSI) in the assisted reproductive technology (ART) treatment of patients with unexplained infertility significantly increases the pregnancy rate.

15. Which of the following are considered benefits of using recombinant follicle-stimulating hormone (FSH) in COH?

   1. There is increased batch-to-batch consistency in potency.
   2. The subcutaneous route of administration of recombinant FSH is preferred by most patients.
   3. Absence of LH is hypothesized to result in decreased androgen production and may be particularly beneficial in patients with PCOS who have significant hyperandrogenism.
   4. The absolute purity of recombinant FSH produced is particularly beneficial for women with FSH-receptor variants.

16. Which of the following is/are not strategies to reduce the risks of ovarian hyperstimulation syndrome and multiple gestation in COH/IUI treatment with gonadotropins in women with PCOS?

   1. Down-regulation with gonadotropin-releasing hormone (GnRH) agonist
   2. Pretreatment and concomitant treatment with *metformin hydrochloride*
   3. Pretreatment with laparoscopic ovarian drilling
   4. Concomitant treatment with *clomiphene citrate*

17. Which of the following is/are established or potential strategies to decrease the risk of HOMG in IVF–embryo transfer (ET)?

1. Use of preimplantation genetic diagnosis to identify nonaneuploidic embryos for transfer
2. Extended culture and transfer of one to two blastocysts
3. Following strict guidelines to limit the number of embryos to be transferred
4. Limiting the number of freshly retrieved oocytes to be fertilized *in vitro*

18. Which of the following is/are risk factors of higher order multiple gestation?

1. Infertility treatment using gonadotropins in COH/IUI
2. Increased maternal age
3. Infertility treatment with ART
4. The use of ICSI over IVF to achieve fertilization in ART

19. Which of the following is/are considered complications of ART?

1. Ovarian hyperstimulation syndrome
2. Tuboovarian abscess
3. Heterotopic ectopic pregnancy
4. Failure to obtain oocytes

20. Which of the following statements is/are true regarding the success rate of ART according to the 1997 Society for Assisted Reproductive Technology (SART) data?

1. The overall delivered-pregnancy rate per oocyte retrieval in 1997 was above 25%.
2. Despite the use of ICSI, the pregnancy rates of couples with male infertility alone remain lower than average.
3. Age of the woman was a significant determinant of success rate in ART.
4. The overall delivered-pregnancy rate for cryopreserved embryo transfer in 1997 was also above 25%.

Answers

1. D

Fecundability is the probability of achieving pregnancy within a single menstrual cycle, and *fecundity* is the probability of achieving a live birth within a single cycle. The fecundability of a normal couple has been estimated at 20% to 25%. On the basis of this estimate, approximately 90% of couples should conceive after 12 months.
Reference: Page 973

2. A

The risk of infertility after a single bout of PID is surprisingly high and increases rapidly with subsequent episodes. In fact, the incidence of tubal infertility has been reported to be 12%, 23%, and 54% after one, two, and three episodes of PID, respectively. Still, approximately 50% of patients with documented tubal damage have no identifiable risk factors for tubal disease. Most of these women are presumed to have had subclinical *Chlamydia* infections.
Reference: Page 1,002

3. C

For males with azoospermia, couples with significant male-factor infertility who do not desire ART, or women seeking pregnancy without a male partner, therapeutic donor insemination offers an effective option. A number of important issues surround the use of this form of artificial insemination. First, despite reports that the use of fresh donor semen is associated with higher pregnancy rates than the use of frozen specimens, both the Centers for Disease Control and Prevention (CDC) and the American Society for Reproductive Medicine recommend the use of frozen samples. This recommendation stems from the increasing incidence of human immunodeficiency virus (HIV) infection in the general population and the lag between HIV infection and seroconversion. Currently, semen donors are screened for HIV infection, hepatitis B, hepatitis C, syphilis, gonorrhea, *Chlamydia* infection, and cytomegalovirus infections, all of which may be transmitted through the semen vector. All cryopreserved samples are quarantined for 6 months, and the donor is retested for HIV before clinical use of the specimen. Donors are likewise questioned concerning a family history of genetically transmitted disorders, both mendelian (e.g., hemophilia, Tay-Sachs disease, thalassemia, cystic fibrosis, congenital adrenal hyperplasia, and Huntington's disease) and polygenic/multifactorial disorders (e.g., mental retardation, diabetes, heart malformation, spina bifida). Those with positive family histories are eliminated as donor candidates.

A second issue surrounding the use of therapeutic donor insemination—that which is most important to the patient—is the success rate of treatment. In patients younger than 30 years who have no other infertility factors, conception rates approach 62% after 12 cycles of treatment with frozen sperm.

IUI was superior to ICI for donor insemination in several prospective randomized or crossover trials. Overall, the cycle fecundity rates ranged from 9.7% to 24% for IUI to 3.9% to 17.9% for ICI. A metaanalysis concluded that IUI had a significantly higher cycle fecundity rate when compared to ICI (odds ratio [OR] 2.4; 95% confidence interval [CI], 1.5–3.8). Moreover, the concomitant use of *clomiphene citrate* or gonadotropin (human menopausal gonadotropin [HMG]) for COH did not result in higher fecundity rates.

The length of recommended treatment must also be addressed. When frozen donor semen is used, more than 80% of consequent pregnancies will occur during the first 12 months of treatment. Thus, patients who do not conceive within 6 to 12 months should be assessed for female factors and be encouraged to terminate treatment or move to alternative forms of therapy.

Last, but not least, one must consider the psychosocial aspects of pregnancies involving donor gametes. Among patients without a male partner, the potential repercussions of becoming a single mother and the issue of telling others about the father of the child must be discussed. It is imperative that the husband of a couple using donor gametes is aware of the process, and most programs require that the husband sign a consent form. A skilled infertility social worker or psychologist can be helpful in addressing these concerns.
Reference: Pages 985–986

4. E

The indications for ICSI have evolved since its introduction. They will most likely continue to evolve as more is learned about risks and benefits of ICSI. One absolute indication for ICSI is severe male-factor infertility as demonstrated by total progressively motile sperm counts higher than 500,000/mL and <3% normal morphology according to strict Tygerberg criteria. Sperm counts of less than 0.5×10^6/mL are associated with poor fertilization rates in IVF, and this too is an indication for ICSI. Other indications for ICSI include the sole presence of spermatozoa lacking an acrosome or those that are completely immotile, as well as the utilization of surgically recovered epididymal or testicular sperm. Other absolute indications for ICSI are not related to male infertility and include a history of two previous fertilization failures with conventional IVF and the fertilization of oocytes prior to preimplantation genetic diagnosis. The benefit of combined IVF/ICSI in ART for unexplained infertility is described in the section on unexplained infertility.
Reference: Pages 987–988

5. D

Ovarian reserve screening tests that have been proposed include serum day-3 FSH, CCCT, serum inhibin B, and transvaginal ultrasound for antral follicle number or ovarian size. Measurement of day-3 FSH is based on evidence that small increases in basal serum FSH levels correlate with the decreased fecundability seen among women in their late 30s. Clomiphene citrate is thought to have antiestrogenic effects in the hypothalamic–pituitary axis, resulting in a decrease in suppression of FSH production by the pituitary. In the CCCT, serum FSH is drawn on day 3, and again on day 10 after administration of clomiphene citrate 100 mg orally daily from days 5 through 9. Levels will vary depending on the assay used and the population being screened; therefore, each ART center will typically set its own reference range for evaluating the results of a CCCT. In a general infertility patient population, the incidence of an abnormal CCCT rises from <10% under age 35 to 26% in patients older than 40 years. However, the results of day-3 FSH levels and CCCT must be interpreted with caution. These tests have mainly been studied in women with subfertility. Among these patients, day-3 FSH testing has a sensitivity of 8% in identifying women who will not conceive with subsequent IVF treatment. Day-3 FSH and CCCT each display a high specificity (96%) in predicting IVF outcome; however, addition of the CCCT to a day-3 FSH only increases the sensitivity of prediction to 26%. Although abnormal results of a CCCT portend a poor prognosis for pregnancy independent of age, older patients with normal CCCT results still have significantly decreased pregnancy rates. Because among older patients even a normal CCCT does not provide reassurance for a good prognosis, chronological age must still be considered a salient, independent predictor of treatment outcome.

A great deal of emotional, physical, temporal, and financial effort is involved in the process of fertility treatments involving ART. Day-3 FSH and CCCT results can be used to counsel patients regarding their potential for pregnancy with IVF treatment. In one study, 5% of 435 women beginning their first IVF cycle had a day-3 FSH level higher than 15 IU/L. These women were 3.9 times more likely to have an unsuccessful treatment cycle. Similarly, among 175 IVF cycles involving women older than 40 years, no pregnancies resulted when testing revealed a day-3 FSH of greater than 11.1 mIU/ml or a day-10 FSH greater than 13.5 mIU/ml after CCCT. Therefore, it is reasonable to advise women with advanced age (>40 years) and abnormal day-3 FSH or CCCT to strictly limit the number of IVF cycle attempts because their overall prognosis is poor. These tests should not, however, be used as the sole basis to exclude women from IVF treatment.

Recently, serum inhibin B has also been proposed as a potential screening test for ovarian reserve. Inhibin B is produced by ovarian granulosa cells predominantly during the follicular phase of the menstrual cycle. Inhibin B suppresses the production of FSH by the pituitary gland. The normal rise in circulating levels of FSH associated with menopause is thought to be secondary to the decrease in inhibin B production accompanying the age-related depletion of functional ovarian follicles. In fact, in the CCCT, the main mechanism by which FSH is normally suppressed is via inhibin B production by granulosa cells. Women with decreased ovarian reserve have a lower rise in the day-10 serum inhibin B levels in response to the CCCT. In addition, women who have clinical evidence of diminished ovarian reserve and normal day-3 FSH levels have been found to have decreased day-3 inhibin B levels. This observation suggests that a decrease in day-3 serum inhibin B levels may precede detectable changes in day-3 FSH levels. Although the degree of elevation in serum inhibin B levels 24 hours after administration of exogenous FSH appears to be positively predictive of good ovarian response, clinical application of serum inhibin B still requires further evaluation. In particular, basal inhibin B levels do not provide additional age-independent prognostic value for predicting pregnancy outcomes after ART. One possible reason for this is that levels of inhibin B may reflect granulosa cell function and thereby forecast only ovarian response in ART. While granulosa cell competence is certainly associated with oocyte quality, clinical application of serum inhibin B testing will also depend on whether levels are predictive of normal meiotic division of the oocyte, considering that fetal karyotype is an important determinant of pregnancy outcome.

Reference: Pages 991–993

6. C

One major cause of the increase in spontaneous losses among older women is their increased incidence of chromosomally abnormal fetuses. A cytogenetic analysis of 750 spontaneous abortions revealed that the increase in chromosomally abnormal conceptus seen with increased maternal age was mainly due to an increase in chromosomal trisomies. In particular, the incidence of trisomies 16, 21, 22, 18, and 20 were significantly increased, with 18 and 20 being the most dramatic. In contrast, the risks of monosomy X and polypoidy did not increase with advanced maternal age. In conclusion, an increased spontaneous loss rate, coupled with a reduced conception rate, significantly decreases the chance of a live birth among women older than 40 years.
Reference: Page 994

7. A

Documentation of the LH surge represents a remarkably reproducible method of predicting ovulation. Ovulation occurs 34 to 36 hours after the onset of the LH surge and approximately 10 to 12 hours after the LH peak. Commercially available kits for documenting the LH surge are generally accurate, quick, convenient, and relatively inexpensive with ELISA using 40 mIU/mL as the threshold for detection. The positive and negative predictive values of these kits have been described to be 90% and 96%, respectively. The finding of a 100% correlation between urinary LH prediction of ovulation and transvaginal ultrasound diagnosis of ovulation has further confirmed urine LH detection kits to be the best method for in-home ovulation detection. Still, there may be up to 5% to 10% of women for whom the ELISA test cannot detect urinary LH, probably either because of failed recognition by the antibody used or because their peak urinary LH concentration does not rise above the threshold set by the kit manufacturers. Serum LH measurements may be necessary to predict ovulation in such cases.
Reference: Page 994

8. C

There are several excellent reasons for recommending weight loss among overweight infertile patients. Using hypocaloric diets, weight loss of 20 kg (mean pretreatment weight, 77 kg) in one study and 10 kg (mean pretreatment BMI, 32 kg/m^2) in another study, has resulted in a decrease in plasma testosterone, androstenedione, LH, and fasting insulin levels. Significant improvement in these parameters, which are thought to function in the pathogenesis of PCOS, helps restore spontaneous ovulation in many patients. In a study of 67 overweight women who had a mean weight loss of 10.2 kg/m^2, spontaneous ovulation and pregnancy occurred in 90% and 30%, respectively. Obese patients are at increased risk for medical conditions such as diabetes, hypertension, and cardiovascular disease. Obesity is also a risk factor for obstetric complications: thus, it is in the interest to both the obstetrician-gynecologist and the infertility patient to reduce weight. As with any other lifestyle change, promotion of weight loss can be difficult and frustrating for both patient and practitioner. Weight loss often requires multidisciplinary efforts, including the involvement of an experienced dietician and promotion of an effective exercise program. Because many women may be discouraged by the time it takes to reduce their weight and the uncertainty of successful weight reduction, it is reasonable to pursue medical options in parallel with lifestyle changes.

Despite the high therapeutic success rates of *clomiphene citrate* in most anovulatory women, treatment has relatively low success in inducing ovulation in women with PCOS and insulin resistance in whom obesity or elevated BMI are also evident. Before initiating therapeutic changes in such women, the differential diagnoses should be reviewed and endocrinologic investigations repeated if necessary. *Dexamethasone,* 0.5 mg at bedtime, combined with typical clomiphene citrate regimens may induce ovulation in patients who have elevations in serum dehydroepiandrosterone sulfate (DHEAS). At this low dosage, *dexamethasone* therapy is associated with minimal adverse effects.

Alternatively, there is now increasing evidence that insulin sensitizers are particularly effective in inducing ovulation in women with PCOS with insulin resistance.

PCOS is currently viewed as a disease that can result from different genotypes with possible modification by environmental factors. In a subset of PCOS patients characterized by increased BMI, hyperinsulinemia, and significant hyperandrogenism, insulin resistance is thought to play a central role in the pathogenesis of their disease. *Metformin hydrochloride* and *troglitazone* are the best-studied of the insulin sensitizers used for ovulation induction.

Metformin hydrochloride is an oral biguanide that is approved by the U.S. Food and Drug Administration for the treatment of non–insulin-dependent diabetes. *Metformin hydrochloride* acts via several mechanisms, including inhibition of gluconeogenesis in the liver and an increase in the uptake of glucose in the periphery. When women with PCOS, hyperandrogenism, and hyperinsulinemia are treated with *metformin hydrochloride* for 12 weeks, their fasting insulin and total testosterone levels, free testosterone index, BMI, waist–hip ratio, hirsutism, and acne all decrease significantly. Moreover, among women who have PCOS, a BMI higher than 28 kg/m^2, and hyperandrogenemia, 89% will ovulate after treatment with a combination of *metformin hydrochloride* and clomiphene citrate. This rate is significantly higher than the 12% of patients who ovulated during combined treatment with placebo and clomiphene citrate. Similarly, *troglitazone,* an insulin sensitizer in the category of thiazolidinediones, has beneficial effects on plasma androgen and fasting insulin levels, and increases the rate of spontaneous ovulation in obese women with hyperandrogenemia and insulin resistance, even in the absence of weight loss. *Troglitazone,* however, has recently been withdrawn from the market, because it carries a 1 in 50,000 chance of fatal liver failure. In contrast, *metformin hydrochloride* has an excellent safety profile. Gastrointestinal complaints are its most common side effects, although isolated cases of fatal lactic acidosis have been reported in patients with underlying renal compromise.
Reference: Pages 996–1,000

9. **E**

In addition to the usual risks associated with laparoscopic surgery, laparoscopic ovarian diathermy involves the rare but potential risk of surgically induced premature ovarian menopause via inadvertent disruption of ovarian vascular supply. More common, however, is the possible formation of adnexal adhesions, which may further compromise fertility. One study reported that 19% of the patients who had a second-look laparoscopy procedure after laparoscopic ovarian diathermy had adhesions. In a series of 112 patients with PCOS, filmy adhesions confined to the ovarian surface were reported in 4 of 15 women who had not conceived at 1 year and who underwent second-look laparoscopy. At present, the impact of such postsurgical adhesion formation on subsequent fertility and defined indications for use of second-look laparoscopy in treated patients remains undetermined.
Reference: Pages 1,000–1,001

10. **C**

It is estimated that infection follows 1% to 3% of hysterosalpingography procedures and occurs almost exclusively in women with hydrosalpinges, or with current or prior pelvic infection. Therefore, known hydrosalpinges, current PID or cervicitis, and palpable adnexal masses or tenderness on bimanual examination all constitute contraindications to hysterosalpingography.
Reference: Pages 1,002–1,003

11. **E**

Approximately 0.2% of women who choose surgical tubal sterilization will request reversal procedures. The success of tubal reanastomosis is dependent on the method

of sterilization, the site of anastomosis, and the presence of other infertility factors. Pregnancy rates are lowest (49%) after the reversal of sterilization procedures involving unipolar electrocautery. In contrast, postprocedure pregnancy rates increase to 67% when the sterilization technique involved Fallope rings or spring-loaded clips and 75% when Pomeroy tubal ligation was used. The prognosis is best when anastomotic sites have no significant differences in tubal diameter (e.g., isthmic–isthmic or cornual–isthmic anastomosis). Tubal length is an important prognostic consideration: Final anastomosed tubal lengths of less than 4 cm are associated with low pregnancy rates. Pregnancy rates higher than 40% have been reported after microsurgical fimbriectomy correction. Laparoscopy to assess surgical prognostic factors—potential final tubal length, site of reanastomosis, method of sterilization (if not previously known), and presence of associated pelvic pathology—often is performed before microsurgical fallopian tubal reanastomosis by laparotomy.
Reference: Pages 1,005–1,006

12. C

For patients with infertility who have not undergone recent imaging tests, it is reasonable to begin their work-up with hysterosalpingography because it has an 85% to 100% sensitivity for detecting tubal pathology among infertility patients. However, hysterosalpingography has only a 44% and a 75% sensitivity in documenting uterine malformations and intrauterine adhesions, respectively.

Sonohysterography appears to be superior to hysterosalpingography in the detection of uterine malformations, correctly identifying 90% of abnormalities among infertile patients. These data are consistent with those observed in patients with abnormal uterine bleeding in the general gynecologic setting, where sonohysterography has sensitivity levels of 87% and 93% in detecting any intrauterine pathology and endometrial polyps, respectively. In women with abnormal bleeding, compared with conventional transvaginal ultrasound, sonohysterography has both higher sensitivity (93% vs. 65%) and specificity (94% vs. 76%) for the detection of endometrial polyps. Sonohysterography also decreases the false-positive and false-negative rates from 25% to 5.4% and 36% to 8%, respectively.

In most practices, diagnostic hysteroscopy remains the best method for the diagnosis of uterine pathology in patients with infertility. However, the ideal imaging test during an infertility workup is relatively noninvasive and has high sensitivity and specificity in the detection of uterine abnormalities as well as tubal blockage. The use of contrast media (i.e., *Echovist*) instead of saline during sonohysterography has been reported to have sensitivity comparable to that of hysterosalpingography and laparoscopic chromotubation in the detection of tubal blockage. This test has great potential for generalized use in infertility investigations but presently lacks prospective comparison to the combined use of hysterosalpingography and diagnostic hysteroscopy in women with infertility.
Reference: Pages 1,009–1,010

13. B

In a retrospective analysis, 131 women with more than 2 years of unexplained infertility were managed expectantly while awaiting IVF. Their pregnancy rate was only 0.9% per exposure cycle, whereas a similar group of 119 women receiving IVF treatment had a 17% pregnancy rate per cycle. The low spontaneous pregnancy rates in these patients promote the abandonment of expectant management and the rapid initiation of empiric therapies. These therapies are all aimed at increasing the chances of conception by increasing the available numbers and proximity of healthy gametes. More specifically, this typically involves superovulation (more female gametes); collection, washing, and concentrating the semen (more healthy sperm); and bypassing a potential cervical factor using intrauterine inseminations Superovulation with *clomiphene citrate* and intrauterine insemination is usually the initial treatment regimen. This combination is efficacious in many couples with unexplained infertility, and is less invasive, less expensive, and associated with fewer complications than other forms of treatment. However, if *clomiphene citrate* with IUI is unsuccessful after 3 months of treatment, COH using gonadotropins should be undertaken in conjunction with IUI (COH/IUI). If both of these approaches fail to result in pregnancy, IVF or ICSI can be performed.

The rationale for using *clomiphene citrate* to increase the fecundity rate in ovulatory women with unexplained infertility is that of superovulation. IUI has become a standard part of the *clomiphene citrate* regimen in treating these women. The degree of superovulation using *clomiphene citrate* is mild, and most commonly results in the release of two eggs in ovulatory women. This low degree of superovulation limits complications such as multiple gestations, but also limits efficacy. In fact, multiple pregnancy occurs in only 10% of patients treated with clomiphene citrate, and most of these are twin pregnancies. A recent metaanalysis of six randomized controlled trials showed that the use of *clomiphene citrate* in women with unexplained infertility to be superior to placebo in increasing the clinical pregnancy rates per patient (OR, 2.37; CI, 1.22–4.62) and per treatment cycle (OR, 2.5; CI, 1.35–4.62).
Reference: Pages 1,016–1,017

14. A

The National Cooperative Reproductive Medicine Network reported that the pregnancy rate is significantly higher in couples who were treated with COH/IUI (33%) than that in IUI alone (18%), COH/ICI (19%), or ICI alone (10%). However, the multiple pregnancy rates were concomitantly increased.

Pregnancy rates using IVF have been reported to be higher than those using COH/IUI in the treatment of unexplained infertility. However, the risks and costs associated with IVF treatment are appreciably higher, making it standard practice to treat these couples with COH/IUI before any IVF attempts. It has been recommended that patients with unexplained infertility experience no more than three to six COH/IUI cycles before therapy is discontinued or changed. One investigation recommended a maximum of three trials of COH/IUI based on the cycle fecundity and cumulative pregnancy rates observed in their prospective study with historical controls involving 594 patients with unexplained infertility. In that study, the investigators reported a mean fecundity rate per cycle of 16.4% and a cumulative pregnancy rate of 39.2% during the first three COH/IUI cycles. Cycles four to six yielded a mean fecundity rate of 5.6% and a cumulative pregnancy rate of 48.5%, a value only 9.3% higher than the rate achieved with three cycles. In contrast, a historical control group consisting of 131 patients who failed three cycles of COH/IUI had a cycle fecundity rate of 36.6% in their first attempt of IVF/ICSI treatment.

The fact that a significant proportion of these patients will exhibit complete failure of *in vitro* fertilization of oocytes suggests that some of the "unexplained" infertility patients who do poorly using COH/IUI actually have demonstrable defects in fertilization. The rates of complete failure of fertilization for conventional IVF have been reported to be 11.4% and 17.6% in two studies on couples with unexplained infertility. The overall pregnancy rate, however, is not increased with the use of ICSI as compared to IVF in patients with unexplained infertility in a prospective, randomized trial. Nevertheless, IVF treatment might be considered diagnostic in identifying those patients with fertilization defects. In short, due to their high risk of complete failure to fertilize in conventional IVF protocols, it is reasonable to offer combined IVF and ICSI on sibling oocytes within a single cycle for couples with unexplained infertility. This approach would prevent the tremendous disappointment and 0% chance of pregnancy faced by couples with total fertilization failure discovered in the first IVF cycle.
Reference: Pages 1,017–1,018

15. A

One of the advantages of using recombinant FSH is an improved batch-to-batch consistency, allowing a more consistent response to the same gonadotropin dosage.

An additional benefit of recombinant FSH is its subcutaneous route of administration, which is preferred over intramuscular injections by most patients.

The absence of LH in recombinant FSH preparations may minimize the amount of androgen production within the theca cells of the follicles, which presumably results in improved follicular quality. This property may be particularly desirable in the subset of PCOS patients who have an elevated LH: FSH ratio. A metaanalysis of prospective, randomized trials comparing purified FSH and HMG in the induction of ovulation among *clomiphene citrate*–resistant women with PCOS showed no differences in clinical pregnancy rates. However, a lower rate of moderate-to-severe ovarian hyperstimulation syndrome (OHSS) appeared to be associated with the use of purified FSH (OR, 0.2; 95% CI, 0.09–0.46). Therefore, both purified FSH and recombinant FSH may be especially beneficial in the ovulation induction of women with PCOS.

The relative efficacies of HMG, purified FSH, highly purified FSH, and recombinant FSH have been studied predominantly in ART cycles. One metaanalysis of randomized, controlled trials found that purified FSH or highly purified FSH was associated with significantly higher clinical pregnancy rates when compared with HMG use in IVF cycles not involving GnRH-agonist down-regulation. However, the same study found that there was no difference in clinical outcomes between the two types of gonadotropins in IVF protocols using GnRH-agonist down-regulation. Because GnRH-agonist down-regulation is not included in most COH/IUI cycles, FSH preparations may be particularly beneficial in these regimens.

Another metaanalysis on 12 randomized, controlled trials comparing urinary FSH (purified FSH and highly purified FSH) and recombinant FSH in ART cycles concluded that higher pregnancy rates resulted from recombinant FSH use (OR, 1.20; 95% CI, 1.02–1.42). There is no evidence to suggest a difference in clinical outcomes between the two available recombinant FSH preparations. Overall, recombinant FSH appears to be superior to other gonadotropin preparations and is preferred in COH cycles with or without ART. Nonetheless, there may be subsets of patients who respond better to HMG, perhaps because they need the LH component. Alternatively, the recombinant forms may not elicit optimal response in patients with particular FSH receptor variants. Therefore, if the ovarian response is poor with recombinant FSH, a trial of HMG should be considered. Reference: Pages 1,018–1,020

16. D

Patients with PCOS represent one of the most challenging subpopulations to treat safely and successfully using COH/IUI. The multiple small ovarian antral follicles characteristic of these patients may be very resistant to stimulation, but they are equally likely to respond and grow with minimal increases in gonadotropin dosage. The incidence of multiple pregnancy and ovarian hyperstimulation syndrome is increased in these patients. Up to 30% or more of COH cycles may be cancelled due to excessive follicular development. Several approaches that have been proposed to avoid complications of COH and cycle cancellation include down-regulation with gonadotropin releasing hormone agonists, dual suppression with oral contraceptives and GnRH-agonist, pretreatment with *metformin hydrochloride,* and surgical ovarian drilling. Reference: Page 1,022

17. A

More progress is being made toward reduction of higher-order multiple gestation in the area of ART. One approach would involve greater use of extended embryo culture, in which embryos are allowed to grow to the blastocyst stage *in vitro*. Blastocysts have been shown to have greater developmental potential and higher implantation rates than day-3 embryos, so that even if fewer (maximum, 1–2) blastocysts are transferred, pregnancy rates remain high. Another approach would follow the lead of countries outside the United States in which limits have been set on the maximum number of embryos transferred in a given ART cycle. The American Society of Reproductive Medicine has recently addressed this by publishing guidelines for embryo transfer during ART. A maximum of three, four, and five embryos can be transferred to women with above average prognosis (age, <35 years), average prognosis (age, 35–40 years), and below average prognosis (age, >40 years or multiple failed ART cycles), respectively. In donor oocyte cycles, the age of the donor (not the recipient) should be used to determine the number of embryos to be transferred. Data on the efficacy of this protocol are expected to be available in a few years. Meanwhile, more stringent guidelines have been advocated, promoting the transfer of a maximum of two embryos in ART cycles to minimize the risk of higher-order multiple gestation. Cryopreservation of excess embryos should certainly be encouraged further to promote more cycles involving transfer of cryopreserved embryos. Universal application of such changes will force patients and doctors to emphasize cumulative birth rates rather than pregnancy rate per cycle. By focusing on cumulative birth rates, patients can have more realistic expectations, and the demand to have an excessive number of embryos transferred would decrease. As discussed for non-ART COH, these changes will involve alterations in the entire financial reimbursement structure for ART service. There is no doubt that this approach will present many challenges.

On the scientific front, new technologies such as preimplantation genetic diagnosis may ultimately eliminate the risks of HOMG. Preimplantation genetic diagnosis is a clinical diagnostic procedure that can be performed on the embryo itself to determine whether a genetic abnormality is present before its transfer into the uterus. It has been developed in an effort to improve the chances for having healthy infants among families at high risk of genetic diseases. Preimplantation genetic diagnosis is most frequently performed using blastomere (a cell from a day-3 embryo containing 6–8 cells) biopsy, followed by genetic testing on the cell obtained. The technique chosen for diagnostic testing depends on the type of genetic defect being investigated. For example, fluorescence *in situ* hybridization (FISH) can be used to assess aneuploidy, translocation, and other chromosomal structural defects. FISH can also be used to exclude transmittal of X-linked diseases by identification of X and Y chromosomes, thus allowing transfer of female embryos only. Alternatively, familial single gene mutations can be identified by extracting blastomere DNA, followed by polymerase chain reaction, restriction enzyme digest or sequencing. In a recent study involving 262 ART cycles, the embryos obtained from women with poor prognosis (characterized by age >35 years, previous IVF failures, and karyotype defects) were randomized to preimplantation genetic diagnosis (PGD) for aneuploidy or a control procedure. Those chromosomes commonly involved in aneuploidies (X, Y, 13, 14, 15, 16, 18, 21, 22) were assessed using FISH in the study group. Although fewer embryos were transferred in the preimplantation genetic diagnosis group, higher clinical pregnancy rates (37% vs. 27%) and implantation rates (22.5% vs. 10.2%) were reported when compared with controls. Therefore, PGD may assist in the selection of euploidic embryos, relegating to this technique a tremendous potential to lower the risk of HOMG by decreasing the number of embryos transferred while maintaining pregnancy rates.
Reference: Pages 1,038–1,039

18. A

In recent years, it has been reported that only 20% of higher-order multiple gestation are the result of spontaneous conceptions. The remaining 80% are attributable to reproductive interventions; of theses multiple gestations half are attributable to ART and half to the use of ovulation drugs in non-ART cycles. Because the average age of women attempting pregnancy has risen over the past few decades, and increased maternal age affects the incidence of multiple gestation, rates of HOMG must be adjusted for maternal age when compared across time.
Reference: Page 1,039

19. E

Although transvaginal ultrasound-guided oocyte retrieval is both rapid and minimally invasive, all potential risks, albeit rare, should be clearly explained to the patient before IVF treatment begins. These include:

- Excessive bleeding, possibly requiring blood transfusion.
- Potential needle-induced injury to structures in proximity to the ovaries including bowel, bladder, and major blood vessels. Such injuries may require repair via emergency laparotomy, resulting in an abdominal surgical scar.
- Late infectious complications, such as abscesses in the peritoneum, bowel, ovary, or uterus. These infectious complications may require hospitalization for intravenous antibiotics or surgical interventions. In the specific case of iatrogenic tubo-ovarian abscess, failure of medical treatment may necessitate surgical removal of the tube(s) and ovary(ies).
- Risks associated with intravenous sedation or general anesthesia.
- A remote risk that no oocytes will be obtained or fertilized.

The incidence of ectopic pregnancy is 2% in the general population. However, its incidence is increased in IVF and can be as high as 4%. The main risk factors for ectopic pregnancy in IVF treatment are tubal factor infertility and, possibly, previous myomectomy. The incidence of heterotopic pregnancy, which is normally rare, is particularly high (1%) after IVF treatment. Multiple gestation and high hormonal levels during COH and early pregnancy have been suggested to be possible causes. It is important to have a high index of suspicion for the occurrence of heterotopic pregnancies, as only 40% to 84% of cases can be diagnosed on transvaginal ultrasound at the initial presentation. After treatment of the heterotopic gestation with laparoscopy, laparotomy,

Table 27.8. Protocols for Using Gonadotropin-Releasing Hormone (GnRH) Agonist with Gonadotropins in Controlled Ovarian Hyperstimulation

Protocol	Time of GnRH-α Start	Time of GnRH-α Discontinuation	Comments
Long (follicular downregulation) (389)	Follicular phase of previous cycle or earlier	Day of hCG injection	Theoretical benefit for patients at high risk for OHSS due to increased suppression
Long (luteal downregulation)	Luteal phase of previous cycle (day 21)	Day of hCG injection	Most common protocol (see text)
Short (flare)	Follicular phase of ART cycle (started concurrently with, or just before, gonadotropins)	Day of hCG injection	Flare effect is hypothesized to cause additional stimulatory effects on follicles Theoretical enhancement of ovarian response in poor responders
Ultrashort (390,391)	Day 2 of ART cycle	GnRH-α is given for 3 days only	
Discontinuous (542)	Luteal phase of previous cycle (day 21)	Start day of gonadotropin injection	Theoretically decreased suppression, which may be desired in poor responders
OCP/microdose (543,544)	Low-dose OCP started on day 1 of previous cycle *Leuprolide acetate* 40 μg SC b.i.d started in luteal phase of previous cycle or concurrently with gonadotropins	Day of hCG injection	Reported to enhance ovarian response in poor responders

or ultrasound-guided potassium chloride injection into the extrauterine pregnancy, the overall delivery rate for the intrauterine pregnancy is 66%.
Reference: Pages 1,028–1,029

20. B

Success rates for IVF vary from program to program; within a program, the rates of success vary with patients' diagnoses and ages. The most comprehensive assessment of the efficacy of North American ART programs comes from the database of the SART. The society's data collection began in 1985, and its annual summary is published in an effort to improve the quality of statistical reporting on ART. The database attempts to eliminate the effects of interprogram variation. The most recently published report of the society summarizes the results of ART in the United States and Canada for 1997 and is shown in Table 27.8. Information on SART and registered ART clinics are accessible by the public at *http://www.sart.org*. Significant improvements in the overall ART outcomes have been made when compared with the previously published results. In 1997, a 28.4% (16.8% in 1992) rate of delivered pregnancies was reported per oocyte retrieval for standard IVF, with a cancellation rate of 21.7% (15.4% in 1992), a pregnancy loss rate of 18.1% (20% in 1992), and an ectopic pregnancy rate of 0.9% (1.2% in 1992) per transfer. The delivered pregnancy rate for cryopreserved embryo

Table 27.9. Reported Outcomes for Assisted Reproductive Technology Procedures Performed in 1997 in the United States[a]

	Standard IVF	IVF Plus ICSI	GIFT	ZIFT	Donor Oocyte Transfer[c]	CPE Transfer	CPE Transfer with Donor Oocyte	Host Uterus Transfer
No. of cyles or procedures[b]	33,032	18,312	1,943	1,104	4,616	10,181	1,584	600
Cancellations (%)	21.7	NA	14.4	10.4	6.2	6.0	4.3	6.2
No. of retrievals	25,878	18,292	1,663	989	NA	NA	NA	563
No. of transfers	24,027	17,243	1,640	911	4,122	9,165	1,467	540
Transfers per retrieval (%)	92.8	94.3	98.6	92.1	NA	NA	NA	95.9
No. of clinical pregnancies	8,975	6,072	627	346	1,978	2,185	400	226
Pregnancy loss (%)	18.1	18.5	20.4	19.9	16.6	21.3	18.8	17.3
No. of deliveries	7,353	4,949	499	277	1,650	1,719	325	187
Deliveries per retrieval (%)	28.4	27.1	30.0	28.0	NA	NA	NA	33.2
Singelton (%)	59.6	62.9	66.9	66.4	56.5	74.4	65.8	83.3
No. of ectopic pregnancies (EP)	220	102	16	11	21	60	10	1
EP transfer (%)	0.9	0.6	1.0	1.2	0.5	0.7	0.7	0.2
Abnormal neonates (%)[e]	1.6	1.7	1.9	1.6	1.9	1.8	2.0	1.9

IVF, *in vitro* fertilization; ICSI, intracytoplasmic sperm injection; GIFT, gamete intrafallopian transfer; ZIFT, zygote intrafallopian transfer; CPE, cryopreserved embryo; NA, not applicable. See text for discussion.
[a] Except combination (n = 1,173), research (n = 40), embryo banking (n = 258), and other (n = 226) cycles.
[b] Includes all cycles regardless of maternal age and infertility diagnosis.
[c] Includes known or anonymous but not host uterus transfer or surrogate.
[d] Cryopreserved embryo transfer cycles not done in combination with fresh embryo transfer and not with donor egg or embryo.
[e] Reporting of structural and functional abnormality is problematic. See text for discussion.
From **Adamson D.** ASRM/SART registry 1997 results. *Fertil Steril* 2000;74:641–653, with permission.

transfer was 18.8% in 1997 (11.6% in 1992). Rates of birth defects were no higher among babies conceived using ART than in the general population.

The age of the woman was a significant determinant of success in ART (see Table 27.9). Women aged 41 years and above had a delivery rate per retrieval of only 9.4%. The increase in cancellation rates with age—most likely the result of poor ovarian response—was consistent with significantly decreased ovarian reserve in older women. With the high efficacy of ICSI as a treatment for male factor infertility, the delivery rates per retrieval among couples with male factor infertility are comparable with those achieved in couples without male factor for a given female age group.
Reference: Pages 1,032–1,033

28

Recurrent Pregnancy Loss

Joseph A. Hill
Bum Chae Choi

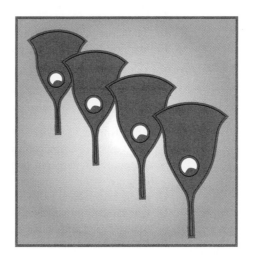

Learning Objectives

1. Be able to describe the potential mechanisms involved in recurrent spontaneous abortion.

2. Be able to differentiate the diagnostic tests and therapies that are potentially useful and effective in treating recurrent spontaneous abortion from those that are not.

3. Be aware of the prognosis for viable birth following documentation of early fetal cardiac activity, as a function of the number of prior pregnancy losses (up to four), and in relation to the potential causes of loss.

4. Develop a caring, empathetic attitude toward the couple experiencing reproductive failure to ameliorate the emotional distress these couples often encounter and to facilitate a rational, cost-effective assessment leading to appropriate consultation and, ultimately, to therapy.

Questions

1. Which of the following is not considered a cause of recurrent early spontaneous pregnancy loss?

    A. Structural chromosomal abnormalities in one or both of the parents
    B. Luteal phase insufficiency
    C. Incomplete intrauterine septum resorption
    D. Sexual intercourse during the first trimester of pregnancy
    E. Inappropriate maternal immune recognition of the implanting fetus

2. Which of the following statements concerning genetic causes of recurrent pregnancy loss is true?

    A. Robertsonian translocations typically involve reciprocal exchange of genetic material between chromosomes.
    B. The more spontaneous pregnancy losses a couple has experienced, the more likely they are to display parental chromosomal abnormalities.
    C. Some sperm have isolated chromosomal abnormalities.
    D. Unbalanced translocations are the most common structural chromosomal abnormality found among parents with genetic-factor recurrent pregnancy loss.
    E. Chromosomal monosomies are better tolerated than chromosomal trisomies.

3. Heritable thrombophilias have been associated with recurrent pregnancy loss. Which of the following should not lead to increased thrombosis?

    A. Genetic mutations in folate-metabolizing enzymes, including methylenetetrahydrofolate reductase (MTHFR)
    B. Genetic mutations in factor V resulting in resistance to activated protein C
    C. Deficiencies in antithrombin III
    D. Mutations in plasminogen that result in increased conversion to plasmin
    E. Heritable deficiencies in protein S

4. Congenital and acquired defects of the reproductive tract have been associated with recurrent spontaneous pregnancy loss. Which of the following factors should not be linked with pregnancy wastage?

    A. Incomplete uterine septum resorption
    B. Intrauterine exposure to diethylstilbesterol (DES)
    C. Transverse vaginal septum
    D. Severe Asherman's syndrome (intrauterine synechiae)
    E. Cervical incompetence

5. Which of the following does not characterize immune phenomena at the maternal–fetal interface?

    A. There is a large accumulation of natural killer–like cells at sites of implantation.
    B. Both T-cell receptor (TCR)-α and β and TCR-γ and δ cells populate the reproductive tract in early pregnancy.
    C. Major histocompatibility complex (MHC) class I molecules are detected on placental tissues.
    D. Hormonal regulation may alter the reactivity of immune cells at the maternal–fetal interface.
    E. MHC class II molecules are up-regulated in placental tissues.

6. Which of the following is useful in diagnosing antiphospholipid antibody syndrome (APAS) using the Sapporo criteria?

   A. A history of fetal death at 16 weeks of gestation
   B. A history of severe preeclampsia in a prior pregnancy leading to delivery at 36 weeks of gestation
   C. Positive identification of antiphosphatidlyserine antibodies in patient sera
   D. A history of a single false-positive test for syphilis
   E. Identification of serum antithyroid antibodies

7. Which of the following inquiries is potentially useful when obtaining a history from a couple with recurrent spontaneous pregnancy loss?

   A. History of uncomplicated pregnancy terminations
   B. The interval between diagnosis of prior fetal demise and pregnancy expulsion
   C. Paternal history of mumps orchitis
   D. History of infertility
   E. Amount of time spent at computer terminals

8. Which of the following tests does not need to be performed during the initial evaluation of a couple who have experienced recurrent early spontaneous pregnancy losses?

   A. Evaluation of the intrauterine cavity
   B. Bleeding time
   C. Maternal karyotyping
   D. Endometrial biopsy
   E. Paternal karyotyping

9. Evaluating the utility of potential testing and interventions among patients with recurrent pregnancy loss is hindered by all of the following **except**

   A. Placebo effects are not significant with most interventions.
   B. Most studies have been small.
   C. Most women with recurrent pregnancy loss will have a viable infant with their next pregnancy regardless of intervention.
   D. Our understanding of the cause of most recurrent pregnancy loss remains limited.
   E. Animal models for recurrent pregnancy loss are limited.

10. Therapies for genetic factor recurrent pregnancy loss includes all of the following **except**

   A. Use of donor gametes (oocytes and sperm or both)
   B. Use of *in vitro* fertilization and preimplantation diagnosis of single gene defects
   C. Genetic screening of sperm prior to use for fertilization
   D. Antithrombotic therapy for patients with inherited thrombophilias
   E. Use of *in vitro* fertilization, preimplantation blastocyst sex determination, and replacement of only female offspring for X-linked disorders

11. All of the following are presently utilized or under investigation for the treatment of women with endocrine factor recurrent pregnancy loss except

   A. Use of hormone replacement therapy involving estrogen receptor modulators among women with premature ovarian failure and recurrent pregnancy loss
   B. Use of insulin-sensitizing agents among some women with polycystic ovary syndrome (PCOS) and recurrent pregnancy loss
   C. Use of ovulation induction in women with PCOS and recurrent pregnancy loss

D. Use of tight glycemic control for women with overt type I diabetes mellitus and recurrent pregnancy loss

E. Use of thyroid hormone replacement among women with hypothyroidism and recurrent pregnancy loss

12. Which of the following therapies has proved to be safe and effective in the treatment of women with the antiphospholipid antibody syndrome (APAS) and recurrent pregnancy loss?

A. *Prednisone*

B. *Prednisone* and *aspirin*

C. *Aspirin* alone

D. *Heparin* and *aspirin*

E. None of the above

13. It is now thought that human leukocyte antigen (HLA) typing is not useful among patients with recurrent pregnancy loss from the general population because

A. Maternal immune cells do not recognize placental antigens

B. There are no HLA antigens expressed at the site of implantation so immune-mediated fetal rejection is impossible

C. HLA sharing is not associated with pregnancy wastage

D. Most couples share a significant portion of chromosome 6, which is the site of the HLA locus

E. None of the above

14. The use of progesterone as a means to regulate immune function at the maternal–fetal interface in women with recurrent pregnancy loss

A. Should be limited to women with unexplained recurrent pregnancy loss

B. Should be administered intravaginally

C. Is unlikely to modulate immune responsiveness

D. Does not require further study

E. None of the above

15. Which of the following has not been associated with the use of low-molecular weight heparins (LMWHs) when compared with the use of unfractionated heparins?

A. Less frequent dosing

B. Less frequent monitoring

C. Fewer side effects

D. Improved patient compliance

E. None of the above

Answers

1. D

Etiologies for recurrent pregnancy loss (recurrent pregnancy loss) can be subclassified, although the precise proportion of patients who belong to each classification varies among the population studied. Even after a thorough diagnostic workup, many couples with a history of recurrent pregnancy loss will have no identifiable etiology. Classification systems for recurrent pregnancy loss typically include the following categories: genetic, anatomic, endocrine, infectious, immunologic, and other miscellaneous factors. From a therapeutic standpoint, it may be of some use to add a new category—thrombotic factors—that would encompass some genetic (heritable thrombophilias) and some immunologic (APAS) factors.

Miscellaneous factors include environmental exposures, medications, and a variety of lifestyle factors. Although it has been hypothesized that coitus may be associated with recurrent pregnancy loss, in the absence of cervical incompetence there is no evidence that sexual intercourse during early pregnancy is in any way harmful.
Reference: Table 28.1; Pages 1,067–1,068

2. C

Genetic causes of recurrent pregnancy loss probably account for less than 5% of cases. They may be subdivided into parental structural chromosomal abnormalities, genetic mosaicism, single gene mutations, and multifactorial genetic disorders. The most common parental structural chromosomal disorder detected among couples with recurrent pregnancy loss is a balanced translocation (all chromosomal material is present, albeit rearranged to some extent). Translocations can be classified as either reciprocal or nonreciprocal, and Robertsonian translocations are one form of nonreciprocal translocation.

The only fetuses that survive with monosomy are those exhibiting monosomy of the X chromosome. Those with trisomy of chromosomes 13, 18, and 21 may live 1 or more years. Some patients with trisomy 21 may have nearly normal lifespans. In combination, these data seem to indicate that chromosomal trisomies are better tolerated than chromosomal monosomies. Genetic mosaicism may, however, be implicated. It has been reported that the greater the number of spontaneous pregnancy losses, the less likely a known etiology for recurrent pregnancy loss will be demonstrated. This is certainly true for parental chromosomal etiologies. Finally, advances in genetic screening have demonstrated that while most sperm in a single semen specimen may be genetically normal, isolated sperm may carry genetic abnormalities. Unfortunately, aneuploid sperm may be particularly motile.
Reference: Pages 1,068–1,069

3. D

The final steps in the pathways toward clot formation (thrombosis) are balanced by control mechanisms that either limit thrombosis or promote clot destruction. These limiting mechanisms include the actions of antithrombin III, protein C, and protein S. Antithrombin III inhibits the activity of factor IIa (thrombin), IXa, Xa, XIa, and XIIa. Proteins C and S limit the procoagulant actions of factors IXa and Xa. The conversion of prothrombin to thrombin involves factor Xa and factor V. Heritable genetic mutations in factor V (e.g., factor V Leiden) may inhibit antithrombotic interactions between protein C and factor V. For factor V Leiden, this is referred to as "activated protein C resistance," and it is associated with increased thrombotic potential. Deficiencies in protein S should have similar prothrombotic consequences.

The conversion of plasminogen to plasmin is catalyzed by tissue plasminogen activator. Plasmin antagonizes the prothrombotic effects of fibrin, so increased conversion of plasminogen to plasmin should limit clot formation.

MTHFR is an enzyme involved in folate metabolism and, indirectly, in homocysteine metabolism. Genetic mutations in MTHFR are associated with elevations in plasma homocysteine and with thrombosis.
Reference: Figs. 28.1–28.2; Pages 1,071–1,072

4. C

Anatomic anomalies of the reproductive tract may be either congenital or acquired. Congenital anomalies typically result from incomplete fusion of the müllerian ducts (duplication defects), or from incomplete resorption of the intervening uterine septum (resorption defects). Both duplication and resorption defects have been linked to fetal wastage, much of which occurs during the second trimester of pregnancy. Formation

Table 28.1. Proposed Etiologies for Recurrent Spontaneous Abortion

Etiology	Proposed Incidence (%)
Genetic Factors 1. Chromosomal 2. Single gene defects 3. Multifactorial	3.5–5

Anatomic Factors
 1. Congenital
    a. Incomplete müllerian fusion or septum resorption
    b. DES exposure
    c. Uterine artery anomalies
    d. Cervical incompetence
 2. Acquired
    a. Cervical incompetence
    b. Synechiae
    c. Leiomyomas
    d. Adenomyosis
	12–16

Endocrine Factors 1. Luteal-phase insufficiency 2. Polycystic ovarian syndrome, including insulin resistance and hyperandrogenism 3. Other androgen disorders 4. Diabetes mellitus 5. Thyroid disorders 6. Prolactin disorders	17–20
Infectious Factors 1. Bacteria 2. Viruses 3. Parasites 4. Zoonotic 5. Fungal	0.5–5

Immunologic Factors
 1. Cellular mechanisms
    a. Suppressor cell or factor deficiency
    b. Alterations in major histocompatibility antigen expression
    c. Alterations in cellular immune regulation
      i. T_H1 immune responses to reproductive antigens (embryo or trophoblast)
      ii. T_H2 cytokine or growth factor deficiency
      iii. Hormonal—progesterone and estrogen
      iv. Tryptophan metabolism
 2. Humoral Mechanisms
    a. Antiphospholipid antibodies
    b. Antithyroid antibodies
    c. Antisperm antibodies
    d. Antitrophoblast antibodies
    e. Blocking antibody deficiency
	20–50

Thrombotic Factors
 1. Heritable thrombophilias
    a. Single gene defects (*fVL, MTHFR,* factor deficiencies)
    b. Antibody-mediated thromboses (APAS, anti-β_2G1)
	Most are included among other categories (e.g., immune, genetic)

Other Factors
 1. Altered uterine receptivity (integrins, adhesion molecules)
 2. Environmental
    a. Toxins
    b. Illicit drugs
    c. Cigarettes and caffeine
	10

Table 28.1.—continued

3. Placental abnormalities (circumvallate, marginate)
4. Medical illnesses (cardiac, renal hematologic)
5. Male factors
6. Coitus
7. Exercise
8. Dyssynchronous fertilization

of the vagina results from fusion of the müllerian ducts (upper vagina) with the lower vagina, which arises from the vaginal plate. Defects in this process can result in a transverse vaginal septum, which would be associated with infertility, rather than recurrent pregnancy loss. *In utero* exposure to DES also results in a variety of anatomic defects of the reproductive tract. All have been linked to spontaneous pregnancy loss.

Acquired anomalies of the reproductive tract that have been associated with recurrent pregnancy loss include submucous leiomyomas (fibroids), intrauterine adhesions

Figure 28.1   Homocysteine metabolism. Dietary methionine is metabolized either to cystathione or back into methionine. Conversion of homocysteine to methionine requires transfer of a methyl group from methyltetrahydrofolate. The conversion of folate to methyltetrahydrofolate is a multistep process requiring vitamin B_{12} and a functional enzyme, MTHFR. Vitamin B_6 is also required for metabolism of sulfur-containing amino acids such as methionine.

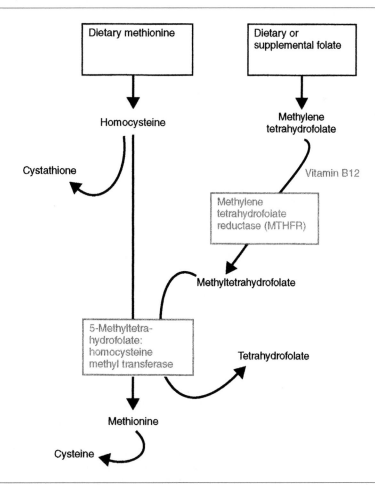

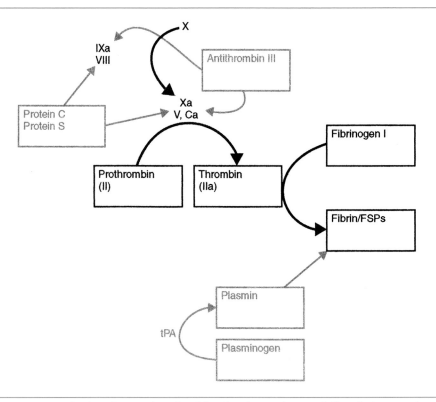

Figure 28.2 Final pathways involved in clot formation and dissolution. Pathways in black are part of the clotting cascade and are prothrombotic. Pathways in red limit or inhibit clot formation and aid in clot dissolution. FSP, fibrin split products; TPA, tissue plasminogen activator.

(Asherman's syndrome), and some forms of cervical incompetence. The latter often results in second trimester losses or preterm births.
Reference: Pages 1,069–1,072

5. E

The human reproductive tract has a variety of immune characteristics that distinguish it from other tissues. Resident immune cells within the reproductive tract, particularly within the endometrium at the site of implantation (decidua), include very distinctive cellular populations. For instance, large granular lymphocytes or decidual natural killer (NK) cells are abundant at the site of implantation. In fact, the presence of these cells within the decidua at the site of implantation represents the single largest accumulation of NK cells in human health or disease. The T cells of the reproductive tract differ from those of the peripheral immune compartment (e.g., spleen and peripheral blood) in that a significant proportion of these cells express the $\gamma\delta$ TCR rather than the $\alpha\beta$ TCR. TCR$\gamma\delta$ $^+$ cells also accumulate in the reproductive tract during early pregnancy.

Characteristics of antigen presentation at the maternal–fetal interface are also quite distinct from those in most other tissues. MHC class II molecules are not expressed in placental tissues in the physiologic state. The MHC class I antigens, HLA-A and -B, are also not expressed in the placenta. Rather, certain placental cells express an unusual combination of MHC class I products—HLA-C, -E, and -G.

Immune phenomena at the site of implantation may be regulated by the milieu in which the resident immune cells develop and act. This may include regulation by the cytokine and growth factor microenvironment, as well as by immunoreactive hormones such as estrogen, progesterone, and human chorionic gonadotropin. These potential hormonal

---

Table 28.2. Concepts in Reproductive Immunology

Cellular Immunity
1. Resident endometrial and decidual cells
   a. Few B cells
   b. TCR-$\alpha\beta^+$ and TCR-$\gamma\delta^+$ cells are present, TCR-$\gamma\delta^+$ cells increase in early pregnancy
   c. NK-like, large granular lymphocytes (decidual NK cells) accumulate at sites of implantation
   d. NKT cells and suppressor macrophage
2. Immune cell education and homing
   a. Thymic versus extrathymic education
   b. Possible *in situ* education and maintenance
   c. Integrins and vascular ligand pairs and mucosal homing
3. Antigen presentation
   a. Class II MHC molecules are not expressed in the placenta
   b. Classic class I MHC molecules HLA-A and HLA-B are not expressed in the placenta
   c. Extravillous cytotrophoblast cells express HLA-C, HLA-E, and HLA-G
4. *In situ* immunoregulation
   a. T_H1 and T_H2 cytokine microenvironments and dysregulation
   b. Hormonal immunomodulation
      i. Progesterone
      ii. Estrogen
      iii. Human chorionic gonadotropin (hCG)
      iv. Others
   c. Tryptophan metabolism and indolamine 2,3-dioxygenase (IDO)
   d. Leukemia-inhibiting factor (LIF)

Humoral Immunity
1. Fetal antigens are recognized by the maternal immune system, and humoral responses are mounted
2. Organ nonspecific autoantibodies
   a. Anticardiolipin antibodies
   b. Lupus anticoagulant
   c. Anti-β_2 glycoprotein 1 and (anti-β_2G) antibodies
   d. Antiphosphatidlyserine antibodies
3. Organ-specific autoantibodies
   a. Antithyroid antibodies
   b. Antisperm antibodies
   c. Antitrophoblast antibodies
      i. Blocking antibodies
      ii. HLA sharing
      iii. Trophoblast and lymphocyte cross-reactive antibodies (TLX)

TCR, T-cell receptor; NK, natural killer; MHC, major histocompatibility complex; HLA, human leukocyte antigen.

regulators may occur at particularly high concentrations at the level of the decidua during early pregnancy.

Reference: Table 28.2; Pages 1,074–1,076

6. A

A new set of criteria for diagnosing APAS was recently introduced during a workshop following the Eighth International Symposium on Antiphospholipid Antibodies held in Sapporo, Japan, in 1998. These criteria are quite specific and utilize a combination of clinical and laboratory criteria for APAS. Complications of pregnancy have been included as clinical diagnostic criteria. A history of three or more spontaneous pregnancy losses prior to 10 weeks of gestation or one or more fetal deaths at greater than 10 weeks of gestation are clinical criteria for the diagnosis of APAS. One or more preterm deliveries secondary to severe preeclampsia or placental insufficiency have also been included as criteria, but deliveries must be at 34 weeks of gestation or less. Laboratory criteria include only the presence of anticardiolipin antibodies or the lupus anticoagulant. The presence of antithyroid antibodies, while indicative of autoimmune disease and linked to recurrent pregnancy loss, is not helpful for the diagnosis of APAS. A false-positive test for syphilis may indicate the presence of anticardiolipin antibodies;

however, anticardiolipin antibodies must be documented on two occasions, 6 or more weeks apart, to meet the Sapporo criteria.
Reference: Pages 1,091–1,092

7. D

The history and physical examination are particularly important for couples with recurrent pregnancy loss. Knowledge of the causes of recurrent pregnancy loss continue to expand; attention should be more directed in our history taking and more specific in our physical examination of patients with recurrent losses.

Unless therapeutic pregnancy terminations have been complicated by excessive bleeding, postprocedure infection, performance at very late gestational ages, or forceful cervical dilatation (posing risk for cervical laceration), a history of therapeutic terminations is seldom useful in defining the cause of recurrent pregnancy loss. Excessive concentration on this history may only serve to bring undue guilt to an already stressful situation.

Interval from fetal demise to pregnancy expulsion is seldom helpful. This timing often varies with patient or practitioner desires and expectations, including plans for tissue karyotyping. A history of paternal mumps orchitis is predictive of poor semen quality and possible male-factor infertility, but has not been linked to recurrent pregnancy loss. Exposure to computer terminals has never been conclusively linked to recurrent pregnancy loss.

A history of subfertility or infertility is potentially useful. Some etiologic factors may be associated with both infertility and recurrent pregnancy loss. In addition, because many pregnancies are lost before or near the time of missed menses, a history of infertility may actually reflect a history of recurrent preclinical losses.
Reference: Table 28.3; Pages 1,084–1,085

8. B

Many laboratory tests have been suggested for use among couples experiencing recurrent pregnancy losses. A number of these have been shown to be useful in the initial evaluation of these couples. Other tests are still under investigation and still others have never been demonstrated to be of value. Parental karyotyping (both maternal and paternal) may be useful to rule out structural, heritable chromosomal disorders. An endometrial biopsy should be performed and repeated if the diagnosis of luteal phase insufficiency is suspected on initial biopsies. Evaluation of the intrauterine cavity with hysterosalpingography, sonohysterography, or office hysteroscopy is usually warranted. Evaluation for thrombotic disorders is typically limited to testing for anticardiolipin antibodies, the lupus anticoagulant, and an assessment of platelets using a peripheral blood count. Assessment of the bleeding time is not necessary during the initial evaluation of a couple with a history of recurrent pregnancy loss.
Reference: Table 28.3; Pages 1,085–1,087

9. A

Study of the causes and treatment of recurrent pregnancy loss has been voluminous but somewhat unfocused. The wide variety of potential causes for recurrent pregnancy loss, but the dearth of proven interventions demonstrates this lack of focus. A number of factors contribute to this discrepancy. Our understanding of the causes of recurrent pregnancy loss remains limited despite intensive study. This most definitely reflects the fact that many differing causes can result in the same outcome—spontaneous pregnancy loss.

There are no good generalizable animal models for recurrent pregnancy loss. We may, in fact, need to develop a variety of animal models for separate causes. Most studies have

---

Table 28.3. Investigative Measures Useful in the Evaluation of Recurrent Early Pregnancy Loss

---

History

1. Pattern, trimester and characteristics of prior pregnancy losses
2. History of subfertility or infertility
3. Menstrual history
4. Prior or current gynecologic or obstetric infections
5. Signs or symptoms of thyroid, prolactin, glucose tolerance, and hyperandrogenic disorders (including PCOS)
6. Personal or familial thrombotic history
7. Features associated with the antiphospholipid syndrome (thrombosis, false-positive test results for syphilis)
8. Other autoimmune disorders
9. Medications
10. Environmental exposures, illicit and common drug use (particularly caffeine, alcohol, cigarettes, and *in utero* DES exposure)
11. Genetic relationship between reproductive partners
12. Family history of recurrent spontaneous abortion, obstetric complications, or any syndrome associated with embryonic or fetal losses
13. Previous diagnostic tests and treatments

Physical Examination

1. General physical examination with particular attention to:
   a. Obesity
   b. Hirsuitism and acanthosis
   c. Thyroid examination
   d. Breast examination and galactorrhea
   e. Pelvic examination
      • Anatomy
      • Infection
      • Trauma
      • Estrogenization

Laboratory

1. Parental peripheral blood karyotype
2. Hysterosalpingography, followed by hysteroscopy or laparoscopy, if indicated
3. Luteal-phase endometrial biopsy
4. Thyroid-stimulating hormone level, serum prolactin level if indicated
5. Anticardiolipin antibody level
6. Lupus anticoagulant (activated partial thromboplastin time or Russell viper venom)
7. Complete blood count with platelets

---

involved small numbers of patients, have been retrospective, and have been improperly controlled. The fact that most patients with recurrent pregnancy loss will have a viable infant with their next pregnancy necessitates use of very large numbers of patients to ensure statistical significance. It also makes use of placebo treatments appear effective. In fact, placebo effects are often very similar to interventional outcomes.
Reference: Page 1,088

10. C

Therapies for genetic factor infertility may take a number of approaches. They may address the effects of the genetic abnormality. This is true for the antithrombotic therapies used in patients with inherited thrombophilias (e.g., hyperhomocystinemia secondary to mutations in folate-metabolizing enzymes). Other approaches aim to circumvent the transmission of genetic abnormalities by utilizing donor gametes that substitute for gametes from the affected parent. Donor gametes are particularly useful for carriers of genetic abnormalities that always result in embryonic aneuploidy. Finally, some approaches aim to identify genetically altered embryos and to select for uterine transfer only those embryos that will not create children who will be affected by a given heritable disease. Use of preimplantation genetic diagnosis allows the identification of some genetic diseases within a given embryo. Preimplantation genetic diagnosis typically involves genetic evaluation of a single cell obtained from a blastocyst derived using

in vitro fertilization (a blastomere from a blastocyst biopsy). If a single gene defect is identified, the affected embryo is not chosen for transfer to the uterus. For X-linked disorders in which only one parent is a carrier, blastomeres may be evaluated for sex chromosome status and only female embryos will be used. This would allow some offspring to be carriers, but none to be affected by the disease. Genetic testing on sperm has not been used despite the fact that semen specimens may have isolated genetic defects within specific sperm. In general, genetic testing of a particular sperm would negate its use for fertilization.
Reference: Page 1,089

11. A

Endocrine abnormalities with potential links to recurrent pregnancy loss include: luteal phase defects, hypothyroidism, PCOS and other hyperandrogenic or insulin-resistant states, diabetes mellitus, and hyperprolactinemia. Although many of the therapies for endocrine-factor recurrent pregnancy loss have not been evaluated in properly designed studies, their use is provocative. In an effort to create better quality embryos and possibly an improved luteal endometrium, women with PCOS and recurrent pregnancy loss have been treated using ovulation induction. Some have proposed that the addition of central hormonal down-regulation with ovulation induction might also be beneficial for these women. Those patients with PCOS, recurrent pregnancy loss, and known insulin resistance have been treated with insulin-sensitizing agents, often in a more directed effort to induce ovulation. It has been suggested that women with type I diabetes mellitus have very tight glycemic control before attempts at conception. This is true for those with and without a history of recurrent pregnancy loss. Women with recurrent pregnancy loss and hypothyroidism may benefit from thyroid hormone replacement. Although decreased ovarian reserve has been associated with poor pregnancy outcome, those women with true premature ovarian failure would present with infertility rather than recurrent pregnancy loss. Standard hormone replacement therapy has no utility in the treatment of recurrent pregnancy loss.
Reference: Page 1,090

12. D

APAS has been definitively linked to recurrent pregnancy loss and, in fact, complications of pregnancy are now considered defining criteria for APAS diagnosis. Proposed therapies for APAS-related pregnancy losses have addressed the resultant hyperthrombotic state, although some immunosuppressive approaches have been utilized as well. Leukocyte immunization has not been used successfully in the treatment of APAS, nor has use of aspirin alone. Combinations of *prednisone* and low-dose *aspirin* and of *heparin* and low-dose *aspirin* have each been demonstrated to effectively improve reproductive outcome among patients with APAS and recurrent pregnancy loss. The combination of prednisone and aspirin, however, is associated with maternal diabetes and hypertension, as well as with premature deliveries among treated women. Its use among women with APAS and recurrent pregnancy loss has been largely abandoned.
Reference: Pages 1,092–1,093

13. E

Human chromosome 6 contains the HLA region, an incredibly polymorphic segment of DNA that encodes for MHC molecules (MHC molecules classes I and II) and a variety of related proteins. It has been hypothesized that if the HLA regions were too similar among couples attempting pregnancy, pregnancy loss might result. Immunologic mechanisms for this hypothesis have been proposed. It has recently been demonstrated that complete sharing of the entire HLA region is indeed linked to recurrent pregnancy losses. However, the study that demonstrated this finding involved a very inbred population. The likelihood of complete HLA sharing among couples who are not members of this or similar populations is exceedingly rare. Because the HLA region is so polymorphic, most couples do not display significant HLA sharing. Therefore, HLA typing is not recommended for recurrent pregnancy loss couples in the general population.

Maternal immune cells recognize placental antigens and evidence of a response to these antigens has been documented. Placental cells (trophoblasts) do not express MHC class II antigens in the physiologic state, nor do they express the classical MHC class I antigens HLA-A and -B. These cells do, however, express a rather unusual subset of MHC class I products—HLA-C, -E, and -G.
Reference: Table 28.2; Pages 1,078–1,080

14. B

Progesterone has been called "nature's immunosuppressant," and therapeutic use of progesterone has been promoted for patients with immunologic factor recurrent pregnancy loss. It is known that progesterone acts as an immunomodulator. Its effects include alterations in T-cell effector function and proliferation and alterations in local T_H1/T_H2 cytokine profiles. It is known that circulating levels of progesterone are elevated during pregnancy. Local levels of *progesterone* at the maternal–fetal interface exceed those in the circulation. Vaginal progesterone supplementation during early pregnancy may recapitulate this physiologic state by delivering *progesterone* more closely (and in higher levels) to its proposed site of action. Higher levels of progesterone can be achieved in the uterus with vaginal suppositories than through other routes of administration.

The use of *progesterone* supplementation in women with immune-mediated recurrent or unexplained pregnancy loss has not been adequately studied. The necessary large, prospective, randomized trial is now being performed.
Reference: Pages 1,072–1,074

15. E

Antithrombotic therapy for women with APAS and recurrent pregnancy loss has been proven useful, with combination unfractionated *heparin* and *aspirin* demonstrably safer than combinations of *prednisone* and *aspirin*. Use of antithrombotic therapies is now being extended to include patients with heritable thrombophilias. The introduction of low-molecular-weight forms of heparin has brought with it a number of improvements over treatment with conventional, unfractionated *heparins*. *LMWHs* have been used in a variety of nonobstetric situations. Extension of their use to pregnancies complicated by thrombosis and to patients with hypercoagulable states and recurrent pregnancy loss is just now being investigated. Safety issues concerning use during pregnancy are being addressed.

LMWH has a number of potential advantages over its unfractionated counterparts, including less frequent dosing and the necessity for less frequent monitoring. Both of these factors improve patient compliance. *LMWHs* also appear to be associated with fewer side effects than unfractionated heparin, including bleeding complications, osteoporosis, and thrombocytopenia.
Reference: Pages 1,092–1,093

29

Menopause

William W. Hurd
Lawrence S. Amesse
John F. Randolph, Jr.

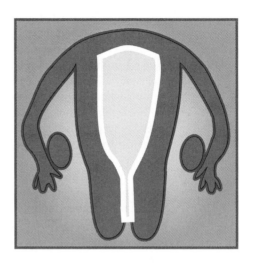

Learning Objectives

1. Understand the perimenopausal phases, including the most common presenting symptoms and health implications.

2. Be aware of the physiologic basis of the symptoms that occur in the perimenopausal period.

3. Understand the relative and absolute contraindications to estrogen replacement therapy.

4. Be aware of the common approaches to hormone replacement therapy.

Questions

1. The following statements are true about the perimenopause **except**

   A. During the period that immediately precedes menopause, hormonal changes may lead to menstrual irregularity and/or subtle signs of relative estrogen deficiency.
   B. The menopause usually occurs at approximately 51 years of age as a result of a genetically determined depletion of ovarian follicles that are able to respond to gonadotropins.
   C. The menopause occurs earlier in smokers, and women who have never had children.
   D. The loss of ovarian function results in absolute estrogen deficiency.
   E. Hormonal replacement therapy is one of the primary concerns of women's health after the menopause.

2. Which one of the following statements is true about perimenopausal symptoms?

   A. During the climacteric, the concerns that a woman has may be markedly different from the primarily medical concerns that gynecologists may have.
   B. Depression and irritability occurring in the perimenopausal period are usually related to low estrogen levels.
   C. Irregular, heavy, or prolonged uterine bleeding are common but of little medical concern in the perimenopause period.
   D. A decrease in libido is an extremely common symptom after surgical menopause.
   E. Skin changes seen during the perimenopause are solely related to age rather than to hypoestrogenemia.

3. The following statements are true about estrogen replacement therapy contraindications **except**

   A. In women with a history of breast cancer, estrogen replacement therapy should be used only with extreme caution.
   B. Estrogen replacement therapy should never be used in a patient with a history of endometrial cancer.
   C. Unopposed estrogen replacement therapy should be avoided in a patient who has undergone a hysterectomy for severe endometriosis.
   D. Estrogen replacement therapy is relatively safe in women with well-controlled hypertension.
   E. A history of thrombophlebitis is not a contraindication to estrogen replacement therapy.

4. Which one of the following statements is true about hormone replacement therapy?

   A. Oral estrogen is used only when the patient cannot tolerate the transdermal or vaginal route of administration.
   B. *Medroxyprogesterone* is by far superior to other available progestins.
   C. There are occasions when unopposed estrogen is appropriate in a woman with a uterus.
   D. Androgen therapy should be considered whenever hormone replacement therapy is prescribed.
   E. Continuous low-dose progestin therapy is associated with a significant risk of endometrial hyperplasia.

5. Which of the following is not a recommended therapy for the prevention or treatment of postmenopausal osteoporosis?

   A. *Calcium*
   B. *Alendronate*

    C. *Estrogen*
    D. *Fluoride*
    E. *Raloxifene*

6. Risk factors for postmenopausal osteoporosis include all of the following **except**

    A. Being black
    B. Family history
    C. Surgical menopause
    D. Low lifetime calcium intake
    E. Being elderly

7. Documented mechanisms by which estrogen may decrease the risk of cardiovascular disease include all **except**

    A. Increased high-density lipoprotein (HDL)
    B. Decreased low-density lipoprotein (LDL)
    C. Vasodilation of coronary vessels
    D. Antioxidant effect
    E. Decreased coagulability at high doses

8. The endometrium should be sampled in all the following scenarios **except**

    A. After 2 years of irregular, variable bleeding in a perimenopausal woman.
    B. When a vaginal ultrasound measures an endometrial "stripe" of 3 mm.
    C. With the onset of spotting 2 years after beginning continuous daily estrogen/progestin hormone replacement therapy (HRT).
    D. Before beginning estrogen/progestin HRT in women with a history of endometrial hyperplasia.
    E. Before a hysterectomy for persistent heavy bleeding on HRT.

9. Which of the following statements are true about the evaluation of postmenopausal bleeding?

    A. The goal of screening tests with postmenopausal bleeding is to achieve the absolute accuracy regardless of risk or expense.
    B. Vaginal ultrasound will never be considered an established first step in the evaluation of perimenopausal bleeding.
    C. In the postmenopausal women, saline injection is of no help for vaginal ultrasound.
    D. An endometrial stripe less than 5 mm thick is associated with an extremely low risk of endometrial cancer.
    E. Endometrial biopsy performed in the office is not as accurate as dilatation and curettage.

10. Which of the following questions about surgical treatment of abnormal perimenopausal bleeding is true?

    A. When endometrial polyps are determined to be the cause of abnormal uterine bleeding, curettage is rarely therapeutic.
    B. Little workup is required prior to hysterectomy, because removal of the uterus is the most common and effective surgical treatment for abnormal uterine bleeding.
    C. It should not be standard practice to remove the ovaries when postmenopausal women undergo hysterectomy.
    D. Endometrial ablation is a relatively new and potentially advantageous approach to dysfunctional uterine bleeding during the menopausal transition.
    E. There is no risk of uterine malignancy after any endometrial ablation.

Answers

1. D

A is true. The period that precedes menopause is characterized by a varying degree of somatic and psychological changes that reflect alterations in the normal cyclic functioning of the ovary. Early recognition of symptoms and the use of appropriate screening tests can minimize the impact of this potentially disruptive period.

B and **C** are true. The menopause occurs at a median age of approximately 51 years. The age of menopause appears to be determined genetically and does not seem to be affected by nutritional status. Menopause occurs earlier in cigarette smokers, in some women who have had hysterectomies, and in nulliparous women.

D is false. The loss of ovarian function does not result in an absolute estrogen deficiency. Because of peripheral conversion of androgens of both ovarian and adrenal origin, some women are less affected by estrogen deficiency than others.

E is true. Even though the long-term health impact of estrogen deficiency may be similar to that of thyroid or adrenal deficiencies, relatively little attention has been paid to this problem. This may be because the health problems associated with estrogen deficiency tend to be chronic rather than acute. For example, osteoporosis is usually not clinically apparent until decades after the menopause, when it is harder to treat. The impact of estrogen deficiency on cardiovascular disease is often confused with age-related changes.
Reference: Page 1,110

2. A

A is true. The loss of fertility and menstrual function that accompany natural and surgical menopause may have an impact on a woman's sense of well-being. The physician should be sensitive to the potentially significant emotional stress faced by these women and be prepared to offer psychological support.

B is false. Studies have failed to show a relationship between clinical depression and hormonal status, suggesting that many psychiatric symptoms that occur during this period may be more related to psychosocial events such as changes in relationships with children, marital status, and other life events. Many women report an increase in anxiety and irritability during the perimenopausal period; thus, these symptoms have become a prominent part of what is sometimes termed the "climacteric syndrome." It is commonly accepted by the lay public that anxiety and irritability are the result of estrogen deficiency. Despite this, multiple studies have found no evidence that most psychological symptoms experienced during the menopausal transition are related to estrogen deficiency or that they resolve with estrogen replacement therapy. The increased anxiety and irritability associated with the perimenopausal period is more clearly associated with psychosocial factors than with estrogen status. It is important to investigate and treat the hormonal status of women who complain of a constellation of symptoms that occur during the menopausal transition. Psychological intervention may be helpful in some women.

C is false. During the climacteric, it has been estimated that menstrual irregularity occurs in more that half of all women. In most cases, uterine bleeding is related to anovulatory cycles. However, pregnancy should also be considered in any menstruating women, because pregnancies are still reported in the late 40s. Of more concern is endometrial cancer, with an incidence of approximately 10% in women with abnormal uterine bleeding. This risk is increased at least fivefold in women with a history of unopposed estrogen use and decreased by more than two thirds in women taking a combination of estrogen and a progestin.

D is false. A major concern is a decrease in libido or a decrease in sexual satisfaction that may occur with natural or surgical menopause. However, sexual activity remains relatively stable in women before and after the menopause. Although only one half of menopausal women report being sexually active, this may be related to the relative decrease in the number of men in the aging population.

E is false. *Estrogen* therapy after menopause has been shown to maintain skin thickness. Although mechanisms underlying this effect are poorly understood, a major factor may be the ability of estrogen to both prevent and restore age-related loss of skin collagen. Because changes in collagen may be the major determinant in skin aging, these effects of estrogen may be important.
Reference: Pages 1,113–1,114

3. B

A is true. The limited data available suggest no increased risk of recurrent breast cancer among postmenopausal estrogen users. Until more long-term data are available, estrogen should be used with caution in women with a history of breast cancer. In a woman with nonmetastatic (node-negative) estrogen-receptor–positive breast cancer, particularly if she has a strong family history of osteoporosis and heart disease, the benefits of estrogen may outweigh the low theoretic risk that the hormone will predispose her to the development of recurrent cancer.

B is false. Although, theoretically, estrogen and progestin therapy should not increase the risk of recurrent endometrial cancer, there are few data regarding estrogen and progestin therapy in women who have been treated for endometrial cancer. Progestins have been used to treat recurrent endometrial cancer. One study of women successfully treated for a stage I endometrial cancer revealed that a combination of estrogen and progestin therapy does not increase the risk of recurrence. Because of the limited information available, any woman with a history of endometrial cancer should be informed of the unknown risk of recurrence with hormonal therapy.

C is true. There have been anecdotal reports of recurrent endometriosis or malignant transformation of endometriosis in women with endometriosis that take estrogen replacement therapy following bilateral oophorectomy. Therefore, these women should be treated with continuous estrogen and a progestin. In women with severe endometriosis, especially when bowel, bladder or ureter are involved, a hormone-free period for up to 6 months immediately after surgery may also be advisable prior to instituting combined estrogen and progestin therapy.

D is true. The doses of conjugated estrogens used for estrogen replacement therapy have little effect on blood pressure. Because chronic hypertension is a well-established risk factor for myocardial infractions and stroke, women with this disorder should be encouraged to maintain low blood pressure levels and to take advantage of the protective effect of estrogen replacement therapy for cardiovascular disease.

E is true. There appears to be no increased risk of thrombophlebitis associated with estrogen replacement therapy. However, no study has addressed the risk of recurrent thrombophlebitis of women taking estrogen. Therefore, women who have a history of thrombophlebitis should be offered estrogen therapy with the understanding that it is unlikely, but uncertain, that this therapy alters the risk of recurrent thrombophlebitis.
Reference: Pages 1,026–1,028

4. C

A is false. In general, oral estrogens are used as the first line of therapy in most women. Transdermal estradiol patches have also been found to be an effective method for hormone administration. However, there are several potential drawbacks to this approach. On a physiologic level, it is uncertain whether the same benefit is achieved in terms of reduction of cardiovascular disease risks, because changes in lipoprotein profiles do not occur as rapidly as with oral therapy. Transdermal patches are more expensive than oral preparations and result in some skin irritation at the site of placement in a third of the users. In women in whom oral estrogen therapy does not alleviate symptoms, is poorly tolerated, or in whom oral preparations create a problem with hypertriglyceridemia, estrogen patches may offer some advantage.

B is false. The most common progestin used is *medroxyprogesterone* given orally. However, many progestin formulations have been evaluated for the treatment of irregular bleeding and found to be effective. No single progestin is clearly superior to another. If a woman has significant side effects with one progestin dose, a lower dose or a different progestin formulation should be given.

C is true. Some women requiring estrogen replacement therapy experience intolerable side effects from progestin therapy. If no dose or formulation of progestin can be found that has acceptable side effects for an individual woman, unopposed estrogens may be given. A reasonable approach is the use of the lowest effective dose of estrogen daily coupled with yearly surveillance of the endometrium, because administration of unopposed estrogen is associated with an increased incidence of endometrial hyperplasia and cancer.

D is false. Studies of testosterone administration have shown mixed results in terms of libido improvement. One 6-month study of the oral preparation showed an adverse effect on the estrogen-induced changes in lipoproteins. Because of a lack of long-term studies of any of these agents, the effects on heart disease and other organ systems are unknown. Until large studies establish a benefit for this type of therapy, androgens should be prescribed with caution. For women who experience decreased sexual responsiveness, appropriate counseling appears to be the most effective therapy.

E is false. Because cyclic progestin therapy may result in symptoms such as breast tenderness, fluid retention, and edema, and psychological symptoms such as anxiety, irritability or depression, regimens utilizing lower doses of progestins given daily have been developed. Daily progestin therapy (2.5–5.0 mg *medroxyprogesterone acetate* or equivalent) protects against endometrium hyperplasia to that of cyclic administration at higher doses.
Reference: Fig. 29.2; Pages 1,129–1,130

5. D

A is true. Calcium can slow bone loss but does not increase bone mass, and adequate calcium intake of 1,200 mg daily is considered a mainstay of both prevention and treatment of osteoporosis.

B is true. In a randomized study, *alendronate* was given orally 5 to 20 mg/d for 3 years or 20 mg/d for 2 years followed by 5 mg/d for the third year, along with 500 mg/d of calcium. Compared with placebo, the rate of vertebral fracture was approximately one half: 3.2% for those receiving *alendronate* versus 6.2% for the placebo group.

C is true. In addition to estrogen, calcium, vitamin D, calcitonin, and bisphosphanates, especially *etidronate* and *alendronate,* have been used for the treatment of postmenopausal osteoporosis.

D is false. Fluoride is the only known agent that can stimulate bone formation and substantially increase bone density, but the bone formed is actually more fracture-prone and fluoride is not recommended therapy.

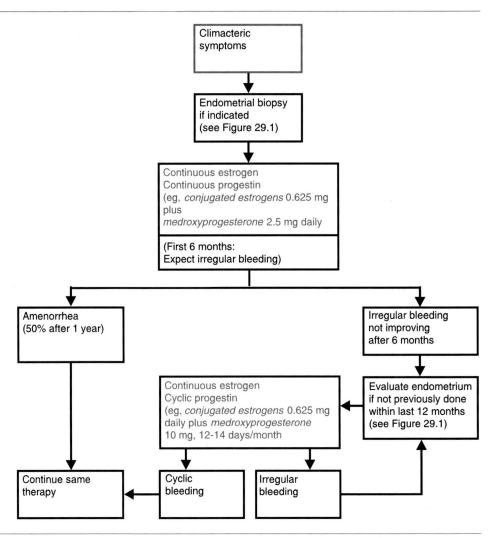

Figure 29.2   Administration of hormone replacement therapy.

E is true. Raloxifene appears to slow bone loss about half as well as conventional HRT (), but may be comparable in reducing fracture risk.
Reference: Pages 1,130–1,133

6. A

A is incorrect. On average, black women have a higher bone mass than white women, and this may explain the low risk of osteoporosis-related bone fractures observed in blacks.

B is correct. A family history of osteoporosis is a strong risk factor.

C is correct. Depending on the age at surgery, surgical menopause poses a higher risk than natural menopause because of the longer period with low estrogen.

D is correct. Dietary calcium, primarily in the form of dairy products, has been shown to be associated with decreased bone loss in premenopausal women.

E is correct. Age is the most important factor associated with bone loss. All women begin losing bone mass in their early thirties, and this loss continues throughout their lives.
Reference: Pages 1,122–1,123

7. E

    A and **B** are true. Estrogen decreases circulating levels of LDLs and increases HDLs. Both the absolute decrease in total cholesterol and the increase in the HDL/LDL ratio appear to retard progression of coronary artery disease. Although these effects are attenuated by concomitant progestin use, this effect appears to decrease over time.

    C is true. A third beneficial effect is that of vasodilation. There appears to be a direct effect on blood vessel endothelial cells that results in immediate vasodilatation, perhaps mediated by estrogen receptors.

    D is true. Estrogen appears to be an antioxidant that decreases the formation of lipid peroxidases, which may decrease arteriosclerosis by minimizing the oxidation of LDL cholesterol, a potent inducer of plaque formation in vessels.

    F is false. A final effect of estrogen is on coagulation. Low doses of estrogen (i.e., 0.625 mg daily of conjugated estrogens) result in a subclinical decrease in coagulability by decreasing platelet aggregation and fibrinogen and by inhibiting plasminogen formation. This effect appears to be lost with higher doses of estrogen (i.e., 1.2 mg of conjugated estrogens). At even higher doses, equivalent to those used in oral contraceptives, there is an increase in coagulability.
Reference: Pages 1,124–1,125

8. B

    A is true. Malignant precursors such as complex endometrial hyperplasia become more common during the menopausal transition. Because early diagnosis is the most effective way to improve a woman's prognosis, perimenopausal women with abnormal uterine bleeding should undergo an endometrial biopsy to exclude a malignant condition.

    B is false. Preliminary studies indicate that if the endometrial stripe is less than 5 mm thick, the risk of endometrial hyperplasia or cancer is extremely small. A thickened endometrial lining or an obvious intrauterine lesion is an indication for more thorough evaluation.

    C is true. It is reasonable to consider a baseline endometrial biopsy for anyone on this protocol who has irregular bleeding.

    D is true. Malignant precursors such as complex endometrial hyperplasia become more common during the menopausal transition. Because early diagnosis is the most effective way to improve a woman's prognosis, perimenopausal women with abnormal uterine bleeding should undergo an endometrial biopsy to exclude a malignant condition.

    D is true. Before recommending hysterectomy, an adequate preoperative evaluation must include endometrial sampling and an adequate trial of hormonal therapy to control the bleeding.
Reference: Pages 1,115–1,116

9. D

    A is false. The goal of evaluation of abnormal uterine bleeding is to achieve the greatest accuracy with the least risk and expense for the patient. In the past, when few diagnostic options were available, this situation was routinely approached with in-patient uterine curettage. However, with the development of less invasive office procedures and more accurate outpatient surgical approaches, uterine curettage without hysteroscopy is seldom part of the standard approach.

    B is false. With the advent of newer diagnostic modalities, vaginal ultrasound has become an established first step in the evaluation of perimenopausal bleeding. In the premenopausal women, vaginal ultrasound is extremely useful for identifying leiomyomata and endometrial asymmetry suggestive of endometrial polyps.

C is false. In the postmenopausal women, vaginal ultrasound with saline injection (sono-hysterography) is helpful for accurately visualizing polyps and other focal intrauterine lesions. A thickened or asymmetric endometrial lining or an obvious intrauterine lesion is an indication for hysteroscopy and curettage.

D is true. In the postmenopausal women, an endometrial stripe less than 5 mm thick by vaginal ultrasound has been shown to be associated with an extremely low risk of endometrial hyperplasia or cancer.

E is false. It is well accepted that endometrial biopsy performed in the office is just as accurate as dilatation and curettage, and certainly more economical. Dilatation and curettage in the operating room should be reserved for patients with abnormal endometrial biopsies or for conditions that preclude performing an office biopsy, such as cervical stenosis.
Reference: Pages 1,115–1,116

10. D

A is false. Removal of endometrial polyps by curettage is often both therapeutic and diagnostic. Because polyps can be missed by curettage alone, it has been recommended that diagnostic hysteroscopy be performed before uterine curettage for abnormal uterine bleeding. Unfortunately, with the exception of endometrial polyps, uterine curettage has not been shown to have any long-term benefit in the treatment of abnormal uterine bleeding.

B is false. Although removal of the uterus is the most common and effective surgical treatment for abnormal uterine bleeding, hysterectomy is associated with a certain degree of morbidity and cost, and therefore should be preceded in every case by a careful preoperative evaluation for treatable causes of bleeding.

C is false. It is appropriate to remove the ovaries in postmenopausal women undergoing hysterectomy to avoid the subsequent risk of ovarian cancer, which remains difficult to diagnose in a timely manner.

D is correct. Endometrial ablation is a relatively new and potentially advantageous approach to dysfunctional uterine bleeding during the menopausal transition since it is a relatively minor surgical procedure which involves destroying the functioning endometrium. However, the long-term efficacy of this approach remains unproven.

E is false. The risk of uterine malignancy after endometrial ablation remains uncertain. The concern is that glandular tissue buried under scar tissue could develop into a malignancy, but might not result in uterine bleeding, thus delaying the diagnosis.
Reference: Pages 1,117–1,118

GYNECOLOGIC ONCOLOGY

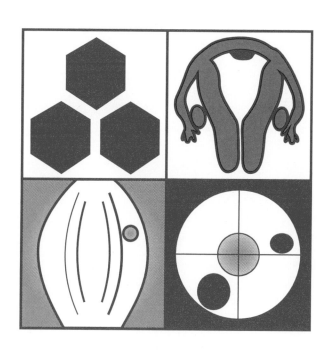

30

Uterine Cancer

John R. Lurain

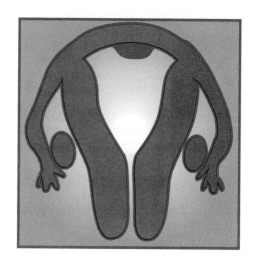

Learning Objectives

1. Understand the epidemiology, risk factors, screening principles, and methods for diagnosis of uterine cancers.

2. Know the different types of endometrial hyperplasias, cancers, and sarcomas, and their natural history.

3. Learn the International Federation of Gynecology and Obstetrics (FIGO) surgical staging system for endometrial cancers and be able to identify important prognostic factors.

4. Develop a logical plan for the surgical and postoperative management of endometrial cancers and sarcomas.

Questions

1. "Estrogen-independent" endometrial cancers are associated with all but which of the following:

   A. Older age
   B. Thin body habitus
   C. Tamoxifen use
   D. Asian race
   E. Atrophic endometrium

2. Risk factors for endometrial cancer include all of the following **except**

   A. Obesity
   B. Diabetes mellitus
   C. Unopposed estrogen therapy
   D. Hypertension
   E. Nulliparity

3. A 32-year-old woman presents with irregular menses and infertility. An endometrial biopsy shows complex hyperplasia with minimal cytologic atypia. The most appropriate therapy for this patient would be

   A. Observation
   B. Ovulation induction
   C. Cyclic estrogen-progestin therapy
   D. Continuous progestin therapy
   E. Hysterectomy

4. What percentage of women with postmenopausal uterine bleeding will have endometrial cancer?

   A. 2%
   B. 10%
   C. 25%
   D. 60%

5. A 62-year-old woman on continuous combined hormone replacement therapy presents with a two-week history of irregular vaginal bleeding. The most appropriate first step in management would be

   A. Change her hormone therapy to cyclic estrogen-progestin
   B. Endometrial aspiration biopsy
   C. Hysteroscopy, dilation and curettage (D & C)
   D. Transvaginal ultrasound
   E. Pap test

6. Variants of endometrioid adenocarcinoma of the endometrium include each of the following **except**

   A. Adenosquamous
   B. Papillary villoglandular
   C. Secretory
   D. Clear cell

7. In addition to a complete history and physical examination, routine pretreatment evaluation of a patient with endometrial cancer should include which one of the following tests:

   A. Serum cancer antigen 125 (CA125)
   B. Chest x-ray

C. Intravenous pyelogram

D. Colonoscopy

E. Computed tomography (CT) scan of the abdomen and pelvis

8. A 72-year-old woman is found to have a well-differentiated endometrial adenocarcinoma on endometrial biopsy done to evaluate postmenopausal bleeding. Physical examination reveals a normal-sized uterus, which sounds to 7 cm. Findings on chest x-ray are within normal limits. The patient should undergo surgery with at least each of following procedures **except**

    A. Peritoneal cytology

    B. Biopsy of any suspicious intraperitoneal lesion

    C. Resection of any enlarged pelvic or paraaortic lymph nodes

    D. Omental biopsy

    E. Extrafascial hysterectomy

9. Abdominal exploration on the above patient was negative. Surgical pathology revealed a moderately differentiated endometrioid adenocarcinoma with one-third myometrial invasion and extension into the lower uterine segment and endocervical mucosa; peritoneal cytology and adnexa were negative for malignancy. According to the 1988 FIGO staging system, the patient's endometrial cancer is classified as stage

    A. IaG1

    B. IbG2

    C. IIaG2

    D. IIIaG2

    E. IIIbG2

10. The incidence of lymph node metastasis in clinical stage I endometrial cancer is approximately

    A. 1%

    B. 5%

    C. 10%

    D. 20%

11. Prognostic variables having an adverse effect on endometrial cancer survival include all of the following **except**

    A. Young age

    B. Grade 3 tumor

    C. Deep myometrial invasion

    D. Lymph–vascular space invasion (LVSI)

    E. Extrauterine disease spread

12. The most commonly used postoperative treatment plan for a patient with stage IbG2 endometrial cancer is

    A. Careful follow-up

    B. Vaginal vault irradiation

    C. External pelvic irradiation

    D. Whole abdominal irradiation

    E. Progestins

13. A 58-year-old woman undergoes exploratory laparotomy with peritoneal washings, total abdominal hysterectomy, bilateral salpingo-oophorectomy, and selective pelvic and paraaortic lymphadenectomies for grade 2 endometrial adenocarcinoma. She is found to have a grade 3 endometrioid tumor with deep ($>\frac{1}{2}$) myometrial invasion and LVSI

but no evidence of disease spread outside the uterus including negative lymph nodes and negative peritoneal cytology. She subsequently receives pelvic and vaginal vault irradiation. Five-year survival for her surgical stage of disease (IcG3) is approximately

A. 90% to 95%
B. 75% to 80%
C. 65% to 70%
D. 40% to 50%

14. At the time of cesarean delivery, a 32-year-old woman is found to have nodules scattered throughout the peritoneal cavity. The most likely diagnosis is

A. Intravenous leiomyomatosis
B. Benign metastasizing leiomyoma
C. Disseminated peritoneal leiomyomatosis
D. Leiomyoblastoma

15. Low-grade endometrial stromal sarcoma or endolymphatic stromal myosis differs from high-grade or undifferentiated endometrial stromal sarcoma by each of the following **except**

A. Lower mitotic rate
B. Rarely extends beyond the uterus
C. Responds to progestin therapy
D. Better prognosis

Answers

1. C

There appear to be two different pathogenetic types of endometrial cancer. The most common type occurs in younger, perimenopausal women with a history of exposure to unopposed estrogen, either endogenous or exogenous. In these women, tumors begin as hyperplastic endometrium and progress to carcinoma. These "estrogen-dependent" tumors tend to be better differentiated and have a more favorable prognosis then tumors that are not associated with hyperestrogenism. The other type of endometrial carcinoma occurs in women with no source of estrogen stimulation of the endometrium. These spontaneously occurring cancers are not associated pathologically with endometrial hyperplasia, but may arise in a background of atrophic endometrium. They are less differentiated and associated with a poorer prognosis than estrogen-dependent tumors. These "estrogen-independent" tumors tend to occur in older, postmenopausal, thin women and are present disproportionately in black and Asian women.
Reference: Pages 1,143–1,144

2. D

Several risk factors for the development of endometrial cancer have been identified (see Table 30.1). Most of these risk factors are related to prolonged, unopposed estrogen stimulation of the endometrium. The risk of endometrial cancer is increased 3 times for women who are 21 to 50 lb overweight and 10 times for those more than 50 lb overweight (excess estrone as a result of peripheral conversion of adrenally derived androstenedione by aromatization in fat). Nulliparous women have 2 to 3 times the risk of parous women. Menopausal estrogen replacement therapy without progestins increases the risk of endometrial cancer 4 to 8 times. This risk is greater with higher doses and more prolonged use and can be reduced to essentially baseline levels by the addition of progestin.

Diabetes mellitus increases a women's risk of endometrial cancer by 1.3 to 2.8 times. Other medical conditions such as hypertension and hypothyroidism have been

Table 30.1. Risk Factors for Endometrial Cancer

Characteristic	*Relative Risk*
Nulliparity	2–3
Late menopause	2.4
Obesity	
21–50 lb overweight	3
>50 lb overweight	10
Diabetes mellitus	2.8
Unopposed estrogen therapy	4–8
Tamoxifen therapy	2–3
Atypical endometrial hyperplasia	8–29

associated with endometrial cancer, but a causal relationship has not been confirmed. Other factors leading to long-term estrogen exposure, such as anovulatory menstrual cycles, late menopause, polycystic ovary syndrome, and functioning ovarian tumors, are also associated with an increased risk of endometrial cancer.
Reference: Pages 1,144–1,145

3. **D**

Endometrial hyperplasias usually evolve within a background of proliferative endometrium as a result of protracted estrogen stimulation in the absence of progestin influence. Endometrial hyperplasias are important clinically because they may precede or occur simultaneously with endometrial cancer. The risk of endometrial hyperplasia progressing to carcinoma occurs in 1% of patients with simple hyperplasia, 3% of patients with complex hyperplasia, 8% of patients with atypical simple hyperplasia, and 29% of patients with atypical complex hyperplasia (see Table 30.2). Therefore, observation would not be appropriate.

For women with endometrial hyperplasia without atypia, ovulation induction, cyclic progestin therapy, or continuous progestin therapy all seem to be effective therapies. Continuous progestin therapy with megestrol acetate 40 mg daily is probably the most reliable treatment for reversing complex or atypical hyperplasia. Therapy should be continued for 2 to 3 months, and endometrial biopsy should be performed 3 to 4 weeks after completion of therapy to assess response. Approximately 25% of patients with atypical complex hyperplasia detected on endometrial biopsy or curettage will already have an associated well-differentiated endometrial carcinoma. Therefore, hysterectomy is advised for patients with complex hyperplasia with significant cytologic atypia, a high mitotic rate, and marked cellular stratification.
Reference: Pages 1,144–1,147

4. **B**

Possible causes of postmenopausal uterine bleeding include endometrial atrophy, endometrial polyps, estrogen replacement therapy, hyperplasia, and cancer (see Table 30.3). Endometrial atrophy is the most common endometrial finding in women with postmenopausal bleeding, accounting for 60% to 80% of such bleeding. Women with

Table 30.2. Classification of Endometrial Hyperplasias

Type of Hyperplasia	*Progression to Cancer (%)*
Simple (cystic without atypia)	1
Complex (adenomatous without atypia)	3
Atypical	
Simple (cystic with atypia)	8
Complex (adenomatous with atypia)	29

From **Kurman RJ, Kaminski PF, Norris HJ.** The behavior of endometrial hyperplasia: a long term study of "untreated" hyperplasia in 170 patients. *Cancer* 1985;56:403–412, with permission.

Table 30.3. Causes of Postmenopausal Uterine Bleeding	
Cause of Bleeding Frequency	*Percentage*
Endometrial atrophy	60–80
Estrogen replacement therapy	15–25
Endometrial polyps	2–12
Endometrial hyperplasia	5–10
Endometrial cancer	10

endometrial atrophy have usually been menopausal for about 10 years, endometrial biopsy often yields insufficient tissue or only blood and mucous, and there is usually no additional bleeding after biopsy. Endometrial polyps account for 2% to 12% of postmenopausal bleeding. Polyps are often difficult to identify with office endometrial biopsy or curettage. Hysteroscopy, transvaginal ultrasonography, or both may be useful adjuncts in identifying endometrial polyps. Unrecognized and untreated polyps may be a source of continued or recurrent bleeding. Estrogen therapy is an established risk factor for endometrial hyperplasia and cancer, and it may be responsible for 15% to 25% of all causes of postmenopausal uterine bleeding. Endometrial biopsy should be performed to assess unscheduled bleeding or annually in women not taking a progestin. Endometrial hyperplasia occurs in 5% to 10% of women with postmenopausal uterine bleeding. Approximately 10% of women with postmenopausal bleeding have endometrial cancer.
Reference: Pages 1,147–1,148

5. B

Postmenopausal estrogen therapy is an established risk factor for endometrial hyperplasia and cancer. Endometrial assessment should be performed in any woman on hormone replacement therapy with nonscheduled bleeding. Office endometrial aspiration biopsy is the accepted first step in evaluating a patient with abnormal uterine bleeding. The diagnostic accuracy of office based endometrial biopsy is 90% to 98% when compared to subsequent findings at D & C or hysterectomy. Hysteroscopy and D & C should be reserved for situations in which cervical stenosis or patient tolerance does not permit adequate evaluation by aspiration biopsy, bleeding recurs after a negative endometrial biopsy, or the specimen obtained is inadequate to explain the abnormal bleeding. Transvaginal ultrasound may be a useful adjunct to endometrial biopsy for evaluating abnormal uterine bleeding and selecting patients for additional testing. The findings of an endometrial thickness greater than 4 mm, a polypoid endometrial mass, or a collection of fluid within the uterus requires further evaluation. More data are needed before the ultrasound finding of an endometrial thickness less than 5 mm eliminates the need for endometrial biopsy in a symptomatic patient. A Pap test is an unreliable diagnostic test—only 30% to 50% of patients with endometrial cancer will have abnormal Pap test results.
Reference: Pages 1,147–1,148

6. D

Endometrioid-type adenocarcinomas account for approximately 80% of endometrial carcinomas (see Table 30.4). The clinical behavior of these tumors is generally related to their differentiation expressed as grade, which is determined by architectural growth pattern and nuclear features. Approximately 15% to 25% of endometrioid carcinomas have areas of squamous differentiation. The behavior of these adenosquamous tumors is largely dependent on the grade of the glandular component. A villoglandular configuration is present in approximately 2% of endometrioid carcinomas. These are always well-differentiated lesions that behave like the regular endometrioid carcinomas and should be distinguished from papillary serous carcinomas. Secretory carcinomas are rare variants of endometrioid carcinoma that account for about 1% of cases. Generally, they occur in early postmenopausal women and have an excellent prognosis.

Table 30.4. Classification of Endometrial Carcinomas

Endometrioid adenocarcinoma
  Usual type
  Variants
    Villoglandular or papillary
    Secretory
    With squamous differentiation

Mucinous carcinoma

Papillary serous carcinoma

Clear cell carcinoma

Squamous carcinoma

Undifferentiated carcinoma

Mixed carcinoma

The tumors are composed of well-differentiated glands with intracytoplasmic vacuoles similar to early secretory endometrium, and, therefore, must be distinguished from the very aggressive clear cell carcinomas, which also have predominantly clear cells.
Reference: Pages 1,149–1,151

7. **B**

After establishing the diagnosis of endometrial cancer, a complete history and physical examination is of utmost importance to determine the best and safest approach to management of the disease. Patients with endometrial carcinoma are often elderly and obese and have a variety of medical problems, such as diabetes mellitus and hypertension, which affect surgical management. Any abnormal symptoms should be evaluated and attention directed to enlarged or suspicious-feeling lymph nodes, abdominal masses, and possible areas of cancer spread within the pelvis on physical examination.

Routine preoperative studies should include electrocardiogram, complete blood and platelet counts, serum chemistries (including renal and liver function tests), blood type and screen, and urinalysis. A chest x-ray should be performed to rule out pulmonary metastasis and to evaluate the cardiorespiratory status of the patient. Other preoperative or staging studies are neither required nor necessary for most patients with endometrial cancer. Studies such as cystoscopy, colonoscopy, intravenous pyelography, barium enema, and CT scanning of the abdomen and pelvis are not indicated unless dictated by patient symptoms, physical findings, or other laboratory tests. Serum CA125 level is elevated in most patients with advanced or metastatic endometrial cancer and may be useful as a tumor marker in assessing response to therapy, but is rarely helpful in the preoperative management of patients with apparently localized disease.
Reference: Page 1,155

8. **D**

Most patients with endometrial cancer should undergo surgical staging (see Fig. 30.7). At a minimum, the surgical procedure should include sampling of peritoneal fluid for cytologic evaluation, exploration of the abdomen and pelvis with biopsy or excision of any extrauterine lesions suggestive of metastatic cancer, extrafascial hysterectomy, and bilateral salpingo-oophorectomy. The uterine specimen should be opened and tumor size, depth of myometrial invasion, and cervical extension assessed. Any suspicious pelvic and paraaortic lymph nodes should be removed for pathologic evaluation. Omental biopsy or partial omentectomy is not indicated unless there is gross evidence of intraperitoneal disease spread or specific histologic tumor subtype with a propensity

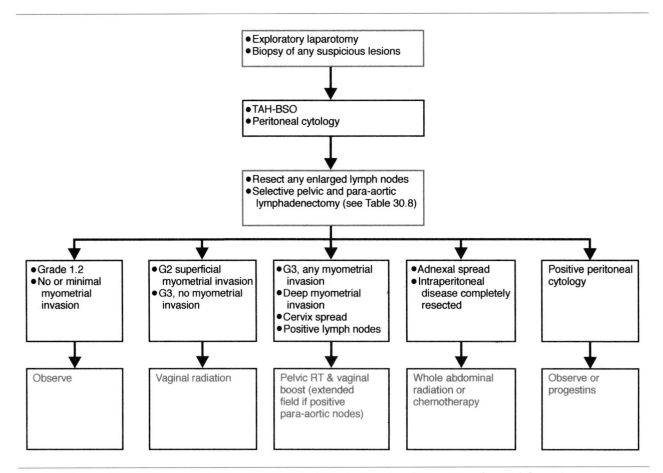

Figure 30.7   Management of patients with clinical stage I and stage II endometrial carcinoma.

for intraabdominal spread, such as papillary serous, clear cell, or mixed müllerian tumors.
Reference: Pages 1,155–1,157

9. C

Clinical staging of endometrial carcinoma according to FIGO 1971 (see Table 30.6) should be performed only in patients who are deemed unsuitable candidates for surgery because of their poor medical condition or because of spread of their disease. This

Table 30.6. FIGO Clinical Staging of Endometrial Carcinoma (1971)

Stage	Characteristic
I	Confined to the corpus
Ia G123	Uterine cavity <8 cm
Ib G123	Uterine cavity >8 cm
II	Involves the corpus and cervix but has not extended outside the uterus
III	Extends outside the uterus but not outside the true pelvis
IV	Extends outside the true pelvis or obviously involves the mucosa of the bladder or rectum
IVa	Spread to adjacent organs
IVb	Spread to distant organs

FIGO, International Federation of Gynecology and Obstetrics.

Table 30.7. FIGO Surgical Staging for Endometrial Carcinoma (1988)

Stage	Finding
Ia G123	No myometrial invasion
Ib G123	$< \frac{1}{2}$ Myometrial invasion
Ic G123	$> \frac{1}{2}$ Myometrial invasion
IIa G123	Extension to endocervical glands
IIb G123	Cervical stromal invasion
IIIa G123	Positive uterine serosa, adnexa, and/or peritoneal cytology
IIIb G123	Vaginal metastasis
IIIc G123	Metastasis to pelvic and/or paraaortic lymph nodes
IVa G123	Tumor invasion of bladder and/or bowel mucosa
IVb	Distant metastasis including intraabdominal and/or inguinal lymph nodes

FIGO, International Federation of Gynecology and Obstetrics.

patient has clinical stage IaG1 disease based on her preoperative assessment. In 1988, FIGO adopted a surgical staging system (see Table 30.7) because of the poor correlation between the preoperative clinical staging evaluation and the surgical–pathologic findings.

This patient has moderately differentiated (G2) endometrial tumor extending into the endocervical mucosa but not invading the cervical stroma or extending outside of the uterus, therefore, stage IIaG2. Superficial ($< \frac{1}{2}$) myoinvasion without cervical mucosal involvement would be stage Ib. Criteria for stage IIIa disease are positive peritoneal cytology, extension to the uterine serosa, or adnexal spread. Stage IIIb indicates vaginal metastasis in the absence of retroperitoneal disease (IIIc) or tumor spread beyond the pelvic reproductive system (IV).
Reference: Pages 1,156–1,157

10. **C**

The overall incidence of lymph node metastasis in clinical stage I endometrial cancer is approximately 10%, including 3% in grade 1, 9% in grade 2, and 18% in grade 3 tumors (see Table 30.9). Fewer than 5% of patients with no or superficial ($< \frac{1}{2}$) myometrial invasion have lymph node metastasis, compared with about 20% of patients with deep ($> \frac{1}{2}$) myometrial invasion (see Table 30.10). Cervical involvement is associated with about a 15% risk of pelvic or paraaortic lymph node metastasis. The incidence of lymph node metastasis also correlates with tumor size (<2 cm = 4%, >2 cm = 15%, entire cavity = 35%). Extrauterine spread of disease including adnexal spread and positive peritoneal cytology increases the risk of nodal metastasis to 32% and 25%, respectively. Therefore, patients with grade 3 tumors, deep myometrial invasion, isthmus–cervix

Table 30.9. Relationship of Grade to Lymph Node Mestastasis in Clinical Stage I Endometrial Carcinoma

Grade	No.	Pelvic Nodes		Aortic Nodes	
		No.	%	No.	%
1	180	5	3	3	2
2	288	25	9	14	5
3	153	28	18	17	11

From **Creasman WT, Morrow CP, Bundy BN, et al.** Surgical pathologic spread patterns of endometrial cancer. *Cancer* 1987;60:2035–2041, with permission.

Table 30.10. Relationship of Myometrial Invasion to Lymph Node Metastasis in Clinical Stage I Endometrial Carcinoma

Myometrial Invasion	No.	Pelvic Nodes		Aortic Nodes	
		No.	%	No.	%
None	87	1	1	1	1
Inner third	279	15	5	8	3
Middle third	116	7	6	1	1
Outer third	139	35	25	24	17

From **Creasman WT, Morrow CP, Bundy BN, et al.** Surgical pathologic spread patterns of endometrial cancer. *Cancer* 1987;60:2035–2041, with permission.

extension, tumor size more than 2 cm, and/or extrauterine disease should have selective pelvic and paraaortic lymph node dissection.
Reference: Pages 1,157–1,159

11. A

Although stage of disease is the most significant variable affecting survival, a number of other individual prognostic factors for disease recurrence or survival have been identified including patient age, tumor grade, histopathology, depth of myometrial invasion, and surgical–pathologic evidence of extrauterine disease spread.

In general, younger women with endometrial cancer have a better prognosis than older women. Five-year survival rates are approximately 95% for patients younger than 50 years, 75% for patients 50 to 75 years, and 50% for patients older than 75 years. Histologic grade of the endometrial tumor is strongly associated with prognosis. Patients with grade 3 tumors are more than 5 times more likely to have recurrence then are patients with grades 1 and 2 tumors. The 5-year disease-free survival rate for patients with grades 1 and 2 tumors is about 90% compared with 65% for patients with grade 3 tumors. Although nonendometrioid histologic subtypes account for only 10% of endometrial cancers, they carry an increased risk for recurrence and distant spread. In contrast to the approximate 90% survival rate for patients with endometrioid tumors, the overall survival rate for patients with one of the more aggressive subtypes, such as papillary serous or clear cell, is only 33%. Because access to lymphatics increases as cancer invades into the outer half of the myometrium, increasing depth of myoinvasion has been associated with increasing likelihood of extrauterine spread, recurrence and death. Patients with noninvasive or superficially invasive tumors have an 80% to 90% 5-year survival, whereas those with deeply invasive tumors have a 60% survival rate. LVSI appears to be an independent risk factor for recurrence and death from all types of endometrial cancer. The 5-year survival rate is approximately 85% for patients without demonstrable LVSI compared with a 65% survival rate for these in whom LVSI is present. Lymph node metastasis is probably the most important prognostic factor in clinical early-stage endometrial cancer. Patients with lymph node metastases have almost a sixfold higher likelihood of developing recurrent cancer than patients without lymph node metastases. The 5-year disease-free survival for patients with lymph node metastasis is approximately 50% compared with 90% for patients without lymph node metastasis. Other extrauterine spread to the adnexa and peritoneum also significantly affects survival.
Reference: Pages 1,160–1,163

12. B

Postoperative therapy should be based on prognostic factors determined by surgical–pathologic staging (see Table 30.14 and Fig. 30.7). Patients with grades 1 and 2 lesions with no or minimal myometrial invasion have an excellent prognosis and require no further therapy. Vaginal vault irradiation can reduce the incidence of local recurrence in patients with tumors apparently confined to the uterus from as high as 15% to as

Table 30.14. Postoperative Management of Endometrial Carcinoma Based on Surgical-Pathologic Findings and Stage

Surgical-Pathologic Findings	Stage	Postoperative Treatment
Low risk		
G1, G2, no myoinvasion	Ia G1, 2	None
No cervix/isthmus invasion		
Negative peritoneal cytology		
No LVSI		
No evidence of metastasis		
Intermediate risk		
G1, G2, <50% myoinvasion	Ib G1, 2	Vaginal cuff irradiation
G3, no myoinvasion	Ia G3	
G3, <50% myoinvasion	Ib G3	Pelvic versus vaginal cuff irradiation
G1, G2 isthmus/cervix extension	IIa G1, G2	
G1, G2, G3 >50% myoinvasion	Ic G1, G2, G3	Pelvic irradiation plus vaginal cuff boost
G3, isthmus/cervix extension	IIa G3	
G1, G2, G3 cervix invasion	IIb G1, G2, G3	
LVSI		
Positive peritoneal cytology	IIIa (+ cytology)	Progestin/^{32}P
High risk		
Adnexal/serosal/parametrial spread	IIIa G1, G2, G3	Pelvic and vaginal irradiation (Extended-field radiation therapy if positive aortic/common iliac lymph nodes)
Vaginal metastasis	IIIb G1, G2, G3	
Lymph node metastasis	IIIc G1, G2, G3	
Bladder/rectal invasion	IVa	Pelvic and vaginal irradiation
Intraperitoneal spread	IVb	Whole-abdomen irradiation; systemic chemotherapy

LVSI, lymph–vascular space invasion.

low as 1% to 2%. Patients most likely to benefit from vaginal irradiation are those who have surgical stage I grade 1 and 2 tumors with superficial ($< \frac{1}{2}$) myometrial invasion (stage IbG1,2) or grade 3 tumors with no or minimal invasion (stage IaG3) and some patients with IIa disease who otherwise meet the aforementioned criteria. Postoperative external pelvic irradiation decreases the risk of pelvic recurrence and may improve survival in certain high-risk groups. Patients found to benefit most from adjuvant postoperative whole pelvis irradiation are those with cervical involvement, pelvic lymph node metastases, pelvic disease outside the uterus, and patients with clinical stage I disease who are at significant risk of nodal metastasis (e.g., grade 3 tumor with any degree of myometrial invasion; grades 1 and 2 tumors with more than $\frac{1}{2}$ myometrial invasion; large [>2 cm] grade 2 tumors with superficial myometrial invasion; and any grade tumor with LVSI). Whole abdominal radiation therapy is usually reserved for patients with adnexal or upper abdominal disease that has been completely excised and patients who are at very high risk for intraabdominal recurrence, such as those with papillary serous tumors. There is no apparent benefit to the use of adjuvant progestin therapy.
Reference: Pages 1,164–1,168

13. C

Patients with stage I endometrial cancer who have grade 3 tumors, deep myometrial invasion, and/or LVSI should receive postoperative external pelvic and vaginal cuff irradiation. The pelvic failure rate is significantly reduced and disease-free survival is improved by the use of postoperative pelvic irradiation in this high-risk group of patients.

Survival in surgical stage I disease ranges from more than 90% for stage IaG1,2 and IbG1,2 to 63% for stage IcG3 (see Table 30.17). Five-year survival is

Table 30.17. Surgically Staged Endometrial Cancer: Acturial 5-Year Survival Rate (%) by Histologic Grade and Stage

	Grade		
Stage	1	2	3
Ia	93	90	69
Ib	90	93	84
Ic	89	81	63
IIa	91	78	57
IIb	78	75	58
IIIa	79	69	44
IIIb	77	40	21
IIIc	61	61	44
IVa	—	—	19
IVb	35	27	7

Adapted from **Creasman WT, Odicino F, Maisonneuve P, et al.** Carcinoma of the corpus uteri. FIGO Annual Report on the Results of Treatment in Gynecological Cancer. *J Epidemiol Biostat* 2001;6:45–86, with permission.

approximately 75% for surgical stage II, 60% for surgical stage III, and 18% for surgical stage IV. Overall 5-year survival in endometrial cancer is about 76% (see Table 30.16).
Reference: Pages 1,177–1,178

14. C

Disseminated peritoneal leiomyomatosis is a rare clinical entity characterized by benign smooth muscle nodules scattered throughout the abdomen on peritoneal surfaces. This condition probably arises as a result of metaplasia of subperitoneal mesenchymal stem cells to smooth muscle, fibroblasts, myofibroblasts, and decidual cells under the influence of estrogen and progesterone. Most reported cases have occurred in 30- to 40-year-old women who are or have recently been pregnant or have a long history of oral contraceptive use. Intriguing features of the disease are its grossly malignant appearance, benign histology, and favorable outcome. Removal of the source of excess estrogen or treatment with progestins or both usually results in regression of tumor masses.
Reference: Page 1,183

Table 30.16. Carcinoma of The Endometrium: Stage Distribution and Actuarial Survival by Stage (Surgical and Clinical)

	Patients Treated		Survival (%)	
Stage	No.	%	3-Year	5-Year
Surgical				
I	3,996	70	92	87
II	709	12	82	76
III	758	13	66	59
IV	231	4	23	18
Clinical				
I	232	61	63	54
II	64	16	53	41
III	54	14	30	23
IV	33	8	12	12
TOTAL	6,260	100	82	76

Adapted from **Creasman WT, Odicino F, Maisonneuve P, et al.** Carcinoma of the corpus uteri. FIGO Annual Report on the Results of Treatment in Gynecological Cancer. *J Epidemiol Biostat* 2001;6:45–86, with permission.

15. B

Low-grade endometrial stromal sarcoma is distinguished from high-grade or undifferentiated endometrial stromal sarcoma by a lower mitotic rate of less than 10 mitotic figures/10 high-power microscopic fields, a diploid DNA context, and a low proliferative index. Low-grade stromal sarcoma has extended beyond the uterus in 40% of cases at the time of diagnosis, but the extrauterine spread is confined to the pelvis most of the time. Although recurrences occur in almost 50% of cases of low-grade stromal sarcoma, the clinical course is much more protracted and the prognosis is better than for high-grade sarcomas. Low-grade stromal sarcomas, unlike high-grade sarcomas, are often responsive to progestin therapy.

Reference: Pages 1,179–1,181

31 Cervical and Vaginal Cancer

Thomas C. Krivak
John W. McBroom
John C. Elkas

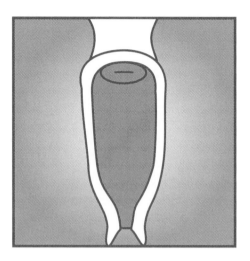

Learning Objectives

1. Be able to identify the histologic characteristics of cervical cancer.

2. Understand the role of colposcopy in the evaluation of cervical lesions.

3. Know the International Federation of Gynecology and Obstetrics (FIGO) staging of cervical cancer.

4. Be able to articulate the different treatment modalities for cervical cancer, as well as the advantages and disadvantages of each.

5. Know how to diagnose vaginal cancer.

6. Know the FIGO staging of vaginal cancer.

7. Be able to articulate the different treatment modalities for vaginal cancer, as well as the advantages and disadvantages of each.

Questions

1. Which of the following studies is *not* permitted by FIGO in the determination of stage in patients with cervical cancer?

    A. Intravenous pyelogram (IVP)
    B. Barium enema (BE)
    C. Chest x-ray (CXR)
    D. Computed tomography (CT)
    E. Cervical conization

2. Which of the following types of hysterectomy is a hysterectomy in which the uterine artery is ligated at its origin and the uterosacral and cardinal ligaments are completely removed?

    A. Extrafascial or type I hysterectomy
    B. Modified radical or type II hysterectomy
    C. Radical or type III hysterectomy
    D. Extended radical or type IV hysterectomy
    E. Partial exenteration or type V hysterectomy

3. Which of the following factors has *not* been clearly shown to influence survival after radical hysterectomy and pelvic lymphadenectomy?

    A. The status of the lymph nodes
    B. Tumor size
    C. Involvement of paracervical tissues
    D. Depth of invasion
    E. The presence or absence of lymph vascular space invasion (LVSI)

4. Which of the following treatment modalities is most appropriate in the treatment of a 30-year-old woman diagnosed with a stage Ia2 squamous cell carcinoma of the cervix?

    A. Cervical conization
    B. Type I hysterectomy
    C. Type II hysterectomy without pelvic lymph node dissection
    D. Type II hysterectomy with pelvic lymph node dissection
    E. Radiation therapy

5. Which of the following statistics regarding the treatment of stage Ib cervical cancer is false?

    A. The 5-year survival is comparable with primary radical surgery versus primary radiation therapy.
    B. There is a significantly higher urologic fistula rate with radical surgery compared with that of radiation therapy.
    C. The surgical mortality from radical surgery is approximately the same as that for intracavitary radiation therapy.
    D. Chronic bladder atony occurs in approximately 3% of patients after radical surgery.
    E. Radiation fibrosis of bowel and bladder occurs in 6% to 8% of patients.

6. In the staging of a patient with vaginal carcinoma, extension to the subvaginal tissues is consistent with which of the following stages?

    A. Stage I
    B. Stage II
    C. Stage III
    D. Stage IVa
    E. Stage IVb

7. Which of the following correctly reflects the histologic subtypes of vaginal cancer from most frequent to least frequent?

   A. Squamous cell, adenocarcinoma, melanoma, sarcoma
   B. Squamous cell, melanoma, adenocarcinoma, sarcoma
   C. Adenocarcinoma, squamous cell, melanoma, sarcoma
   D. Adenocarcinoma, squamous cell, sarcoma, melanoma
   E. Squamous cell, sarcoma, melanoma, adenocarcinoma

8. A tumor involving the lower one third of the vagina and extending to the vulva should be staged as follows:

   A. Stage II vaginal cancer
   B. Stage III vaginal cancer
   C. Stage IVa vaginal cancer
   D. Stage IVb vaginal cancer
   E. At least stage III vulvar carcinoma (T3 lesion)

9. All of the following statements regarding vaginal carcinoma are true **except:**

   A. Approximately 30% of patients with vaginal carcinoma have a history of cervical cancer treated within the previous 5 years.
   B. Any vaginal cancer diagnosed at least 5 years after a cervical cancer diagnosis should be considered a new primary.
   C. The most common site of vaginal carcinoma is the upper one third of the vagina on the anterior wall.
   D. Most patients are diagnosed in stages II through IV rather than stage I.
   E. The most common mode of spread is by direct extension.

10. Which of the following statements regarding cervical cancer in pregnancy is false?

    A. Diagnosis is often delayed during pregnancy because bleeding may be attributed to obstetric causes.
    B. If absolutely indicated, cervical conization in pregnancy should be performed in the second trimester.
    C. Patients with more than 5 mm of invasion should undergo immediate surgical intervention without consideration of the gestational age.
    D. In advanced stages of disease, radiation therapy should be undertaken, and in the first trimester, spontaneous abortion should be anticipated before the delivery of 4,000 cGy.
    E. The diagnosis of cervical cancer in the postpartum period has been associated with more advanced disease and therefore, decreased survival.

11. A 24-year-old woman undergoes a cervical conization after a colposcopically directed biopsy reveals a carcinoma *in situ,* and rules out a microinvasive carcinoma. The cone shows 2-mm invasion of a well-differentiated squamous carcinoma. There is no lymph–vascular involvement and the margins are free of disease. She wants to preserve her fertility. The best therapeutic option is

    A. Observation
    B. Hysterectomy
    C. Repeated conization
    D. Modified radical hysterectomy
    E. Radical hysterectomy

12. A 32-year-old woman has a 5-cm cervical lesion. The biopsy shows a poorly differentiated squamous cell carcinoma of the cervix. On clinical assessment, the tumor extends into the right parametrium. The most appropriate therapy is

    A. Pelvic radiation therapy
    B. Radical hysterectomy and lymphadenectomy

C. Concurrent pelvic radiation and chemotherapy
D. Pelvic radiation therapy followed by radical hysterectomy
E. Radical hysterectomy followed by pelvic radiation therapy

13. A 48-year-old woman underwent pelvic radiation therapy for a stage IIb cervical cancer 2 years ago, and now presents with vaginal bleeding. The vaginal examination reveals a 3-cm central pelvic mass at the vaginal apex. The biopsy is consistent with a recurrent squamous carcinoma. Metastatic evaluation shows no clinical evidence that the disease has spread. The most effective subsequent therapy is

    A. Chemotherapy
    B. Radiation therapy
    C. Pelvic exenteration
    D. Radiation plus chemotherapy
    E. Radical hysterectomy and radiation

14. The infectious agent that is involved in the development of cervical cancer is

    A. Herpes virus
    B. *Chlamydia*
    C. Syphilis
    D. Human papilloma virus (HPV)
    E. None

15. In a patient a stage Ib1 squamous cell cervical cancer who underwent a type III radical hysterectomy for therapy, risk factors for development of recurrent cancer include:

    A. Positive pelvic lymph nodes
    B. Positive parametrial spread
    C. Positive surgical margins
    D. All the above

Answers

1. **D**

   Cervical cancer and vaginal cancer are the two gynecologic malignancies that are staged clinically rather than surgically. Once a patient has been assigned to a particular stage, the stage should not be changed. The stage distribution in cervical cancer is as follows: stage I, 38%; stage II, 32%; stage III, 26%; and stage IV, 4%. CT scan, lymphangiography, ultrasonography, magnetic resonance imaging (MRI), radionuclide scanning, and laparoscopy may all be used in planning treatment but are not allowed by FIGO in the determination of stage. These studies are not universally available throughout the world and, therefore, are not practical for staging because cervical cancer is the most common gynecologic malignancy worldwide. All of the other diagnostic modalities listed are permissible by FIGO for staging in this malignancy. In addition, physical examination, biopsy, cystoscopy, and proctoscopy are also permitted (see Table 31.2).
   Reference: Pages 1,204–1,206, 1,232–1,233

2. **C (see Fig. 31.9)**

   The radical hysterectomy (type III hysterectomy) described by Meigs in 1944 includes removal of as much of the uterosacral and cardinal ligaments as possible and removal of the upper one third of the vagina. It also includes ligation of the uterine artery at its origin. Pelvic lymphadenectomy is performed. The type II hysterectomy as described by Wertheim is less extensive and involves removal of the medial one half of the uterosacral and cardinal ligaments and ligation of the uterine artery as it traverses the ureter rather

Table 31.2. Staging Procedures

Physical examination[a]	Palpate lymph nodes
	Examine vagina
	Bimanual rectovaginal examination (under anesthesia recommended)
Radiologic studies[a]	Intravenous pyelogram
	Barium enema
	Chest x-ray
	Skeletal x-ray
Procedures[a]	Biopsy
	Conization
	Hysteroscopy
	Colposcopy
	Endocervical curettage
	Cystoscopy
	Proctoscopy
Optional studies[b]	Computerized axial tomography
	Lymphangiography
	Ultrasonography
	Magnetic resonance imaging
	Radionucleotide scanning
	Laparoscopy

[a]Allowed by the International Federation of Gynecology and Obstetrics (FIGO).
[b]Information that is not allowed by FIGO to change the clinical stage.

than at its origin. In a type IV hysterectomy, the periureteral tissue, superior vesicle artery, and up to three fourths of the vagina are removed. The type V hysterectomy, or partial exenteration, is rarely performed today because of the widespread availability of radiation therapy.
Reference: Page 1,212

Figure 31.9   The pelvic ligaments and spaces.

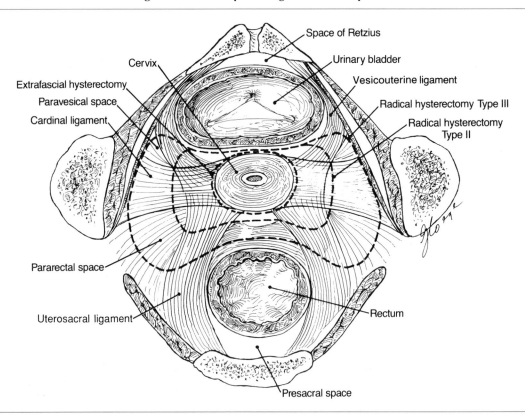

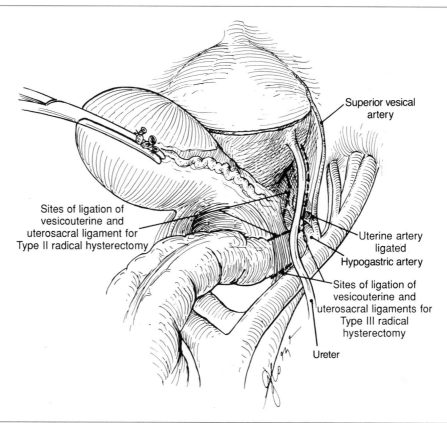

Figure 31.10 labels:
- Superior vesical artery
- Sites of ligation of vesicouterine and uterosacral ligament for Type II radical hysterectomy
- Uterine artery ligated
- Hypogastric artery
- Sites of ligation of vesicouterine and uterosacral ligaments for Type III radical hysterectomy
- Ureter

Figure 31.10   Radical hysterectomy. Uterine artery is ligated, ureter is dissected, and sites for division of the vesicouterine and uterosacral ligaments are shown.

3. E (see Fig. 31.10)

Many studies have shown that the status of the lymph nodes affects survival. The 5-year survival in stage Ib1 cervical cancer is 85% to 90% when the lymph nodes are negative but decreases significantly in the presence of positive nodes. When more than three positive pelvic nodes are present, the recurrence rate is 68% in contrast to 30% to 50% when fewer than three nodes are involved. Lesion size has been shown to be an independent predictor of survival with survival rates of approximately 90% with lesions smaller than 2 cm, in contrast to 60% for lesions larger than 2 cm. The depth of invasion also influences survival: Survival rates significantly decrease when the depth of invasion is more than 1 cm. The 5-year survival is approximately 95% with negative parametrium versus 69% with positive parametrium. The significance of LVSI is somewhat more controversial and may be more a predictor of lymph node metastasis rather than an independent predictor of survival. Future studies are needed to settle this controversy.

Reference: Pages 1,214–1,219

4. D (see Tables 31.3 and 31.4)

In a young patient with a stage Ia1 squamous cell cancer of the cervix with no evidence of lymph–vascular space invasion, conization may be adequate treatment if margins are negative. The incidence of pelvic lymph node metastases in this setting is less than 1%. If the patient does not desire fertility, she may be treated with type I hysterectomy. If LVSI is present, consideration should be given to performing a type II hysterectomy. In the setting of a stage Ia2 lesion, the incidence of pelvic lymph node metastases is nearly 4% and, therefore, pelvic lymph node dissection is required. A type II hysterectomy is most appropriate. If the patient has a stage Ib lesion (either Ib1 or Ib2), a type III hysterectomy with pelvic lymphadenectomy is appropriate with consideration of

Table 31.3. Incidence of Pelvic and Paraaortic Nodal Metastasis by Stage

Stage	No. of Patients	Positive Pelvic Nodes (%)	Positive Paraaortic Nodes (%)
Ia1 (≤3 mm)	179[a]	0.5	0
Ia2 (>3–5 mm)	84[a]	4.8	<1
Ib	1926[b]	15.9	2.2
IIa	110[c]	24.5	11
IIb	324[c]	31.4	19
III	125[c]	44.8	30
IVa	23[c]	55	40

[a]References 42, 47, 69, 70, 75, 79
[b]References 12, 42, 44, 49, 52, 53, 56, 57, 58, 59, 60
[c]References 11, 12, 53, 56, 57, 61, 81

paraaortic lymph node evaluation. Surgery is preferable to radiation therapy in young patients with early-stage disease.
Reference: Pages 1,217–1,218

5. B (see Table 31.5)

The overall 5-year survival is approximately 85% for patients with stages Ib/IIa cervical cancer when treated with either radical surgery or radiation therapy. The choice of treatment is individualized, with surgery generally selected for relatively young patients in good health. The urologic fistula rate is approximately 1% to 2% after radical surgery and is less than 5% overall after radiation therapy and is therefore not significantly higher with radical surgery. Surgical mortality is approximately 1% with both radical surgery and intracavitary implants and is most commonly related to pulmonary embolism. The most common chronic complication after radical hysterectomy is bladder hypotonia or atony and occurs in approximately 3% of patients.
Reference: Pages 1,218–1,219

6. B

Like cervical cancer, vaginal cancer is clinically staged (see Table 31.6). Cancer of the vagina most often spreads via direct extension, and involvement of pelvic lymph nodes may occur in advanced stages of disease. Stage II disease indicates involvement of the subvaginal tissues in the absence of spread to the sidewall of the pelvis. Approximately 75% of patients present in stages II through IV, indicating delay in diagnosis. There is no FIGO category for microinvasive cancer of the vagina as is seen with cervical cancer.
Reference: Pages 1,232–1,233

7. A

Squamous cell carcinoma is the most common histologic subtype, occurring in 80% of vaginal cancers. Like cervical cancer, vaginal carcinoma may have a link to HPV. In some cases, invasive vaginal carcinoma may progress from vaginal intraepithelial neoplasia (VAIN) but the true incidence of this progression is not known. VAIN is

Table 31.4. Surgical Management of Early Invasive Cancer of the Cervix

Stage Ia1	≤3 mm invasion	
	No lymph-vascular space invasion	Conization Type I hysterectomy
	With lymph-vascular space invasion	Type I or II hysterectomy with (?) pelvic lymph node dissection
Stage Ia2	>3–5 mm invasion	Type II hysterectomy with pelvic lymphadenectomy
Stage Ib	>5 mm invasion	Type III hysterectomy with pelvic lymphadenectomy

Table 31.5. Comparison of Surgery versus Radiation for Stage Ib/IIa Cancer of the Cervix

	Surgery	*Radiation*
Survival	85%	85%
Serious complications	Urologic fistulas 1%–2%	Intestinal and urinary strictures and fistulas 1.4%–5.3%
Vagina	Initially shortened, but may lengthen with regular intercourse	Fibrosis and possible stenosis, particularly in postmenopausal patients
Ovaries	Can be conserved	Destroyed
Chronic effects	Bladder atony in 3%	Radiation fibrosis of bowel and bladder in 6%–8%
Applicability	Best candidates are younger than 65 years of age. <200 lb, and in good health	All patients are potential candidates
Surgical mortality	1%	1% (from pulmonary embolism during intracavitary therapy)

not believed to have as great a malignant potential as cervical intraepithelial neoplasia (CIN). Approximately 30% of patients with vaginal cancer have a history of cervical cancer treated within the previous 5 years. Any new vaginal carcinoma diagnosed at least 5 years after a diagnosis of cervical cancer should be considered a new primary.

Adenocarcinoma of the vagina is the second-most-common histologic subtype and comprises approximately 9% of all primary vaginal carcinomas. Adenocarcinomas may arise in wolffian rest elements, periurethral glands, and foci of endometriosis and, in women exposed to *diethylstilbestrol (DES)*, adenocarcinomas may arise in vaginal adenosis. Metastatic adenocarcinoma of the vagina may originate from the colon, endometrium, ovary, pancreas, or stomach; in fact, metastatic vaginal adenocarcinoma is more common than primary vaginal adenocarcinoma.

The next-most-common subtype is melanoma, which is extremely rare. Most of the lesions are deeply invasive at the time of diagnosis and are quite lethal. Vaginal sarcomas are also quite rare and are usually fibrosarcomas or leiomyosarcomas.
Reference: Pages 1,233–1,236

8. E
The FIGO staging system of gynecologic malignancies mandates that a tumor involving both the vagina and cervix be designated as a cancer of the cervix. Similarly, a tumor involving both the vagina and vulva should be classified as a vulvar cancer. Cancer of the vulva is staged surgically but, at a minimum, a vulvar cancer that extends into the vagina is considered a T3 lesion and is therefore at least a stage III vulvar

Table 31.6. FIGO Staging of Vaginal Cancer

Stage 0	Carcinoma *in situ,* intraepithelia carcinoma.
Stage I	The carcinoma is limited to the vaginal wall.
Stage II	The carcinoma has involved the subvaginal tissue but has not extended to the pelvic wall.
Stage III	The carcinoma has extended to the pelvic wall.
Stage IV	The carcinoma has extended beyond the true pelvis or has involved the mucosa of the bladder or rectum.
Stage IVa	Spread of the growth to adjacent organs.
Stage IVb	Spread to distant organs.

FIGO, International Federation of Gynecology and Obstetrics.

carcinoma. It may fall into the category of stage IV depending on the status of the nodes on final pathology. If there is no cervical or vulvar involvement of the vaginal cancer, it should then be considered a vaginal carcinoma and should be staged by the FIGO staging system for vaginal cancer (see Table 31.6).
Reference: Page 1,232

9. C

The diagnosis of vaginal cancer is usually made after abnormal cytology mandates the pursuit of such a diagnosis. It may also be diagnosed after visualization and biopsy of a gross lesion. The most common site for vaginal cancer is the upper one third of the vagina on the *posterior wall.* These tumors may be missed when they are in early stages because they may be obscured by the speculum blades at the time of pelvic examination. Colposcopy should be undertaken with abnormal cytology or in the setting of persistent unexplained vaginal bleeding. Unfortunately, a minority of patients are diagnosed in stage I (75% present with stages II–IV), indicating delays in diagnosis. Cancer of the vagina spreads most frequently by direct extension. Metastases to the pelvic and paraaortic lymph nodes may occur in advanced or late disease as does hematogenous spread to lungs, liver, or bone. Lesions in the lower one third of the vagina may metastasize to the inguinal femoral lymph nodes in addition to the sites described previously.
Reference: Pages 1,233–1,234

10. C

Cervical cancer is estimated to complicate 1 in 2,200 pregnancies. The key to approaching this cancer during pregnancy is individualization with consideration for both mother and fetus. A diagnostic conization may be necessary if there is a high suspicion of malignancy and the diagnosis cannot be made with colposcopy and biopsy. If required, conization should be performed in the second trimester because the abortion rate may be as high as 33% in the first trimester. If a patient is diagnosed with stage Ib cervical cancer in pregnancy (> 5-mm invasion), the timing of treatment depends upon the gestational age of the fetus and wishes of the patient. If the cancer is diagnosed in the third trimester, fetal pulmonary maturity can be assessed via amniocentesis and therapy undertaken with pulmonary maturity. Treatment should probably not be delayed more than 4 weeks and, in the third trimester, consists of cesarean delivery, radical hysterectomy, and pelvic lymphadenectomy. Conversely, when a patient is diagnosed early in pregnancy, treatment should also not be delayed more than 4 weeks and radical hysterectomy is generally accomplished without hysterotomy with the fetus *in situ.* When carcinoma of the cervix is diagnosed in the middle of pregnancy, decisions regarding timing of treatment are less clear and again individualization with regard to the wishes of the patient is a most important consideration.
Reference: Pages 1,226–1,227

11. A

Cervical conization has now become standard treatment for microinvasive carcinoma of the cervix when the patient wishes to preserve fertility. In lesions invasive to less than 3 mm without lymph–vascular invasion, the risk of lymph node metastasis is essentially nil.
Reference: Page 1,217

12. A

The standard treatment for a stage IIb cervical cancer is concurrent chemotherapy with pelvic radiation therapy. Results of recently published clinical trials have shown a survival benefit for patients treated with concurrent chemotherapy and radiation. Surgery is contraindicated in such patients.
Reference: Pages 1,219–1,220, 1,224–1,225

13. C

Pelvic exenteration is used for patients with potentially curable disease that appears confined to the central pelvis. The patient undergoes exploratory surgery to look for any metastatic disease, and if none is found, the exenteration is performed. The uterus, cervix, ovaries, tubes, vagina, bladder, and, if necessary, the rectosigmoid colon are extirpated.

Reference: Pages 1,230–1,232

14. D

Many recent studies have confirmed the presence of HPV in up to 99% of squamous cell cervical cancer. HPV has proteins that interact with the *p53* and *Rb* tumor suppressor genes.

Reference: Page 1,200

15. D

Risk factors for recurrent disease after radical hysterectomy are important to identify so patients may receive adjuvant radiation therapy to decrease the likelihood of recurrence. All these risk factors have been associated with increased rates of recurrent disease. Positive vaginal or parametrial margins, positive pelvic lymph nodes, and parametrial spread of tumor place patients at a higher risk of disease recurrence. A recently published Gynecologic Oncology Group trial has shown an improved survival in patients with these risk factors who receive adjuvant concurrent chemotherapy and pelvic radiation therapy.

Reference: Pages 1,218–1,220

32 Ovarian Cancer

Robert E. Bristow
Jonathan S. Berek

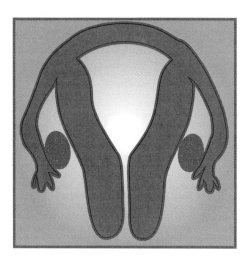

Learning Objectives

1. Understand the principles and surgical techniques involved in staging of epithelial ovarian cancer.

2. Understand the appropriate surgical therapy and indications for surgical staging of germ cell and sex cord–stromal ovarian malignancies.

3. Understand the genetic transmission of and ovarian cancer risk associated with site-specific familial ovarian cancer, breast–ovarian familial cancer syndrome, and Lynch II syndrome.

4. Know the chemotherapeutic agents used in first-line treatment of epithelial, germ cell, and sex cord–stromal ovarian cancer and their associated toxicities.

5. Know the clinical factors influencing the prognosis of advanced epithelial ovarian cancer.

6. Be able to identify, on the basis of clinical factors, those patients with recurrent ovarian cancer who are most likely to benefit from secondary cytoreductive surgery.

Questions

1. Which of the following is *not* part of the diagnostic criteria for an ovarian tumor of low malignant potential?

   A. Epithelial proliferation with papillary formation and pseudostratification
   B. Disease confined to one or both ovaries
   C. Nuclear atypia and increased mitotic activity
   D. Absence of true stromal invasion

2. What is the rate of bilaterality of malignant mucinous carcinomas?

   A. 1% to 2%
   B. 8% to 10%
   C. 20%
   D. 33%

3. What percentage of ovarian neoplasms in postmenopausal women is malignant?

   A. 7%
   B. 20%
   C. 30%
   D. 50%

4. Preoperative testing for a postmenopausal woman with a pelvic mass and suspected ovarian cancer should include all of the following **except**

   A. Hematologic and biochemical assessment
   B. Chest x-ray
   C. Electrocardiogram
   D. Magnetic resonance imaging (MRI) of the abdomen and pelvis

5. Which of the following are independent prognostic variables for ovarian cancer?

   A. Stage of disease
   B. Volume of ascites
   C. Extent of residual disease after primary surgery
   D. All of the above

6. Complete surgical staging of those with apparent stage I or II disease will result in the upstaging of what percentage of patients?

   A. 5%
   B. 15%
   C. 30%
   D. 50%

7. The benefits of primary cytoreductive surgery include

   A. Prolonged progression-free survival
   B. Improved patient comfort
   C. Theoretical enhancement of chemotherapy through cellular kinetic effects
   D. All of the above

8. First-line chemotherapy of choice for advanced epithelial ovarian cancer is

   A. *Cisplatin, paclitaxel*
   B. *Carboplatin, paclitaxel*
   C. *Paclitaxel, cyclophosphamide*
   D. *Cisplatin, cyclophosphamide*

9. A second-look operation is performed after a prescribed course of chemotherapy to determine the response to therapy on a patient who has

   A. No clinical evidence of disease
   B. A palpable tumor mass but a negative cancer antigen 125 (CA125)
   C. No palpable tumor mass but an elevated CA125
   D. A palpable tumor mass and an elevated CA125

10. During the first two decades of life, germ cell tumors account for what percentage of ovarian malignancies?

    A. 10%
    B. 33%
    C. 66%
    D. None of the above

11. Of germ cell malignancies, bilateral ovarian involvement occurs in 10% to 15% of

    A. Dysgerminoma
    B. Endodermal sinus tumor
    C. Immature teratoma
    D. Choriocarcinoma

12. Appropriate management of a premenopausal woman with a dysgerminoma apparently confined to one ovary is

    A. Unilateral salpingo-oophorectomy, ipsilateral pelvic lymph node dissection, and staging
    B. Bilateral salpingo-oophorectomy, bilateral pelvic lymph node dissection, and staging
    C. Karyotype
    D. A and C
    E. B and C

13. Preferred treatment for advanced stage, incompletely resected dysgerminoma is

    A. Three to four cycles of *bleomycin/etoposide/cisplatin* (BEP)
    B. Six cycles of *cisplatin/paclitaxel*
    C. Three cycles of BEP plus three cycles of *vincristine/actinomycin D/ cyclophosphamide* (VAC)
    D. Four cycles of *vinblastine/bleomycin/cisplatin* (VBP)

14. Prognosis of immature teratoma is correlated with the

    A. Amount of undifferentiated neural tissue
    B. Degree of glandular differentiation
    C. Presence of mature teratoma
    D. Presence of sexual pseudoprecosity

15. A 58-year-old woman undergoes an exploratory laparotomy for an irregularly shaped pelvic tumor. An invasive malignant ovarian cancer is found and she undergoes a total abdominal hysterectomy, bilateral salpingo-oophorectomy, omentectomy, and tumor reductive surgery. All of the macroscopic disease is removed (i.e., she has an "optimally" resected tumor). The diagnosis is a stage IIIb serous adenocarcinoma of the ovary. Based on the current data, which of the following chemotherapeutic regimens should be used for this patient?

    A. *Cisplatin, paclitaxel*
    B. *Carboplatin, cisplatin*
    C. *Carboplatin, paclitaxel*
    D. *Cisplatin, cyclophosphamide*

16. A 17-year-old girl undergoes an exploratory laparotomy for a complex 12-cm pelvic tumor. The pathology shows a grade 3 immature teratoma. The staging laparotomy confirms that the disease is a stage Ia tumor. Which of the following chemotherapeutic regimens should be administered to this patient?

A. *Cisplatin*
B. *Cisplatin, etoposide*
C. BEP
D. *Cisplatin, etoposide, bleomycin, methotrexate*

Answers

1. B (see Table 32.1)

Borderline tumors of the ovary, or tumors of low malignant potential, can be unilateral or bilateral. The histologic diagnosis depends on specific criteria, including the presence of papillary formations and pseudostratification. Nuclear atypia is usually seen, as is increased mitotic activity. Lesions lack, however, true stromal invasion, and thus they represent noninvasive, albeit highly proliferative, lesions.
Reference: Pages 1,246–1,249

2. B

The rate of bilaterality varies depending on the histologic type of the tumor and, importantly, on the stage of the tumor. For apparent low-stage tumors, the rate of bilateral serous tumors is about 5%, whereas for mucinous tumors it is 8% to 10%.
Reference: Pages 1,247–1,252

Table 32.1. Epithelial Ovarian Tumors

Histologic Type	Cellular Type
I. Serous A. Benign B. Borderline C. Malignant	Endosalpingeal
II. Mucinous A. Benign B. Borderline C. Malignant	Endocervical
III. Endometrioid A. Benign B. Borderline C. Malignant	Endometrial
IV. Clear-cell "mesonephroid" A. Benign B. Borderline C. Malignant	Müllerian
V. Brenner A. Benign B. Borderline (proliferating) C. Malignant	Transitional
VI. Mixed epithelial A. Benign B. Borderline C. Malignant	Mixed
VII. Undifferentiated	Anaplastic
VIII. Unclassified	Mesothelioma, etc.

From **Seroy SF, Scully RE, Sobin LH.** *International histological classification of tumours no. 9. Histological typing of ovarian tumors.* Geneva: World Health Organization, 1973, with permission.

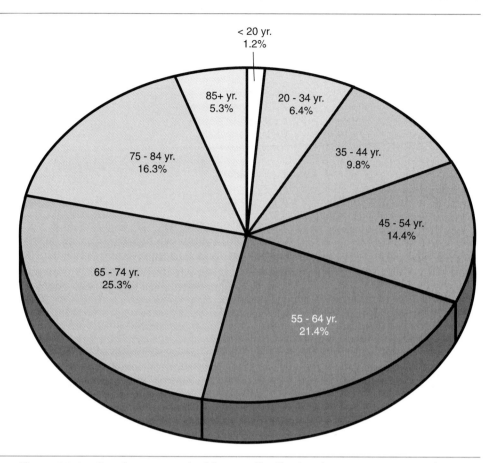

Figure 32.6   Ovarian cancer incidence: distribution by age. (From *J Natl Cancer Inst* 1995;87:1280, with permission.)

3. C (see Fig. 32.6)

More than 80% of epithelial ovarian cancers are found in postmenopausal women. The peak incidence is 62 years. About 30% of ovarian neoplasms found in postmenopausal women are malignant, compared with only 7% in premenopausal women.
Reference: Pages 1,252–1,253

4. D

The preoperative evaluation of a postmenopausal woman with an adnexal mass should be kept to a minimum. With a few exceptions, these patients warrant surgical exploration, and thus, the tests will add little to the preoperative assessment in the vast majority of women.

Expensive scanning and testing should be kept to a minimum, particularly if there is no clinical suspicion that the pelvic tumor is anything other than an adnexal lesion. The yield on computed tomography (CT) and MRI scans is low.
Reference: Pages 1,258–1,259

5. D

These features are each independent variables that have an impact on prognosis. The stage of the disease is highly prognostic, however, within the advanced-stage group, the extent of ascites and the maximum size of the residual disease after cytoreductive surgery correlate with survival. Those patients with stage III disease who have microscopic or small macroscopic (largest tumor diameter <5 mm) disease have a much longer median survival than those patients whose diseases are larger.
Reference: Pages 1,260–1,261, 1,267

Table 32.2. FIGO Staging for Primary Carcinoma of the Ovary

Stage I	Growth limited to the ovaries.	
	Stage Ia	Growth limited to one ovary; no ascites containing malignant cells. No tumor on the external surface; capsule intact.
	Stage Ib	Growth limited to both ovaries; no ascites containing malignant cells. No tumor on the external surfaces; capsules intact.
	Stage Ic[a]	Tumor either stage Ia or Ib but with tumor on the surface of one or both ovaries; or with capsule ruptured; or with ascites present containing malignant cells or with positive peritoneal washings.
Stage II	Growth involving one or both ovaries with pelvic extension.	
	Stage IIa	Extension and/or metastases to the uterus and/or fallopian tubes.
	Stage IIb	Extension to other pelvic tissues.
	Stage IIc[a]	Tumor either stage IIa or IIb but with tumor on the surface of one or both ovaries; or with capsule(s) ruptured; or with ascites present containing malignant cells or with positive peritoneal washings.
Stage III	Tumor involving one or both ovaries with peritoneal implants outside the pelvis and/or positive retroperitoneal or inguinal nodes. Superficial liver metastasis equals stage III. Tumor is limited to the true pelvis, but with histologically proven malignant extension to small bowel or omentum.	
	Stage IIIa	Tumor grossly limited to the true pelvis with negative nodes but with histologically confirmed microscopic seeding of abdominal peritoneal surfaces.
	Stage IIIb	Tumor of one or both ovaries with histologically confirmed implants of abdominal peritoneal surfaces, none exceeding 2 cm in diameter. Nodes negative.
	Stage IIIc	Abdominal implants >2 cm in diameter or positive retroperitoneal or inguinal nodes or both.
Stage IV	Growth involving one or both ovaries with distant metastasis. If pleural effusion is present, there must be positive cytologic test results to allot a case to stage IV. Parenchymal liver metastasis equals stage IV.	

These categories are based on findings at clinical examination or surgical exploration or both. The histologic characteristics are to be considered in the staging, as are results of cytologic testing as far as effusions are concerned. It is desirable that a biopsy be performed on suspicious areas outside the pelvis.
[a]In order to evaluate the impact on prognosis of the different criteria for allotting cases to stage Ic or IIc, it would be of value to know if rupture of the capsule was (a) spontaneous or (b) caused by the surgeon and if the source of malignant cells detected was (a) peritoneal washings or (b) ascites.

6. **C (see Table 32.2)**

   A comprehensive surgical staging should be performed in patients with epithelial ovarian cancer (i.e., a staging laparotomy, including the aspiration of any free peritoneal fluid, obtaining multiple peritoneal washings and peritoneal biopsies, and performing a pelvic and paraaortic lymphadenectomy and an omentectomy). In doing so, about 30% of patients whose disease appears to be confined to the pelvis (apparent stages I and II) will in fact have microscopic evidence of tumor metastasis. About one fifth will have positive lymph node metastasis.
   Reference: Pages 1,261–1,263

7. **D (see Fig 32.9)**

   The role of "debulking" surgery or cytoreductive surgery in advanced-stage epithelial ovarian cancer is to facilitate the response to subsequent chemotherapy and, thus, to improve survival. There are substantial retrospective and limited prospective data that

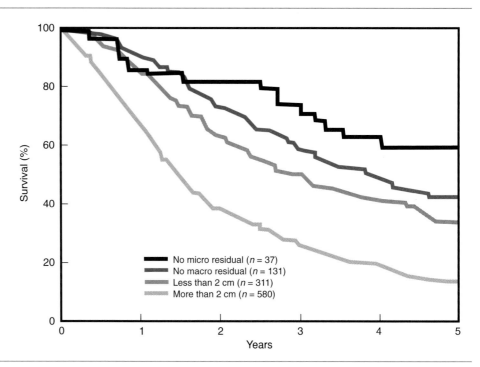

Figure 32.9 Survival of patients with stage IIIc epithelial ovarian cancer based on the maximum size of residual tumor after exploratory laparotomy and tumor resection. (From **Pecoreeli S, Odicino F, Maisonneuve P, et al.** Carcinoma of the ovary: annual report of the results of treatment of gynaecological cancer. *J Epidemiol Biostat* 1998;3:75–102, with permission.)

demonstrate a longer median survival in patients whose disease has been resected so that they have minimal residual, or "optimal" residual, disease at the initiation of or within a few cycles of chemotherapy.
Reference: Pages 1,264–1,267

8. B

Based on large prospective trials, the combination of *carboplatin* plus *paclitaxel* is considered the treatment of choice for stages III and IV epithelial ovarian cancer. These trials compared this treatment to the former standard regimen of *cisplatin* and *paclitaxel*. The survival of the patients was similar for the two regimens, but the toxicity for the carboplatin-containing regimen was lower. The use of these agents in low-stage disease is also being tested.
Reference: Pages 1,272–1,273

9. A

A second-look operation is defined as one performed in a patient who has no clinical evidence of disease after the completion of a planned course of chemotherapy. Such a patient would have a normal CA125, a normal physical examination, and no radiologic evidence of disease. The value of a second-look operation in terms of the prolongation of survival is controversial. Second-look surgery is no longer considered mandatory, but it is used selectively for young patients and those who are on experimental treatment protocols.
Reference: Pages 1,276–1,277

10. C (see Table 32.5)

Germ cell tumors account for about two thirds of all malignancies in the first two decades of life. Epithelial and stromal tumors are less common. Germ cell tumors are rare after the third decade of life.
Reference: Pages 1,282–1,284

Table 32.5. Histologic Typing of Ovarian Germ Cell Tumors

1. Dysgerminoma

2. Teratoma
   A. Immature
   B. Mature
      1) Solid
      2) Cystic
         a. Dermoid cyst (mature cystic teratoma)
         b. Dermoid cyst with malignant transformation
   C. Monodermal and highly specialized
      1) Struma ovarii
      2) Carcinoid
      3) Struma ovarii and carcinoid
      4) Others

3. Endodermal sinus tumor

4. Embryonal carcinoma

5. Polyembryoma

6. Choriocarcinoma

7. Mixed forms

From **Seroy SF, Scully RE, Robin IH.** *Histological typing of ovarian tumors: international histological classification of tumors,* no. 9. Geneva: World Health Organization, 1973, with permission.

11. A (see Fig. 32.14)

Dysgerminomas are frequently bilateral, whereas immature teratomas are rarely bilateral. Endodermal sinus tumors and choriocarcinomas are unilateral lesions. The significance of this issue relates to the need to look for and remove, if necessary, tumors from both ovaries.
Reference: Pages 1,284–1,286

12. D

The surgical management of a unilateral dysgerminoma is the removal of the involved ovary and the performance of a staging laparotomy. These lesions occur in young women for whom the preservation of fertility is important. Because about 5% of dysgerminomas occur in women with dysgenetic ovaries, a karyotype also should be performed.
Reference: Pages 1,286–1,287

13. A (see Fig. 32.17)

The use of combination chemotherapy for women with germ cell tumors is now well established as effective. In addition, this approach permits the preservation of fertility in most of these women because this treatment is given in lieu of radiation therapy that would render the ovary without function.

The BEP combination is the most extensively tested regimen for the treatment of germ cell tumors of the ovary and testes. Three or four cycles appear to be sufficient to produce excellent results and high cure rates.
Reference: Pages 1,287–1,289

14. A

Most patients who present with a diagnosis of immature teratomas have stage I tumors. Within that group, the most important prognostic feature is the extent of immaturity of the elements (i.e., the grade). The element that correlates best with prognosis is the differentiation of the neural tissues.
Reference: Pages 1,290–1,291

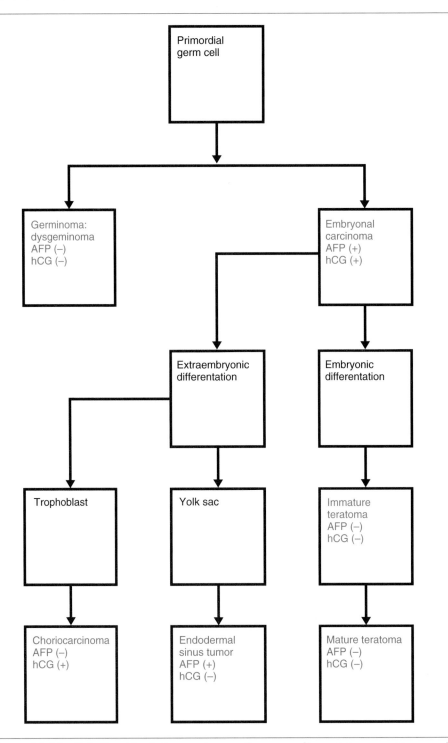

Figure 32.14 Relationship between types of pure malignant tumors. Germ cell tumors and their secreted marker substances. (From **Berek JS, Hacker NF.** *Practical gynecologic oncology.* 3rd ed. Baltimore: Lippincott Williams & Wilkins, 2000:525, with permission.)

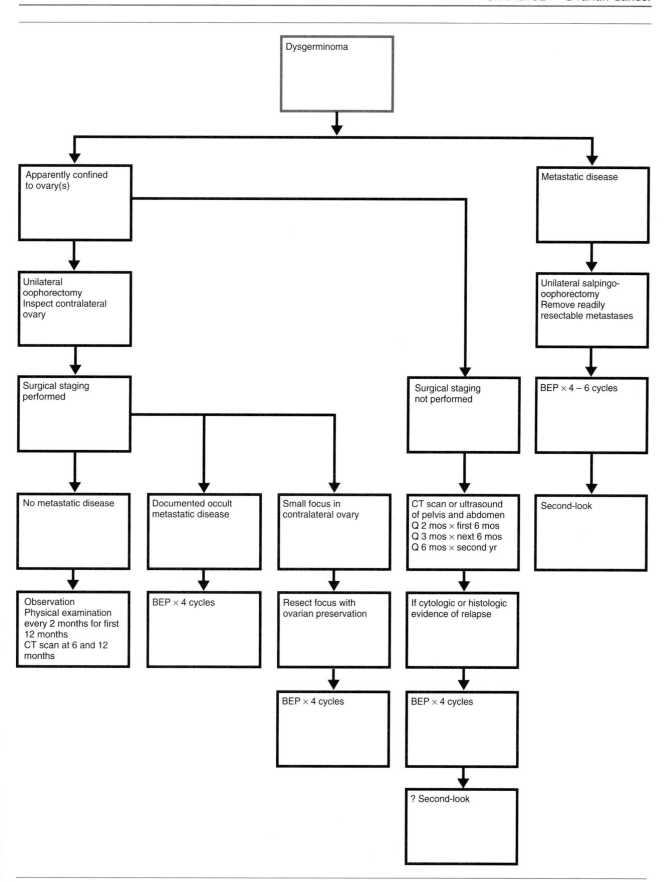

Figure 32.17   Management of dysgerminoma of the ovary. (From **Berek JS, Hacker NF.** *Practical gynecologic oncology.* 3rd ed. Baltimore: Lippincott Williams & Wilkins. 2000:530, with permission.)

15. C

As noted above, in question 8, the treatment of choice in these patients is *carboplatin* and *paclitaxel*.
Reference: Pages 1,272–1,274

16. C

As noted above, in question 13, the BEP regimen is the preferred treatment.
Reference: Pages 1,292–1,293

33

Vulvar Cancer

Christine H. Holschneider
Jonathan S. Berek

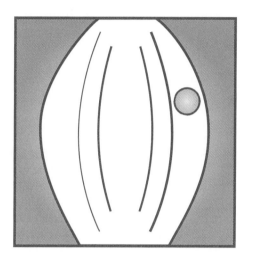

Learning Objectives

1. Know the incidence of and risk factors for invasive vulvar cancer.

2. Understand the histopathology and routes of disease spread, focusing on the implications of lesion size and depth of invasion to lymph node metastasis, which in turn prognosticates patient outcome.

3. Be able to classify patients by the International Federation of Gynecology and Obstetrics (FIGO) surgical staging system.

4. Understand the rationale for individualization of treatment for all patients.

5. Understand the role of conservative surgery, including vulvar conservation, selection of cases for groin dissection, use of separate groin incisions, and elimination of routine pelvic lymphadenectomy.

6. Recognize the role of preoperative radiation to obviate the need for exenteration in patients with advanced disease.

7. Recognize the role of postoperative radiation to decrease the incidence of local groin recurrence in patients with multiple positive groin nodes.

8. Recognize differences in staging and managing patients with vulvar melanoma, as well as treatment of other vulvar malignancies such as Bartholin gland carcinoma, basal cell carcinoma, and vulvar sarcoma.

Questions

1. Risk factors for squamous cell carcinoma of the vulva occurring in patients younger than 50 years include:

   A. Immunosuppression
   B. History of vulvar intraepithelial neoplasia (VIN)
   C. Cigarette smoking
   D. Infection with the human papillomavirus (HPV)
   E. History of other lower genital tract neoplasias
   F. B and D
   G. B, C, and D
   H. A, B, and D
   I. B, D, and E
   J. All of the above

2. A 57-year-old woman has a 3-cm raised papillary lesion at the posterior fourchette, which does not involve the vagina or anus. She has bilateral, palpably enlarged inguinal lymph nodes. Biopsy reveals a squamous cell carcinoma. She undergoes a radical posterior vulvectomy and bilateral inguinofemoral lymphadenectomy. Final pathology reveals a 3-cm, moderately differentiated squamous cell carcinoma. Depth of invasion is 3 mm, resection margins are negative, and the bilateral lymph nodes show no evidence of metastasis. What is the FIGO stage for this patient?

   A. Stage Ia
   B. Stage Ib
   C. Stage II
   D. Stage III
   E. Stage IVa

3. Microinvasive carcinoma of the vulva is an early invasive cancer in which the risk for lymph node metastases is so low that routine lymphadenectomy is not required. This would be defined as a lesion with which of the following characteristics:

   A. Tumor less than 2 cm in diameter with less than 3 mm depth of invasion as measured from the epithelial–stromal junction of the adjacent, most-superficial dermal papilla to the deepest point of invasion.
   B. Tumor less than 2 cm in diameter with less than 1 mm depth of invasion as measured from the epithelial–stromal junction of the adjacent, most-superficial dermal papilla to the deepest point of invasion.
   C. Tumor less than 2 cm in diameter with less than 3-mm tumor thickness as measured from the surface of the tumor epithelium to the deepest point of tumor invasion.
   D. Tumor less than 2 cm in diameter with less than 1-mm tumor thickness as measured from the surface of the tumor epithelium to the deepest point of tumor invasion.
   E. Squamous lesion of the vulva with marked proliferation, numerous mitotic figures, and abnormal maturation of the full-thickness vulvar epithelium with no breakthrough through the basement membrane.

4. Vulvar cancer may spread by direct extension, lymphatic embolization, or hematogenous spread. Which of the following statements regarding lymphatic metastasis is false?

   A. Cloquet's node is the most cephalad of the femoral node group.
   B. Lymphatic drainage of the vulva proceeds from femoral to inguinal to pelvic nodes.
   C. The overall incidence of lymph node metastasis is about 30%.
   D. The incidence of pelvic node metastasis is about 12%.

5. Which of the following lesions would be most appropriately treated by radical local excision alone?

    A. A 2-cm periclitoral lesion with less than 1-mm invasion
    B. A 2-cm right labium minus lesion with less than 1-mm invasion
    C. A 1-cm right labium minus lesion with less than 1-mm invasion in a background of VIN 3
    D. A 1-cm right labium majus lesion with more than 1-mm invasion

6. A squamous cell carcinoma of the vulva located on the right labium majus metastasizes primarily to the following lymph nodes:

    A. Right inguinofemoral lymph nodes
    B. Bilateral inguinofemoral lymph nodes
    C. Pelvic lymph nodes
    D. A and C
    E. B and C

7. A complete inguinofemoral lymphadenectomy carries significant morbidity, especially wound complications and lymphedema. Following appropriate surgery for the primary vulvar lesion, complete inguinofemoral lymphadenectomy can be safely omitted in the following patients with squamous cell carcinoma of the vulva:

    A. Patients with microinvasive carcinoma
    B. Patients with frankly invasive carcinoma if they will instead undergo groin irradiation
    C. Patients with invasive squamous cell carcinoma who had a negative superficial inguinal lymph node dissection
    D. Patients with a T_1 vulvar cancer and palpably normal lymph nodes
    E. All of the above

8. A 67-year-old woman notes a pruritic 3-cm mass on the left labium majus. Radical vulvectomy and bilateral groin lymphadenectomy reveal that two superficial lymph nodes are involved with microscopic disease on the left. Margins of 1 cm are achieved on the primary lesion. The next step in this patient's treatment should involve

    A. Regular examinations and Pap smears every 3 months
    B. Radiation to the site of the primary vulvar lesion
    C. Radiation to the pelvis and bilateral groins
    D. Bilateral pelvic lymph node dissection

9. A 72-year-old woman has a large T_3 lesion involving the lower urethra. Which of the following treatments will provide cure with the least potential for morbidity?

    A. Anterior pelvic exenteration
    B. Radical vulvectomy by *en bloc*/butterfly incision
    C. Radical vulvectomy by separate vulva and groin incisions
    D. Preoperative radiation therapy followed by limited vulvar resection

10. The most common late postoperative complication of inguinofemoral lymphadenectomy is

    A. Recurrent lymphangitis/cellulitis
    B. Chronic leg edema
    C. Femoral hernia
    D. Femoral nerve injury

11. Prognosis and recurrence of vulvar carcinoma both correlate best with

    A. Size of primary tumor
    B. Response of tumor to chemotherapy

C. Number and size of lymph nodes with metastases

D. Preoperative radiation therapy

12. A 78-year-old woman underwent excision of a pigmented vulvar lesion, which revealed melanoma. The tumor was 0.7 cm in diameter, invading to a depth of 1.5 mm from the granular layer, with a tumor thickness of 2 mm. Her disease is best staged as

A. FIGO stage Ia

B. FIGO stage Ib

C. Chung level III

D. Clark level I

E. None of the above

13. Bartholin gland carcinoma may be underdiagnosed if Honan's criteria are strictly followed. Which of the following is not among Honan's criteria?

A. Correct anatomic position

B. Obliteration of normal glandular architecture

C. Overlying skin is intact

D. Tumor is located deep in the labium majus

14. A 49-year-old woman presents with a 3-cm, raised lesion at the posterior fourchette of the vulva. Office biopsy reveals VIN 3. The most appropriate next step in the treatment of this patient is

A. Laser ablation

B. Radical vulvectomy with bilateral inguinofemoral lymphadenectomy

C. Wide local excision

15. Which of the following is the treatment of choice for a large verrucous carcinoma of the vulva with no palpable lymphadenopathy?

A. Radical local excision

B. Radical vulvectomy with bilateral inguinofemoral lymphadenectomy

C. Radiation therapy

D. Radiation therapy with concomitant chemotherapy

Answers

1. **J**

Squamous cell carcinoma of the vulva is of heterogeneous nature, with a bimodal age incidence that is thought to reflect distinct epidemiologic entities. Younger women (average age, 45 years) tend to present with multifocal, VIN-associated disease, which tests HPV-positive in over 90% of cases, and is more common in smokers and patients with immunosuppression. In contrast, squamous cell carcinomas in older women tend to be unifocal and are more frequently associated with lichen sclerosus and squamous hyperplasia.

Reference: Page 1,322

2. **C**

A clinical staging system for vulvar cancer based on the TNM classification was adopted by FIGO in 1969. However, the accuracy of clinical assessment of the lymph node status is poor. Yet, lymph node status is the major prognostic factor for patients with squamous cell carcinoma of the vulva. Therefore, FIGO introduced a surgical staging system in 1988, which was revised in 1995 to its currently used form (see Table 33.4).

Reference: Pages 1,326–1,328

Table 33.4. Revised FIGO Surgical Staging for Vulvar Cancer (36)

FIGO Stage	TNM Classification	Clinical/Pathologic Findings
0	Tis[a]	Carcinoma *in situ*, intraepithelial carcinoma
I	$T_1N_0M_0$	Tumor confined to vulva and/or perineum, ≤ 2 cm in greatest dimension, nodes are negative
Ia[b]		Stromal invasion ≤ 1 mm
Ib		Stromal invasion >1 mm
II	$T_2N_0M_0$	Tumor confined to vulva and/or perineum, >2 cm in greatest dimension, nodes are negative
III	$T_3N_0M_0$ $T_{1-3}N_1M_0$	Tumor of any size with 1. Adjacent spread to lower urethra, vagina, or anus or 2. Unilateral regional lymph node metastases
IVa	$T_4N_{any}M_0$ $T_{any}N_2M_0$	Tumor of any size with 1. Adjacent spread to upper urethra, bladder mucosa, rectal mucosa, pelvic bone or 2. Bilateral regional lymph node metastases
IVb	$T_{any}N_{any}M_1$	Any distant metastases, including pelvic lymph nodes

[a]TNM Classification:

T: Primary tumor
Tx: Primary tumor cannot be assessed
T_0:   No evidence of primary tumor
Tis: Carcinoma *in situ* (preinvasive carcinoma)
T_1:   Tumor confined to the vulva and/or perineum, ≤ 2 cm in greatest dimension
T_2:   Tumor confined to the vulva and/or perineum, >2 cm in greatest dimension
T_3:   Tumor invades any of the following: lower urethra, vagina, anus
T_4:   Tumor invades any of the following: bladder mucosa, rectal mucosa, upper urethra, pelvic bone

N: Regional lymph nodes
       Regional lymph nodes are the femoral and inguinal nodes
Nx   Regional lymph nodes cannot be assessed
N_0 No lymph node metastases
N_1 Unilateral regional lymph node metastases
N_2 Bilateral regional lymph node metastases
M   Distant metastases
Mx   Presence of distant metastases cannot be assessed
M_0 No distant metastases
M_1 Distant metastases (including pelvic lymph node metastases)

[b]The depth of stromal invasion is measured from the epithelial–stromal junction of the adjacent most superficial dermal papilla to the deepest point of invasion.

3. B

The incidence of lymph node metastasis is related to the depth of stromal invasion. As summarized in Table 33.3, when depth of invasion is less than or equal to 1 mm, the incidence of positive nodes is essentially 0%. For depth of invasion 1.1 to 2 mm, 2.1 to 3 mm, 3.1 to 5 mm, and greater than 5 mm, the respective incidences of lymph node metastasis are 7.7%, 8.3%, 26.7%, and 34.2%. Recognition of the substantial increase in the risk of lymph node metastasis with 1- to 2-mm invasion compared to less than 1-mm invasion underscores the importance of adherence to the FIGO definition for microinvasive vulvar cancer and accurate performance of the measurement of depth of invasion. Reference: Page 1,327

Table 33.3. Nodal Status in T_1 Squamous Cell Carcinoma of the Vulva Versus Depth of Stromal Invasion

Depth of Invasion	No.	Positive Nodes	Nodes
≤ 1 mm	163	0	0
1.1–2 mm	145	11	7.7
2.1–3 mm	131	11	8.3
3.1–5 mm	101	27	26.7
>5 mm	38	13	34.2
Total	578	62	10.7

From **Berek JS, Hacker NF.** *Practical gynecologic oncology.* 3rd ed. Philadelphia: Lippincott Williams & Wilkins 2000, pg. 560, with permission.

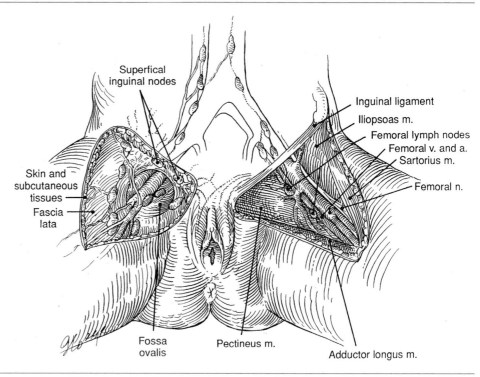

Figure 33.3   Inguinofemoral lymph nodes.

4. B

Lymphatics of the vulva drain first to the superficial inguinal or groin nodes, then to the femoral nodes along the femoral vessels, which in turn drain to the pelvic lymph node chain (see Fig. 33.3). Cloquet's node is the most cephalad of the femoral node group; this is the last node involved before the pelvic lymph nodes.
Reference: Page 1,326

5. B

Radical local excision is advocated for lesions on the lateral or posterior vulva. Local recurrence rates are comparable to those of radical vulvectomy. In periclitoral lesions, alternative treatment with radiation can reduce psychosocial consequences. In cancer arising from a field of VIN, additional superficial local excision beyond radical local excision may be required for the noninvasive component. Regardless of lesion size, all patients with stromal invasion of more than 1 mm require groin node dissection.
Reference: Pages 1,329–1,330

6. A

A lateralized lesion on the vulva metastasizes primarily to the ipsilateral inguinofemoral lymph nodes. Involvement of the contralateral groin nodes or pelvic nodes is extremely rare unless the ipsilateral groin nodes are involved. This has implications for a patient's surgery: Patients with a lateralized lesion can be primarily treated with a radical local excision and ipsilateral inguinofemoral lymphadenectomy, whereas patients with midline lesions require bilateral groin dissections.
Reference: Pages 1,326–1,328

7. A

The only patient with virtually no risk of lymph node metastasis is the one whose tumor invades the stroma to less than 1 mm. All other patients require full inguinofemoral lymphadenectomy. Neither superficial lymphadenectomy nor groin irradiation can substitute for a complete groin dissection. Intraoperative lymphatic mapping for the detection

of the sentinel lymph node is an appealing concept; however, the technique remains to be assessed in large clinical trials.
Reference: Pages 1,327, 1,332

8. C

The presence of one microscopically positive groin node does not worsen prognosis or survival. With two or more microscopically positive nodes or one grossly positive node, groin irradiation improves survival and provides local control of disease recurrence. There are no data to suggest benefit of pelvic radiation over pelvic lymphadenectomy. Enlarged pelvic nodes should be removed because radiation will not cure bulky nodal disease. Postoperative radiation to the vulvar primary site may prevent local recurrence in patients with positive or close (<5 mm) surgical margins.
Reference: Pages 1,332–1,333

9. D

To treat a large primary vulvar cancer involving the urethra, rectovaginal septum, anus, or rectum, radical vulvectomy alone is insufficient to obtain adequate surgical margins. Morbidity from pelvic exenteration surgery can be avoided by combining preoperative radiation with a more limited vulvar resection. If persistent disease is present following preoperative teletherapy, brachytherapy can potentially reduce tumor volume further to minimize the need for radical surgery. Based on limited data on the vulva and extrapolating from data on cervical cancer, radiation therapy should generally be given with concomitant platinum-based chemotherapy.
Reference: Pages 1,334–1,335

10. B

Even with the three incision techniques, approximately 30% of patients will have chronic leg edema. Full groin dissection combined with groin irradiation often results in severe leg edema. About 10% of patients will have recurrent lymphangitis or leg cellulitis. Femoral hernia is an uncommon late complication. Femoral nerve injury is noted as an early postoperative complication and resolves slowly over time.
Reference: Page 1,334

11. C

The number of positive groin lymph nodes is the most important prognostic variable for recurrent disease and survival. If three or more groin lymph nodes are positive for metastatic disease, a high incidence of disease recurrence and a poor prognosis exist. Patients with N_0 or N_1 lesions are reported to have a 78% 2-year survival compared to patients with N_2 or N_3 lesions, who have 52% and 33% 2-year survivals, respectively. Local recurrence is more likely if the primary lesion is greater than 4 cm in size, although this can be treated by further surgical excision. Tumor ploidy also appears to have prognostic implication for survival.
Reference: Page 1,336

12. C

The most significant prognostic factor for patients with vulvar melanoma is the microscopic depth of invasion. There are various microstaging classifications for vulvar melanoma (see Table 33.6). The staging systems used most frequently for the vulva are Chung tumor levels and Breslow tumor thickness. Vulvar melanoma is not staged by the FIGO criteria for vulvar carcinoma.
Reference: Pages 1,339–1,340

13. B

The best criterion to classify a vulvar tumor as a Bartholin gland carcinoma is the transition of normal and malignant tissue. Some recognizable normal gland should be identifiable to clearly characterize a Bartholin gland carcinoma. The deep location of

Table 33.6. Microstaging of Vulvar Melanoma

	Clark Level (117)	Chung Depth of Invasion (115)	Breslow Tumor Thickness (118)
I	Intraepithelial	Intraepithelial	<0.76 mm
II	Into papillary dermis	<1 mm from granular layer	0.76–1.5 mm Superficial invasion
III	Filling dermal papillae	1.1–2.0 mm from granular layer	1.51–2.25 mm Intermediate invasion
IV	Into reticular dermis	>2 mm from granular layer	2.26–3.0 mm Intermediate invasion
V	Into subcutaneous fat	Into subcutaneous fat	>3 mm Deep invasion

the gland may result in delay of diagnosis and necessitate extensive dissection, but stage for stage, prognosis is similar.
Reference: Pages 1,340–1,341

14. C

A reported 10% to 20% of apparent vulvar carcinomas *in situ* harbor an occult invasive component. Preferred treatment of defined VIN 3 lesions, especially if clinically suspicious, should therefore be wide local excision, which produces a specimen for additional histologic evaluation. Laser ablation is adequate therapy for VIN 3 in which colposcopic, histologic evaluations reveal no evidence of invasive disease, and the clinical suspicion is low. Laser ablation is frequently the preferred therapy for biopsy-confirmed periclitoral or perianal VIN 3 lesions.
Reference: Pages 1,324–1,325

15. A

Verrucous carcinoma of the vulva is a variant of squamous cell carcinoma that has been linked to HPV-6 or -11. It is characterized by an exophytic, papillary, or cauliflowerlike lesion. Microscopically, there is invasion in a broad, pushing front, cellular atypia is minimal, and mitoses are few. These tumors are slow-growing and locally invasive. Lymph node metastases are rare. There is no therapeutic benefit to radiation and there are several anecdotal cases in the literature that indicate that radiation may induce an anaplastic transformation in these lesions. There are no data to support the use of chemotherapy in verrucous carcinoma of the vulva.
Reference: Pages 1,343–1,344

34

Gestational Trophoblastic Disease

Ross S. Berkowitz
Donald P. Goldstein

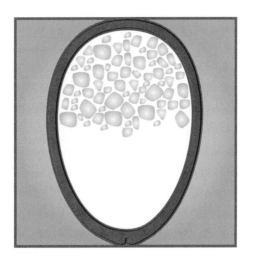

Learning Objectives

1. Understand the histopathologic and cytogenetic differences between complete and partial hydatidiform moles.

2. Understand the natural history of gestational trophoblastic diseases.

3. Understand the principles of management of persistent gestational trophoblastic tumors.

4. Understand later reproductive outcome in patients who are successfully treated for gestational trophoblastic diseases.

Questions

1. Complete molar pregnancy most frequently has the following chromosomal pattern:

   A. 46,XX—One set of paternal chromosomes, one set of maternal chromosomes
   B. 46,XX—Two sets of maternal chromosomes
   C. 46,XX—Two sets of paternal chromosomes
   D. 69,XXY (triploid)—Two sets of maternal chromosomes, one set of paternal chromosomes
   E. 69,XXY (triploid)—One set of maternal chromosomes, two sets of paternal chromosomes

2. Partial molar pregnancy most frequently has the following chromosomal pattern:

   A. 46,XX—One set of paternal chromosomes, one set of maternal chromosomes
   B. 46,XX—Two sets of maternal chromosomes
   C. 46,XX—Two sets of paternal chromosomes
   D. 69,XXY (triploid)—Two sets of maternal chromosomes, one set of paternal chromosomes
   E. 69,XXY (triploid)—One set of maternal chromosomes, two sets of paternal chromosomes

3. The most common site of metastasis in persistent gestational trophoblastic tumor is the

   A. Vagina
   B. Brain
   C. Lung
   D. Liver
   E. Kidney

4. Classical pathologic features of a complete mole include:

   A. Fetal and embryonic tissues
   B. Marked scalloping of chorionic villi
   C. Stromal trophoblastic inclusions
   D. Diffuse swelling of chorionic villi with diffuse trophoblastic hyperplasia
   E. Fetal anomalies consistent with triploidy

5. Pathologic features of partial molar pregnancy include:

   A. Diffuse swelling of chorionic villi
   B. Diffuse trophoblastic hyperplasia
   C. Prominent growth of intermediate trophoblast
   D. Prominent hyaline debris
   E. Fetal and embryonic tissues

6. Following a complete molar pregnancy, about what percentage of patients develop persistent tumor?

   A. 4%
   B. 10%
   C. 20%
   D. 30%
   E. 40%

7. Following a partial molar pregnancy, about what percentage of patients develop persistent tumor?

   A. 4%
   B. 10%

C. 20%

D. 30%

E. 40%

8. Patients with complete mole who have high human chorionic gonadotropin (hCG) levels and excessive uterine size may develop all of the following medical complications **except**

    A. Theca–lutein ovarian cysts

    B. Nephrotic syndrome

    C. Hyperthyroidism

    D. Toxemia

    E. Respiratory insufficiency

9. Following chemotherapy, patients with persistent gestational trophoblastic disease may in general expect in later pregnancy a

    A. Higher incidence of congenital anomalies

    B. Higher incidence of spontaneous abortion

    C. Normal reproductive outcome

    D. Lower fertility

    E. Higher incidence of prematurity

10. Patients with low-risk metastatic gestational trophoblastic disease with pulmonary metastasis may be appropriately treated with

    A. Lung resection

    B. Intensive combination chemotherapy with *methotrexate, actinomycin D,* and *etoposide*

    C. Single-agent chemotherapy with *methotrexate* or *actinomycin D*

    D. Radiation therapy

    E. *Paclitaxel* and *carboplatin*

11. Which of the following statements about vaginal metastases in patients with gestational trophoblastic tumors is not true?

    A. Arteriographic embolization may control bleeding effectively.

    B. Vaginal metastases should be biopsied to confirm the diagnosis.

    C. Vaginal metastases may develop after a complete molar pregnancy.

    D. Vaginal metastases may be cured with chemotherapy, including single-agent chemotherapy, when tumors are small.

    E. Vaginal metastases develop in about 30% of patients with metastatic disease.

12. Which of the following statements about brain metastases in patients with gestational trophoblastic tumors is not true?

    A. Brain metastases require treatment with intensive combination chemotherapy.

    B. Brain metastases frequently occur in the absence of pulmonary involvement.

    C. Brain metastases may be treated with whole-brain irradiation as part of treatment.

    D. Craniotomy may need to be performed to control bleeding or provide acute decompression.

    E. Brain metastases tend to occur in patients with far-advanced disease.

Answers

1. **C (see Fig. 34.2)**

    Cytogenetic studies have demonstrated that complete hydatidiform moles usually have a 46,XX karyotype, and the molar chromosomes are entirely of paternal origin. It

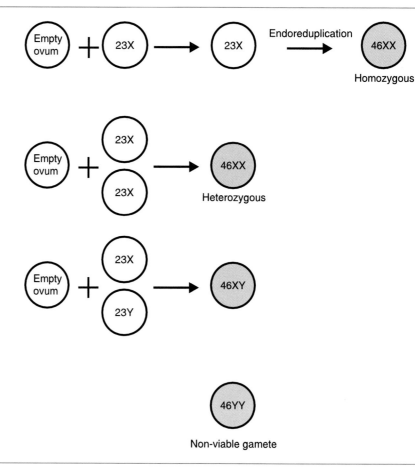

Figure 34.2   The karyotype of complete hydatidiform mole.

appears that complete moles usually arise from an ovum that has been fertilized by a haploid sperm, which then duplicates its own chromosomes. The ovum nucleus may be either absent or inactivated.
Reference: Page 1,355

2. E

Partial moles generally have a triploid karyotype (69 chromosomes); the extra haploid set of chromosomes usually is derived from the father (see Fig. 34.4). One study reported that 93% of partial moles were triploid whereas another found 90% to be triploid.
Reference: Page 1,355

3. C

The most common sites of metastases are the lungs (80%), vagina (30%), pelvis (20%), liver (10%), and brain (10%).
Reference: Page 1,362

4. D

Complete moles lack identifiable embryonic or fetal tissues, and the chorionic villi exhibit generalized hydatidiform swelling and diffuse trophoblastic hyperplasia (see Fig. 34.1).
Reference: Page 1,354

5. E

Partial hydatidiform moles are characterized by the following pathologic features (see Fig. 34.3):

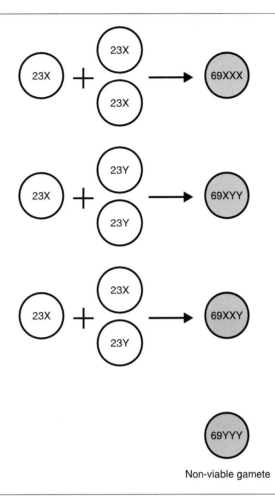

Figure 34.4   The karyotype of partial hydatidiform mole.

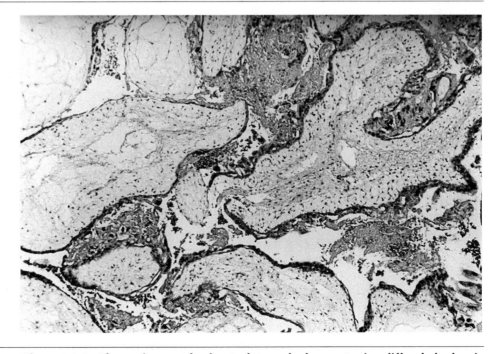

Figure 34.1   Photomicrograph of complete mole demonstrating diffusely hydropic chorionic villi and diffuse trophoblastic hyperplasia.

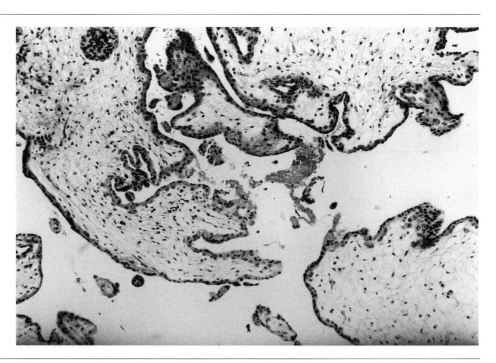

Figure 34.3 **Photomicrograph of partial mole showing varying-sized chorionic villi with focal trophoblastic hyperplasia, stromal trophoblastic inclusions, and villous scalloping.** (From **Berkowitz RS, Goldstein OP.** Gestational trophoblastic diseases. In: **Ryan KJ, Berkowitz R, Barbieri R,** eds. *Kistner's gynecology principles and practice,* 5th ed. Chicago: Year Book Medical Publishers, 1990:433, with permission.)

1. Chorionic villi of varying size with focal hydatidiform swelling, cavitation, and trophoblastic hyperplasia
2. Marked villous scalloping
3. Prominent stromal trophoblastic inclusions
4. Identifiable embryonic or fetal tissues

Reference: Pages 1,355–1,356

6. C

Complete moles have a potential for local invasion and dissemination. After molar evacuation, local uterine invasion occurs in 15% of patients and metastases occur in 4%.
Reference: Page 1,359

7. A

Persistent tumor, usually nonmetastatic, develops in approximately 4% of patients with a partial mole, and chemotherapy is required to achieve remission. Patients who develop persistent disease have no distinguishing clinical or pathologic characteristics.
Reference: Page 1,359

8. B

Patients with complete mole, high hCG levels, and excessive uterine size may develop medical complications including toxemia, theca–lutein ovarian cysts, hyperthyroidism, hyperemesis, and respiratory insufficiency. Theca–lutein ovarian cysts result from hyperstimulation by high serum hCG levels.
Reference: Page 1,358

9. C

Patients with gestational trophoblastic tumor who are treated successfully with chemotherapy can expect normal reproduction in the future. It is particularly reassuring that the frequency of congenital anomalies is not increased.
Reference: Page 1,366

10. C

Of 143 patients treated with stage III (pulmonary) disease, 142 (99%) attained complete remission. Gonadotropin remission was induced with single-agent chemotherapy (*methotrexate* or *actinomycin D*) in 80 (82.5%) of 97 patients with low-risk disease. All patients who were resistant to single-agent treatment subsequently achieved remission with combination chemotherapy.
Reference: Page 1,366

11. B

Vaginal metastases occurs in 30% of patients with metastatic tumor. These lesions are usually highly vascular and may bleed vigorously if biopsied.
Reference: Page 1,366

12. B

Metastatic trophoblastic disease involves the brain in 10% of patients. Cerebral involvement is generally seen in patients with advanced disease; virtually all patients with brain metastases have concurrent pulmonary or vaginal involvement or both.
Reference: Page 1,367

35

Breast Cancer

Armando E. Giuliano
Dean T. Nora

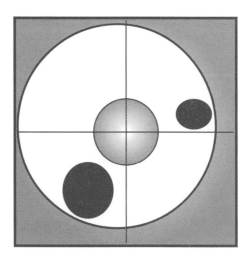

Learning Objectives

1. Know the risk factors for development of breast cancer.

2. Be aware of the methods used to diagnose breast cancer.

3. Be cognizant of the TNM classification for staging breast cancer.

4. Understand the appropriate steps in the preoperative evaluation of breast cancer.

5. Know the treatment options for breast cancer, including the advantages and disadvantages of each.

6. Be aware of the prognosis for different forms of breast cancer.

Questions

1. Which of the following is true regarding risk factors for breast cancer?

    A. Most women who develop breast cancer have a family history.
    B. Having a sister who developed breast cancer postmenopausally significantly increases the risk of personally developing breast cancer.
    C. Menstrual irregularity is clearly an associated risk factor.
    D. Nulliparity increases the risk of breast cancer.

2. Which of the following is true regarding estrogen replacement therapy?

    A. Significantly increases the risk of breast cancer development if used less than 5 years.
    B. Should be discouraged in postmenopausal women.
    C. Can reduce the risk of osteoporosis and heart disease.
    D. Is best given continuously and without progestins.

3. Breast cancer most commonly arises in the

    A. Upper inner quadrant
    B. Lower inner quadrant
    C. Lower outer quadrant
    D. Upper outer quadrant

4. Screening mammography

    A. Contributes to improved survival in women younger than 40 years
    B. Is complementary with physical exam because 10% to 20% of palpable lesions are not seen mammographically.
    C. Along with ultrasound is a standard screening tool for breast cancer.
    D. Is much more sensitive than magnetic resonance imaging (MRI) for the detection of small lesions.

5. Which of the following statements is true regarding breast masses?

    A. Ninety percent of clinically benign masses will be proved benign by biopsy.
    B. Fine-needle aspiration (FNA) is exquisitely sensitive in detecting carcinoma in palpable masses, helps with planning, and has a 0% false-positive rate.
    C. Breast masses can be followed for one or two menstrual cycles if clinically benign in premenopausal women.
    D. When cytology is negative based on FNA, breast masses are considered benign and can be ignored, even in postmenopausal women.

6. Biopsy is indicated in which of the following situations?

    A. A bloody FNA of a palpable mass
    B. A clear aspirate on three occasions of a persistent breast mass
    C. Equivocal findings on FNA of a palpable mass
    D. A palpable mass in a postmenopausal woman
    E. All of the above

7. Which of the following subtypes of breast cancer has the most favorable prognosis?

    A. Medullary
    B. Intraductal
    C. Lobular
    D. Tubular
    E. Papillary

8. A patient with a newly diagnosed breast cancer (5 cm) should have the following tests performed initially **except**

    A. Bone scan
    B. Serum chemistries, including liver function tests
    C. Computed tomography (CT) scan of the chest, abdomen, and pelvis
    D. Chest x-ray
    E. Complete blood count

9. A patient with breast cancer and clinically negative axilla on physical examination undergoing axillary dissection

    A. Has up to a 20% to 30% risk of chronic lymphedema
    B. Will harbor metastasis in two thirds of cases
    C. Should be treated staged with level 1 lymph node sampling
    D. Has a 5% risk of acute complications other than lymphedema

10. Which of the following patients is an appropriate candidate for adjuvant, cytotoxic chemotherapy?

    A. 75-year-old woman with a 1.1-cm ductal carcinoma, estrogen receptor (ER)– and progesterone receptor (PR)–positive, and 0/10 positive lymph nodes
    B. 30-year-old woman with a 0.5-cm lobular carcinoma and 0/8 positive lymph nodes
    C. 70-year-old woman with a 2-cm ER/PR-positive tubular carcinoma and 0/12 positive lymph nodes
    D. 45-year-old man with a 4-cm ductal carcinoma who refuses axillary lymph node sampling

11. The prognosis of a patient with Paget's disease of the breast is most dependent on

    A. The extent of nipple/areolar involvement
    B. Size of the lesion
    C. The associated histologic type of neoplasm

12. *Tamoxifen*

    A. Should be given before cytotoxic chemotherapy and continued afterward.
    B. Reduces the incidence of hot flashes
    C. Decreases the risk of thromboembolic events
    D. Decreases the risk of contralateral breast cancer by up to 50%

13. Inflammatory breast cancer is best treated by

    A. Immediate radical mastectomy
    B. Immediate modified radical mastectomy
    C. Antibiotic therapy initially, followed by surgery
    D. Systemic chemotherapy and radiation therapy followed by salvage mastectomy in select patients

14. All of the following approaches are reasonable therapeutic alternatives for lobular carcinoma *in situ* (LCIS) **except**

    A. *Tamoxifen*
    B. Bilateral mastectomy
    C. Lumpectomy and close observation
    D. Radiation therapy

15. Regarding ductal carcinoma *in situ* (DCIS), which of the following statements is true?

    A. Metastases occur frequently enough to warrant axillary dissection.
    B. It should not be considered a malignancy and does not pose a risk for local recurrence; simple excision with clear margins is adequate therapy.

C. Modified radical mastectomy is a surgical option.

D. It is most common in premenopausal women.

16. Regarding breast cancer in pregnancy, which of the following is true?

A. Radiation therapy cannot be given in the second trimester.

B. Lactation should be suppressed postpartum.

C. Chemotherapy should be administered only after delivery.

D. Subsequent pregnancies should be clearly discouraged in early-stage breast cancer survivors because there is an associated decrease in 5- and 10- year survival rates.

Answers

1. D

Only 20% to 30% of women who develop breast cancer have a family history. Factors that significantly increase risk include nulliparity, personal history of colon or ovarian cancer, early menarche, late menopause, and use of exogenous estrogens over a prolonged period. Having a family member who develops breast cancer postmenopausally does not significantly increase risk. Menstrual irregularity has not been shown to be an associated risk factor.
Reference: Page 1,375

2. C

Estrogen replacement therapy has been shown to increase the risk of breast cancer especially if used over a prolonged period (>10 years). The risk increases if estrogens are not given cyclically or used in conjunction with progestins. The benefits of estrogen replacement therapy such as reductions in bone loss, death from heart disease, and hot flash episodes must be taken into careful consideration.
Reference: Page 1,376

3. D

Breast cancer most commonly arises in the upper outer quadrant. This fact can be partially explained by the fact that there is more breast tissue in this quadrant than in the other quadrants.
Reference: Page 1,377

4. B

Screening mammography is recommended for women older than 40 years. Some women with significant risk factors may be considered for screening at an earlier age. Ultrasound is complementary to mammography but should not be used as a screening tool. Magnetic resonance imaging (MRI) is exquisitely sensitive but has a considerable false-positive rate.
Reference: Page 1,377

5. C

Up to 25% of clinically benign breast masses will be proved malignant with biopsy. FNA is an extremely sensitive diagnostic tool and should be considered as the initial diagnostic modality in palpable masses. However, there is a small but appreciable false-positive rate. Breast masses can be followed carefully for one or two menstrual cycles especially in younger women because a number will regress. Most breast masses in postmenopausal women should be considered malignant until proved otherwise. An equivocal finding on FNA should prompt the use of other biopsy modalities.
Reference: Page 1,378

6. E

FNA can help guide the management of a breast mass. Aspiration of clear or green fluid and subsequent resolution of the mass prevents unnecessary biopsy. If the aspirate is bloody or solid, biopsy is unwarranted. Failure of the mass to resolve after multiple aspirations is also an indication for biopsy. Again, masses in postmenopausal women should elicit a high index of suspicion.
Reference: Page 1,378

7. D

Tubular carcinomas, although uncommon, are well-differentiated tumors with a very favorable prognosis. Lymph node metastasis can still occur, albeit rarely.
Reference: Pages 1,379–1,380

8. C

This patient clearly has a T_2 lesion. A bone scan as well as routine laboratory studies, including liver function tests, complete blood count, and chest x-ray, should be performed. If there is elevation in liver enzymes or abnormalities on chest x-ray, a CT scan can then be ordered to complete staging. There is no role for tumor markers such as cancer antigen 125 (CA125), carcinoembryonic antigen (CEA), or CA27-29 as screening tests. Bilateral diagnostic mammography should always be performed when a breast mass is present.
Reference: Page 1,381

9. A

The risk of chronic lymphedema is significant in women undergoing axillary dissection for breast cancer. This risk is increased with the addition of radiation therapy. Additionally, there is an up to 20% risk of acute complications such as bleeding, infection, or wound problems. Limited lymph node sampling has a high false-negative rate and should be discouraged. A formal level 1 and 2 dissection should be performed. Only one third of patients will be found to have nodal disease. This underscores the utility of sentinel lymph node dissection in the staging of disease.
Reference: Pages 1,383–1,386

10. D

Lymph node metastasis is a significant contributor to risk of death. Most premenopausal women who have positive lymph nodes, regardless of the characteristics of the primary lesion, are offered adjuvant chemotherapy. That is not to say that other characteristics of the primary tumor are not important. Most patients with tumors that are larger than 1 cm or hormone-unresponsive should be considered for adjuvant chemotherapy. For postmenopausal women, adjuvant cytotoxic chemotherapy is about one half as effective as tamoxifen in hormone responsive disease. The risks of chemotherapy must be weighed carefully.
Reference: Page 1,387

11. C

The prognosis of a patient with Paget's disease of the breast is most reliant on the histologic type of neoplasm. Paget's disease is simply involvement of the nipple areolar complex with tumor. Treatment is usually mastectomy or central resection of the nipple and areolar complex.
Reference: Pages 1,391–1,392

12. D

Tamoxifen is effective in reducing the incidence of contralateral breast cancer by up to 50%. There are associated risks of *tamoxifen,* such as increased incidence of hot flashes, vaginal dryness, and thromboembolic events. When used in conjunction with adjuvant chemotherapy, tamoxifen is typically given last.
Reference: Pages 1,389–1,391

13. D

Inflammatory breast cancer is an aggressive form that is best treated initially with high-dose chemotherapy, with or without radiation for control. Immediate mastectomy will lead to a high local recurrence rate. Salvage mastectomy can be performed after chemotherapy is given.
Reference: Page 1,392

14. D

LCIS or lobular neoplasia is not considered a malignancy but rather a marker for risk of developing breast cancer. The risk is bilateral and can include both ductal and lobular forms of cancer. Some women request bilateral mastectomy and this procedure can be performed in special circumstances, especially in high-risk patients. Tamoxifen can reduce the risk of breast cancer in the ipsilateral and the contralateral breasts and is a reasonable option. There is no role for radiation therapy in this tumor type.
Reference: Page 1,392

15. C

DCIS should be considered a premalignant lesion. There is a small risk of lymph node metastasis, but it does not warrant axillary dissection. The role of sentinel node dissection remains to be determined, but studies are ongoing. DCIS should be managed with wide excision to clear margins and mammographic microcalcifications. Postoperative radiation has been shown to reduce the local recurrence rate. Local recurrence can be DCIS or frank carcinoma. For patients with diffuse or multifocal disease, modified radical mastectomy is a reasonable option.
Reference: Pages 1,392–1,393

16. B

Radiation therapy can be given safely as long as the fetus is shielded. It should be discouraged in the first trimester. For patients with high-risk lesions, chemotherapy can be given during the second and third trimesters. Future pregnancies have not been shown to adversely affect survival. In some studies, women with subsequent pregnancies actually fared better. The present data are insufficient to support recommendations to discourage future pregnancies.
Reference: Pages 1,393–1,394

Appendix I: Preventive Health Care by Age Groups

Table 8.3. Periodic Assessment Ages 13–18 Years

Screening	*Evaluation and Counseling*
History	**Sexuality**
Reason for visit	Development
Health status: medical, surgical, family	High-risk behaviors
Dietary/nutrition assessment	Preventing unwanted/unintended pregnancy
Physical activity	—Postponing sexual involvement
Use of complementary and alternative medicine	—Contraceptive options
Tobacco, alcohol, other drug use	Sexually transmitted diseases
Abuse/neglect	—Partner selection
Sexual practices	—Barrier protection
Physical examination	**Fitness and nutrition**
Height	Dietary/nutrition assessment (including eating disorders)
Weight	Exercise: discussion of program
Blood pressure	Folic acid supplementation (0.4 mg/d)
Secondary sexual characteristics (Tanner staging)	Calcium intake
Pelvic examination (yearly when sexually active or beginning at age 18 years) Skin[a]	
Laboratory testing	**Psychosocial evaluation**
Periodic	
Pap testing (yearly when sexually active or beginning at age 18 years)	Interpersonal/family relationships
	Sexual identity
	Personal goal development
	Behavioral/learning disorders
	Abuse/neglect
	Satisfactory school experience
	Peer relationships
High-risk groups [a]	**Cardiovascular risk factors**
Hemoglobin level assessment	Family history
Bacteriuria testing	Hypertension
Sexually transmitted disease testing	Dyslipidemia
Human immunodeficiency virus testing	Obesity
Genetic testing/counseling	Diabetes mellitus
Rubella titer assessment	

Table 8.3. — *continued*

Tuberculosis skin testing

Lipid profile assessment

Fasting glucose testing

Cholesterol testing

Hepatitis C virus testing

Colorectal cancer screening[b]

	Health/risk behaviors
	Hygiene (including dental); fluoride supplementation
	Injury prevention
	—Safety belts and helmets
	—Recreational hazards
	—Firearms
	—Hearing
	Skin exposure to ultraviolet rays
	Suicide: depressive symptoms
	Tobacco, alcohol, other drug use

[a]See Table 8.7.

[b]Only for those with a family history of familial adenomatous polyposis or 8 years after the start of pancolitis. For a more detailed discussion of colorectal cancer screening, see **Byers T, Levin B, Rothenberger D, et al.** American Cancer Society guidelines for screening and surveillance for early detection of colorectal polyps and cancer: update 1997. American Cancer Society Detection and Treatment Advisory Group on Colorectal Cancer. *CA Cancer J Clin 1997;*47:154–160.

From American College of Obstetricians and Gynecologists Committee on Gynecologic Practice. Primary and preventive care: periodic assessments Washington, DC: ACOG; 2000; Committee Opinion No. 246, with permission.

Table 8.4. Periodic Assessment Ages 19–39 Years

Screening	*Evaluation and Counseling*
History	**Sexuality**
Reason for visit	High-risk behaviors
Health status: medical, surgical, family	Contraceptive options for prevention of unwanted pregnancy
Dietary/nutrition assessment	Preconceptional and genetic counseling for desired pregnancy
Physical activity	Sexually transmitted diseases
Use of complementary and alternative medicine	—Partner selection
Tobacco, alcohol, other drug use	—Barrier protection
Abuse/neglect	Sexual function
Sexual practices	
Urinary and fecal incontinence	
Physical examination	**Fitness and nutrition**
Height	Dietary/nutrition assessment
Weight	Exercise: discussion of program
Blood pressure	Folic acid supplementation (0.4 mg/d)
Neck: adenopathy, thyroid	Calcium intake
Breasts	
Abdomen	
Pelvic examination	
Skin[a]	
Laboratory testing	**Psychosocial evaluation**
Periodic	
Pap testing (physician and patient discretion after three consecutive normal tests if low risk)	Interpersonal/family relationships
	Domestic violence
	Work satisfaction
	Lifestyle/stress
	Sleep disorders
High-risk groups [a]	**Cardiovascular risk factors**
Hemoglobin level assessment	Family history
Bacteriuria testing	Hypertension
Mammography	Dyslipidemia
Fasting glucose testing	Obesity
Cholesterol testing	Diabetes mellitus
Sexually transmitted disease testing	Lifestyle
Human immunodeficiency virus testing	
Genetic testing/counseling	

Table 8.4. — *continued*

Rubella titer assessment	
Tuberculosis skin testing	
Lipid profile assessment	
Thyroid-stimulating hormone testing	
Colonoscopy	
Hepatitis C virus testing	
Colorectal cancer screening	
	Health/risk behaviors
	Hygiene (including dental)
	Injury prevention
	—Safety belts and helmets
	—Occupational hazards
	—Recreational hazards
	—Firearms
	—Hearing
	Breast self-examination
	Chemoprophylaxis for breast cancer (for high-risk women ages 35 years or older)[b]
	Skin exposure to ultraviolet rays
	Suicide: depressive symptoms
	Tobacco, alcohol, other drug use

[a]See Table 8.7.

[b]The decision to use tamoxifen should be individualized. For a more detailed discussion of risk assessment and chemoprevention therapy, see American College of Obstetricians and Gynecologists. Tamoxifen and the prevention of breast cancer in high-risk women. ACOG Committee Opinion 224. Washington, DC: ACOG, 1999.

From American College of Obstetricians and Gynecologists Committee on Gynecologic Practice. Primary and preventive care: periodic assessments Washington, DC: ACOG; 2000; Committee Opinion No. 246, with permission.

Table 8.5. Periodic Assessment Ages 40–64 Years

Screening	*Evaluation and Counseling*
History	**Sexuality**[b]
Reason for visit	High-risk behaviors
Health status: medical, surgical, family	Contraceptive options for prevention of unwanted pregnancy
Dietary/nutrition assessment	Sexually transmitted diseases
Physical activity	—Partner selection
Use of complementary and alternative medicine	—Barrier protection
Tobacco, alcohol, other drug use	Sexual functioning
Abuse/neglect	
Sexual practices	
Urinary and fecal incontinence	
Physical examination	**Fitness and nutrition**
Height	Dietary/nutrition assessment
Weight	Exercise: discussion of program
Blood pressure	Folic acid supplementation (0.4 mg/d before age 50 years)
Oral cavity	Calcium intake
Neck: adenopathy, thyroid	
Breasts, axillae	
Abdomen	
Pelvic examination	
Skin[a]	
Laboratory testing	**Psychosocial evaluation**
Periodic	
Pap testing (physician and patient discretion after three consecutive normal tests if low risk)	Family relationships
Mammography (every 1–2 years until age 50 years, yearly beginning at age 50 years)	Domestic violence
Cholesterol testing (every 5 years beginning at age 45 years)	Work satisfaction
Yearly fecal occult blood testing plus flexible sigmoidoscopy every 5 years *or* colonoscopy every 10 years *or* double contrast barium enema (DCBE) every 5–10 years, with digital rectal examination performed at the time of each screening sigmoidoscopy, colonoscopy, or DCBE (beginning at age 50 years)	Retirement planning
Fasting glucose testing (every 3 years after age 45 years)	Lifestyle/stress
	Sleep disorders

Table 8.5.—continued

High-risk groups[a]	Cardiovascular risk factors
Hemoglobin level assessment	Family history
Bacteriuria testing	Hypertension
Fasting glucose testing	Dyslipidemia
Sexually transmitted disease testing	Obesity
Human immunodeficiency virus testing	Diabetes mellitus
Tuberculosis skin testing	Lifestyle
Lipid profile assessment	
Thyroid-stimulating hormone testing	
Colonoscopy	
Hepatitis C virus testing	
Colorectal cancer screening	
	Health/risk behaviors
	Hygiene (including dental)
	Hormone replacement therapy
	Injury prevention
	—Safety belts and helmets
	—Occupational hazards
	—Recreational hazards
	—Sports involvement
	—Firearms
	—Hearing
	Breast self-examination
	Chemoprophylaxis for breast cancer (for high-risk women)[c]
	Skin exposure to ultraviolet rays
	Suicide: depressive symptoms
	Tobacco, alcohol, other drug use

[a]See Table 8.7.

[b]Preconceptional and genetic counseling is appropriate for certain women in this age group.

[c]The decision to use tamoxifen should be individualized. For a more detailed discussion of risk assessment and chemoprevention therapy, see American College of Obstetricians and Gynecologists. Tamoxifen and the prevention of breast cancer in high-risk women. ACOG Committee Opinion 224. Washington, DC: ACOG, 1999.

From American College of Obstetricians and Gynecologists Committee on Gynecologic Practice. Primary and preventive care: periodic assessments Washington, DC: ACOG; 2000; Committee Opinion No. 246, with permission.

Table 8.6. Periodic Assessment Age 65 Years and Older

Screening	Evaluation and Counseling
History	**Sexuality**
Reason for visit	Sexual functioning
Health status: medical, surgical, family	Sexual behaviors
Dietary/nutrition assessment	Sexually transmitted diseases
Physical activity	—Partner selection
Use of complementary and alternative medicine	—Barrier protection
Tobacco, alcohol, other drug use, and concurrent medication use	
Abuse/neglect	
Sexual practices	
Urinary and fecal incontinence	
Physical examination	**Fitness and nutrition**
Height	Dietary/nutrition assessment
Weight	Exercise: discussion of program
Blood pressure	Calcium intake
Oral cavity	
Neck: adenopathy, thyroid	
Breasts, axillae	
Abdomen	
Pelvic examination	
Skin[a]	
Laboratory testing	**Psychosocial evaluation**
Periodic	
Pap testing (physician and patient discretion after three consecutive normal tests if low risk)	Neglect/abuse
Urinalysis	Lifestyle/stress
Mammography	Depression/sleep disorders
Cholesterol testing (every 3–5 years before age 75 years)	Family relationships
Yearly fecal occult blood testing plus flexible sigmoidoscopy every 5 years *or* colonoscopy every 10 years *or* double contrast barium enema (DCBE) every 5–10 years, with digital rectal examination performed at the time of each screening sigmoidoscopy, colonoscopy, or DCBE	Work/retirement satisfaction
Fasting glucose testing (every 3 years after age 45 years)	
High-risk groups[a]	**Cardiovascular risk factors**
Hemoglobin level assessment	Hypertension
Sexually transmitted disease testing	Dyslipidemia
Human immunodeficiency virus testing	Obesity
Tuberculosis skin testing	Diabetes mellitus
Lipid profile assessment	Sedentary lifestyle

Table 8.6. — *continued*

Thyroid-stimulating hormone testing

Colonoscopy

Hepatitis C virus testing

Colorectal cancer screening

Health/risk behaviors

Hygiene (general and dental)

Hormone replacement therapy

Injury prevention

—Safety belts and helmets

—Prevention of falls

—Occupational hazards

—Recreational hazards

—Firearms

Visual acuity/glaucoma

Hearing

Breast self-examination

Chemoprophylaxis for breast cancer (for high-risk women)[b]

Skin exposure to ultraviolet rays

Suicide: depressive symptoms

Tobacco, alcohol, other drug use

[a]See Table 8.7.

[b]The decision to use *tamoxifen* should be individualized. For a more detailed discussion of risk assessment and chemoprevention therapy, see American College of Obstetricians and Gynecologists. *Tamoxifen* and the prevention of breast cancer in high-risk women. ACOG Committee Opinion 224. Washington, DC: ACOG, 1999.

From American College of Obstetricians and Gynecologists Committee on Gynecologic Practice. Primary and preventive care: periodic assessments Washington, DC: ACOG; 2000; Committee Opinion No. 246, with permission.

Table 8.7. High-risk Factors

Intervention	High-risk Factor
Bacteriuria testing	Diabetes mellitus
Cholesterol testing	Familial lipid disorders; family history of premature coronary heart disease; history of coronary heart disease
Colorectal cancer screening[a]	Colorectal cancer or adenomatous polyps in first-degree relative younger than 60 years or in two or more first-degree relatives of any ages; family history of familial adenomatous polyposis or hereditary nonpolyposis colon cancer; history of colorectal cancer, adenomatous polyps, or inflammatory bowel disease
Fasting glucose testing	Obesity; first-degree relative with diabetes mellitus; member of a high-risk ethnic population (e.g., African American, Hispanic, Native American, Asian, Pacific Islander); have delivered a baby weighing more than 9 lb or history of gestational diabetes mellitus; hypertensive; high-density lipoprotein cholesterol level of at least 35 mg/dl; triglyceride level of at least 250 mg/dl; history of impaired glucose tolerance or impaired fasting glucose
Fluoride supplementation	Live in area with inadequate water fluoridation (<0.7 ppm)
Genetic testing/counseling	Exposure to teratogens; considering pregnancy at age 35 or older; patient, partner, or family member with history of genetic disorder or birth defect; African, Acadian, Eastern European Jewish, Mediterranean, or Southeast Asian ancestry
Hemoglobin level assessment	Caribbean, Latin American, Asian, Mediterranean, or African ancestry; history of excessive menstrual flow
Hepatitis A vaccination	International travelers; illegal drug users; people who work with nonhuman primates; chronic liver disease; clotting-factor disorders; sex partners of bisexual men; measles-, mumps-, and rubella nonimmune persons; food service workers; health care workers; day care workers
Hepatitis B vaccination	Intravenous drug users and their sexual contacts; recipients of clotting factor concentrates; occupational exposure to blood or blood products; patients and workers in dialysis units; persons with chronic renal or hepatic disease; household or sexual contact with hepatitis B virus carriers; history of sexual activity with multiple partners; history of sexual activity with sexually active homosexual or bisexual men; international travelers; residents and staff of institutions for the developmentally disabled and of correctional institutions
Hepatitis C virus (HCV) testing	History of injecting illegal drugs; recipients of clotting factor concentrates before 1987; chronic (long-term) hemodialysis; persistently abnormal alanine aminotransferase levels; recipient of blood from a donor who later tested positive for HCV infection; recipient of blood or blood-component transfusion or organ transplant before July 1992; occupational percutaneous or mucosal exposure to HCV-positive blood
Human immunodeficiency virus (HIV) testing	Seeking treatment for sexually transmitted diseases; drug use by injection; history of prostitution; past or present sexual partner who is HIV positive or bisexual or injects drugs; long-term residence or birth in an area with high prevalence of HIV infection; history of transfusion from 1978 to 1985; invasive cervical cancer; pregnancy. Offer to women seeking preconception care.

333

Table 8.7.—*continued*

Influenza vaccination	Anyone who wishes to reduce the chance of becoming ill with influenza; resident in long-term care facility; chronic cardiopulmonary disorders; metabolic diseases (e.g., diabetes mellitus, hemoglobinopathies, immunosuppression, renal dysfunction); health-care workers; day-care workers; pregnant women who will be in the second or third trimester during the epidemic season. Pregnant women with medical problems should be offered vaccination before the influenza season regardless of stage of pregnancy.
Lipid profile assessment	Elevated cholesterol level; history of parent or sibling with blood cholesterol of at least 240 mg/dl; first-degree relative with premature (<55 years of age for men, <65 years of age for women) coronary heart disease; diabetes mellitus; smoking habit
Mammography	Women who have had breast cancer or who have a first-degree relative (i.e., mother, sister, or daughter) or multiple other relatives who have a history of premenopausal breast or breast and ovarian cancer
Measles-mumps-rubella (MMR) vaccination	Adults born in 1957 or later should be offered vaccination (one dose of MMR) if there is no proof of immunity or documentation of a dose given after first birthday; persons vaccinated in 1963–1967 should be offered revaccination (2 doses); health care workers, students entering college, international travelers, and rubella-negative postpartum patients should be offered a second dose.
Pneumococcal vaccination	Chronic illness such as cardiovascular disease, pulmonary disease, diabetes mellitus, alcoholism, chronic liver disease, cerebrospinal fluid leaks, functional or anatomic asplenia; exposure to an environment where pneumococcal outbreaks have occurred; immunocompromised patients (e.g., HIV infection, hematologic or solid malignancies, chemotherapy, steroid therapy); pregnant patients with chronic illness. Revaccination after 5 years may be appropriate for certain high-risk groups.
Rubella titer assessment	Childbearing age and no evidence of immunity
Sexually transmitted disease (STD) testing	History of multiple sexual partners or a sexual partner with multiple contacts; sexual contact with persons with culture-proven STD; history of repeated episodes of STDs; attendance at clinics for STDs; routine screening for chlamydial and gonorrheal infection for all sexually active adolescents and other asymptomatic women at high risk for infection
Skin examination	Increased recreational or occupational exposure to sunlight; family or personal history of skin cancer; clinical evidence of precursor lesions
Thyroid-stimulating hormone testing	Strong family history of thyroid disease; autoimmune disease (evidence of subclinical hypothyroidism may be related to unfavorable lipid profiles)
Tuberculosis skin testing	Human immunodeficiency virus infection; close contact with persons known or suspected to have tuberculosis; medical risk factors known to increase risk of disease if infected; born in country with high tuberculosis prevalence; medically underserved; low income; alcoholism; intravenous drug use; resident of long-term care facility (e.g., correctional institutions, mental institutions, nursing homes and facilities); health professional working in high-risk health care facilities

Table 8.7.— *continued*	
Varicella vaccination	All susceptible adults and adolescents, including health-care workers; household contacts of immunocompromised individuals; teachers; day care workers; residents and staff of institutional settings, colleges, prisons, or military installations; international travelers; nonpregnant women of childbearing age

[a]For a more detailed discussion of colorectal cancer screening, see **Byers T, Levin B, Rothenberger D, et al.** American Cancer Society guidelines for screening and surveillance for early detection of colorectal polyps and cancer: update 1997. American Cancer Society Detection and Treatment Advisory Group on Colorectal Cancer. *CA Cancer J Clin* 1997;47:154–160.
From American College of Obstetricians and Gynecologists Committee on Gynecologic Practice. Primary and preventive care: periodic assessments Washington, DC: ACOG; 2000; Committee Opinion No. 246, with permission.

Table 8.8. Immunizations

Ages 13–18 Years	*Ages 19–39 Years*	*Ages 40–64 Years*	*Age 65 Years and Older*
Periodic			
Tetanus-diphtheria booster (once between ages 11 years and 16 years) Hepatitis B vaccine (one series for those not previously immunized)	Tetanus-diphtheria booster (every 10 years)	Influenza vaccine (annually beginning at age 50 years) Tetanus-diphtheria booster (every 10 years)	Tetanus-diptheria booster (every 10 years) Influenza vaccine (annually) Pneumococcal vaccine (once)
High-risk groups[a]			
Influenza vaccine	Measles-mumps-rubella vaccine	Measles-mumps-rubella vaccine	Hepatitis A vaccine
Hepatitis A vaccine	Hepatitis A vaccine	Hepatitis A vaccine	Hepatitis B vaccine
Pneumococcal vaccine	Hepatitis B vaccine	Hepatitis B vaccine	Varicella vaccine
Measles-mumps-rubella vaccine	Influenza vaccine	Influenza vaccine	
Varicella vaccine	Pneumococcal vaccine Varicella vaccine	Pneumococcal vaccine Varicella vaccine	

[a]See Table 8.7.
From American College of Obstetricians and Gynecologists Committee on Gynecologic Practice. Primary and preventive care: periodic assessments Washington, DC: ACOG; 2000; Committee Opinion No. 246, with permission.

Appendix II: Primary Care Guidelines

Table 9.7. Selected Medications and Dosage for Control of Essential Hypertension

Medication (Class)	Normal Daily Dosage (mg/day) and Interval	Dispensing Unit (mg)
ACE inhibitors		
Enalapril	5–40 (qd, bid)	2.5, 5, 10, 20
Captopril	12.5–150 (bid, tid)	12.5, 25, 50, 100
Calcium channel blockers		
Verapamil, sustained release	120–480 (qd)	120, 180, 240, 360
Diltiazem, sustained release	120–240 (bid)	60, 90, 120
α-Blockers		
Terazosin	1–20 (qd)	1, 2, 5, 10
Mixed α-and β-blockers		
Labetalol	200–800 (bid)	100, 200, 300
Diuretics		
Hydrochlorothiazide	12.5–50 (qd)	25, 50
Triamterene (potassium-sparing)	50–100 (bid)	50, 100
β-Blockers		
Propranolol (lipid soluble)	60–160 (qd)	60, 80, 120, 160
Atenolol (water soluble)	50–100 (qd)	50, 100
Angiotensin receptor antagonists		
Losartan	25–100 (qd)	25, 50, 100

ACE, angiotensin-converting enzyme.

Table 9.8. Initial Classification Based on the Total Cholesterol and HDL Cholesterol Levels

	Initial Classification
Total cholesterol	
<200 mg/dl	Desirable blood cholesterol
200–239 mg/dl	Borderline high blood cholesterol
≥240 mg/dl	High blood cholesterol
HDL cholesterol	
<35 mg/dl	Low HDL cholesterol
Triglycerides	
<200 mg/dl	Normal
200–400 mg/dl	Borderline high
400–1000 mg/dl	High
>1000 mg/dl	Very high

HDL, high-density lipoproteins.
Adapted from The Second Report of the National Cholesterol Education Program (NCEP) Expert Panel on the Detection, Evaluation, and Treatment of High Blood Cholesterol in Adults. *JAMA* 1993;269: 3015–3023.

Table 9.9. Classification of Diabetes Mellitus

1. Type 1 diabetes (characterized by pancreatic destruction leading to insulin deficiency)

   A. Idiopathic

   B. Immune mediated

2. Type 2 diabetes (a combination of insulin resistance and some degree of inadequate insulin secretion)

3. Other types of diabetes

   A. Impaired glucose tolerance (IGT)

   B. Endocrinopathies (Cushing's syndrome, acromegaly, pheochromocytoma, hyperaldosteronism)

   C. Drug- or chemical-induced

   D. Diseases of the exocrine pancreas (pancreatitis, neoplasia)

   E. Infections

   F. Genetic defects of β-cell function and insulin action

   G. Gestational diabetes mellitus

Adapted from The Expert Committee on the Diagnosis and Classification of Diabetes Mellitus. Report of the Expert Committee on the Diagnosis and Classification of Diabetes Mellitus. *Diabetes Care* 2000;23: S4–S42.

Table 9.10. Physician Guidelines in the Therapy of Diabetes Mellitus

- Establish diagnosis and classify type of diabetes mellitus (DM).

- The oral glucose tolerance test (OGTT) is not recommended for routine clinical use because of its higher cost, time requirement, and limited reproducibility.

- Initiate diabetes education classes to learn blood glucose monitoring and diabetic medications, to learn signs and symptoms and complications, and to learn how to manage sick days.

- Place patient on ADA diet with appropriate caloric, sodium, and lipid restrictions.

- Establish cardiac risk factors, evaluate for baseline kidney function (serum creatinine, urine for microalbuminuria).

- If neuropathy is present, refer to a neurologist.

- Establish extent of funduscopic lesion (refer to ophthalmologist as needed).

- Check feet and toenails at each visit.

- Patient to use finger-stick blood glucose for daily diabetic control.

- Follow chronic glycemic control by HbA_{1c} every 2 to 3 months in the office.

- Initial general health evaluation should consist of a complete history and physical examination and the following laboratory tests: CBC with differential, chemistry profile, fasting lipid profile, urinalysis, thyroid function tests, urine for microalbuminuria and ECG (baseline at age 40 or older, repeat yearly).

- Oral hypoglycemic agents (OHA) like the sulfonylureas may be considered if fasting blood glucose does not decline or increase, if the patient has had diabetes for less than 10 years, does not have severe hepatic or renal disease, and is not pregnant or allergic to sulfa drugs.

- While on oral hypoglycemic agents, check the HbA_{1c} every 3 months.

- If the HbA_{1c} is <7% or the postprandial glucose is <200 mg/dl, omit the oral hypoglycemic agents, place on diet therapy alone, and follow every 3 months.

- If the fasting serum glucose is >200 mg/dl consistently or the HbA_{1c} is over 10%, consider starting insulin and referring the patient to an internist.

- Administer the flu vaccine every fall and the pneumococcal vaccine every 6 years.

ADA, American Diabetic Association; HgA_{1c}, hemoglobin A_{1c}; CBC, complete blood count; ECG, electrocardiogram; FSG, fasting serum glucose.
Adapted from The Expert Committee on the Diagnosis and Classification of Diabetes Mellitus. Report of the Expert Committee on the Diagnosis and Classification of Diabetes Mellitus. *Diabetes Care* 2000;23: S4–S42.

Table 9.11. Patient Guidelines for Treatment of Type 2 Diabetes

- Initiate an ADA reducing diet (50% CHO, 30% fat, 20% protein, high fiber) with three meals a day.

- Maintain ideal body weight or reduce weight by 5% to 15% in 3 months if obese.

- Modify risk factors (smoking, exercise, fat intake).

- Check fasting blood glucose by finger stick daily for 2 months. If FBG declines, no other therapy is needed. If FBG does not decline or increases, use of an oral hypoglycemic agent may be considered.

ADA, American Diabetic Association; CHO, carbohydrate; FBG, fasting blood glucose.
Adapted from The Expert Committee on the Diagnosis and Classification of Diabetes Mellitus. Report of the Expert Committee on the Diagnosis and Classification of Diabetes Mellitus. *Diabetes Care* 2000;23: S4–S42.

Table 9.12. Commonly Used Oral Hypoglycemic Agents

OHA	Trade Name	Daily Dose	Duration of Action (hrs)
Tolbutamide	Orinase	750 mg–3.0 g in divided doses	6–12
Tolazamide	Tolinase	200–1000 mg in divided doses	12–24
Acetohexamide	Dymelor	250–1500 mg in a single dose	12–24
Chlorpropamide	Diabinese	100–500 mg in a single dose	up to 60
Glyburide	Micronase, DiaBeta	2.5–20 mg variable dose	10–24
Glipizide	Glucotrol	2.5–40 mg variable dose	3–8
Metformin	Glucophage	500 mg–2.5 grams in 2 or 3 divided doses	6–12

OHA, oral hypoglycemic agent.

Appendix III: Contraception

Table 10.1. Percentage Distribution of Contraceptive Users Aged 15–44 Years, by Current Method, 1982–1995

Method	1982	1988	1995
Sterilization	34.1	39.2	38.6
Female	23.2	27.5	27.7
Male	10.9	11.7	10.9
Pill	28.0	30.7	26.9
Implant	NA	NA	1.3
Injectable	NA	NA	3.0
Intrauterine device	7.1	2.0	0.8
Diaphragm	8.1	5.7	1.9
Male condom	12.0	14.6	20.4
Foam	2.4	1.1	0.4
Periodic abstinence	3.9	2.3	2.3
Withdrawal	2.0	2.2	3.0
Other	2.5	2.1	1.3
Total no. of women	30,142,000	34,912,000	38,663,000

NA, not applicable.
From **Piccinino LJ, Mosher WD.** Trends in contraceptive use in the United States: 1982–1995. *Fam Plann Perspect* 1998;30:4–10, 46, with permission.

Table 10.2. Percentage of Women Experiencing a Contraceptive Failure During the First Year of Use and the Percentage Continuing Use at the End of the First Year

Method	Women Experiencing Accidental Pregnancy within the First Year of Use (%)		Women Continuing Use at 1 Year (%)
	Typical Use	Perfect Use	
Chance	85	85	
Spermicides	21	6	43
Periodic abstinence			67
Calendar		9	
Ovulation method		3	
Symptothermal		2	
Postovulation		1	
Withdrawal	19	4	
Cap			
Parous women	36	26	45
Nulliparous women	18	9	58
Diaphragm	18	6	58
Condom			
Female (Reality)	21	5	56
Male	12	3	63
Pill	3		72
Progestin only		0.5	
Combined		0.1	
Intrauterine device			
Progesterone T	2.0	1.5	81
Copper T380A	0.8	0.6	78
Levonorgestrel T20	0.1	0.1	81
DepoProvera	0.3	0.3	70
Norplant[a]	0.3	0.3	85
Female sterilization	0.4	0.4	100
Male sterilization	0.15	0.10	100

[a] Cumulative 5-year pregnancy rate for pliable tubing, divided by 5.
From **Hatcher RA, Trussell J, Stewart F, et al.** *Contraceptive technology.* 16th ed. New York: Irvington Publishers Inc., 1994:113, with permission.

Table 10.3. Overview of Contraceptive Methods

Method	Advantages	Disadvantages	Risks	Noncontraceptive Benefits
Coitus interruptus	Available, free	Depends on male control	Pregnancy	?Decreased STD risk
Lactation	Available, free	Unreliable duration of effect	Pregnancy	?Decreased breast cancer
Periodic abstinence	Available, free	Complex methodology; motivation is essential	Pregnancy	None
Condoms	Available, no prescription needed	Motivation is essential; must be used each time; depends on male	Pregnancy	Proven to decrease STDs and cervical cancer
Spermicides	Available, no prescription needed	Must be used each time	Pregnancy	Some decrease in STDs
Diaphragm/cap	Nonhormonal	Must be used each time; fitting required	Pregnancy, cystitis	Proven to decrease STDs and cervical cancer
IUD T380A	High efficacy for 10 years, unrelated to coitus	Initial cost; skilled inserter; pain and bleeding	Initial mild risk for PID and septic abortion	None
Levo-Norgestrel T	High efficacy for 5 years; unrelated to coitus	Initial cost; skilled inserter; amenorrhea for some	Initial mild risk for PID and septic abortion	Reduced bleeding; can be used to treat menorrhagia
Progestasert	Reasonable efficacy	Initial cost; skilled inserter; replace every year	Initial mild risk for PID, ectopic pregnancy	Reduced dysmenorrhea and menstrual blood loss
Oral contraceptives	High efficacy	Motivation to take daily; cost	Thrombosis; older smokers have increased risk of MI and stroke	Many benefits (see text)
DMPA	High efficacy, convenience	Injection required; bleeding pattern	Probably none	Many (see text)
Monthly injectable	High efficacy, convenience	Monthly injection	Probably same as orals	Probably same as orals
Implants	High efficacy, convenience	Surgical insertion and removal; initial cost; bleeding pattern	Functional cysts	Unknown
Postcoital hormones	Moderate efficacy	Frequent use disrupts menses; nausea	None	Unknown

STDs, sexually transmitted diseases; IUD, intrauterine device; PID, pelvic inflammatory disease; MI, myocardial infarction; DMPA, depomedroxyprogesterone acetate.

Table 10.10. Ten-year Life-table Cumulative Probability of Pregnancy per 1,000 Procedures with Different Methods of Tubal Sterilization, United States, 1978–1986.

Method	
Unipolar coagulation	7.5
Postpartum partial salpingectomy	7.5
Silastic band (Falope or Yoon)	17.7
Interval partial salpingectomy	20.1
Bipolar coagulation	24.8
Hulka-Clemens clip	36.5
Total: all methods	18.5

From **Peterson HB, Xia Z, Hughes JM, et al.** The risk of pregnancy after tubal sterilization: findings from the U.S. Collaborative Review of Sterilization. *Am J Obstet Gynecol* 1996;174:1164 (Table II) (184), with permission.

Table 10.12. Death to Case Rates for Legal Abortion Mortality by Weeks of Gestation, United States, 1972–1987

Weeks of Gestation	Deaths	Abortions	Rate[a]	Relative Risk
≤8	33	8,673,759	0.4	1.0
9–10	39	4,847,321	0.8	2.1
11–12	33	2,360,768	1.4	3.7
13–15	28	962,185	2.9	7.7
16–20	74	794,093	9.3	24.5
≥21	21	175,395	12.0	31.5

[a] Legal abortion deaths per 100,000 procedures; excludes deaths from ectopic pregnancies or pregnancy with gestation length unknown.
From **Lawson HW, Frye A, Atrash HK, et al.** Abortion mortality, United States, 1972–1987. *Am J Obstet Gynecol* 1994;171:1365–1372, with permission.

Table 10.13. Death to Case Rates for Legal Abortions by Type of Procedure and Weeks of Gestation, United States, 1974–1987[a]

Procedure	≤8	9–10	11–12	13–15	16–20	≥21
Vacuum curettage[b]	0.3	0.7	1.1	—	—	—
Dilation and evacuation	—	—	—	2.0	6.5	11.9
Instillation[c]	—	—	—	3.8	7.9	10.3
Hysterectomy, hysterotomy	18.3	30.0	41.2	28.1	103.4	274.3

[a] Legal induced abortion deaths per 100,000 legal induced abortions.
[b] Includes all suction and sharp curettage procedures.
[c] Includes all instillation methods (saline, prostaglandin).
From **Lawson HW, Frye A, Atrash HK, et al.** Abortion mortality, United States, 1972–1987. *Am J Obstet Gynecol* 1994;171:1365–1372, with permission.

Appendix IV: Medications for PMS and Psychiatric Conditions

Table 12.2. Scientific Basis of Selected Medications Used to Treat PMS

Treatment	Scientific Basis	Advantages	Disadvantages	Notes
Alprazolam	Several double-blind, placebo-controlled, randomized crossover studies. Results were mixed. Placebo was as effective as alprazolam in some studies.	Oral medication appears to be more effective in alleviating depression and anxiety symptoms than physical symptoms.	Potential for dependence, requires tapering; drowsiness reported by many subjects; long-term effects unknown; safety during pregnancy unknown.	The studies involved highly selective groups of women. There was a high dropout rate in one of the positive studies. In one study that found alprazolam effective, 87% of the women had a history of major depression or an anxiety disorder. Different doses were used in the studies (0.75–2.25 mg); the standard effective dosage is unknown.
Fluoxetine (Prozac)	Several double-blind, randomized, placebo-controlled, crossover trials. All found fluoxetine effective.	Well tolerated; single daily oral dose. Significant decrease in psychic and behavioral symptoms.	Long-term effects unknown. Safety during pregnancy unknown. Appears less effective in controlling physical symptoms.	Trials involved very small, highly select groups of women. Duration of treatment did not exceed 3 months. All trials used 20 mg orally daily.
Gonadotropin-releasing hormone agonist	Several small, double-blind, randomized, placebo-controlled, crossover trials. Most patients experienced improvement.	Rapidly reversible; many patients report being virtually symptom-free during therapy.	Produces pseudomenopause; expensive; risk for osteoporosis, hypoestrogenic symptoms. Usually given for only short periods of time.	An add-back regimen of estrogen-progestin in addition to gonadotropin-releasing hormone agonist has been reported. If replicated, it may have potential for an effective, long-term treatment for premenstrual syndrome.
Spironolactone	Several double-blind, randomized, placebo-controlled trials. Mixed results.	May alleviate bloating and improve symptoms related to mood. Oral medication taken once or twice a day. Nonaddictive.	Effectiveness not proven consistently across studies.	Spironolactone is the only diuretic that has shown effectiveness in treating premenstrual syndrome in controlled, randomized trials. Method of action may be antiandrogen properties.
Vitamin B_6	Ten randomized double-blind trials. About one-third of the trials reported positive results, one-third reported negative results, and one-third reported ambiguous results.	—	No conclusive evidence that vitamin B_6 is more effective than placebo.	Doses ranged from 50 to 500 mg. Only one study involved more than 40 subjects. The large multicenter trial (N = 204) reported similar results for placebo and vitamin B_6.

PMS; premenstrual syndrome.
From **The American College of Obstetricians and Gynecologists.** *Committee Opinion.* Washington, DC: ACOG, 1995, with permission.

Table 12.3. Pharmacology of Antidepressant Medications

Drug	Therapeutic Dosage Range (mg/day)	Average (range) of Elimination Half-lives (hours)[a]	Potentially Fatal Drug Interactions
Tricyclics			
Amitriptyline (Elavil, Endep)	75–300	24 (16–46)	Antiarrhythmics, MAO inhibitors
Clomipramine (Anafranil)	75–300	24 (20–40)	Antiarrhythmics, MAO inhibitors
Desipramine (Norpramin, Pertofrane)	75–300	18 (12–50)	Antiarrhythmics, MAO inhibitors
Doxepin (Adapin, Sinequan)	75–300	17 (10–47)	Antiarrhythmics, MAO inhibitors
Imipramine (Janimine, Tofranil)	75–300	22 (12–34)	Antiarrhythmics, MAO inhibitors
Nortiptyline (Aventyl, Pamelor)	40–200	26 (18–88)	Antiarrhythmics, MAO inhibitors
Protriptyline (Vivactil)	20–60	76 (54–124)	Antiarrhythmics, MAO inhibitors
Trimipramine (Surmontil)	75–300	12 (8–30)	Antiarrhythmics, MAO inhibitors
Heterocyclics			
Amoxapine (Asendin)	100–600	10 (8–14)	MAO inhibitors
Bupropion (Wellbutrin)	225–450	14 (8–24)	MAO inhibitors (possibly)
Maprotiline (Ludiomil)	100–225	43 (27–58)	MAO inhibitors
Trazodone (Desyrel)	150–600	8 (4–14)	—
Selective serotin reuptake inhibitors			
Fluoxetine (Prozac)	10–40	168 (72–360)[b]	MAO inhibitors
Paroxetine (Paxil)	20–50	24 (3–65)	MAO inhibitors[c]
Sertraline (Zoloft)	50–150	24 (10–30)	MAO inhibitors[c]
Monoamine oxidase inhibitors (MAO inhibitors)[d]			
Isocarboxazid (Marplan)	30–50	Unknown	For all three MAO inhibitors: vasoconstrictors,[e] decongestants,[e] meperidine, and possibly other narcotics
Phenelzine (Nardil)	45–90	2 (1.5–4.0)	
Tranylcypromine (Parnate)	20–60	2 (1.5–3.0)	

[a] Half-lives are affected by age, sex, race, concurrent medications, and length of drug exposure.
[b] Includes both fluoxetine and norfluoxetine.
[c] By extrapolation from fluoxetine data.
[d] MAO inhibition lasts longer (7 days) than drug half-life.
[e] Including pseudoephedrine, phenylephrine, phenylpropanolamine, epinephrine, norepinephrine, and others.
From **Depression Guideline Panel.** *Depression in primary care: detection, diagnosis, and treatment.* Quick reference guide for clinicians, No. 5. Rockville, MD: U.S. Department of Health and Human Services, Public Health Service, Agency for Health Care Policy and Research; 1993:15; AHCPR pub no 93-0552, with permission.

Table 12.4. Side-Effect Profiles of Antidepressant Medications

	Side Effect[a]						
		Central Nervous System		*Cardiovascular*			
	Anticholinergic[b]	*Drowsiness*	*Insomnia/ Agitation*	*Orthostatic Hypotension*	*Cardiac Arrhythmia*	*Gastrointestinal Distress*	*Weight Gain (over 6 kg)*
Amitriptyline	4+	4+	0	4+	3+	0	4+
Desipramine	1+	1+	1+	2+	2+	0	1+
Doxepin	3+	4+	0	2+	2+	0	3+
Imipramine	3+	3+	1+	4+	3+	1+	3+
Nortriptyline	1+	1+	0	2+	2+	0	1+
Protriptyline	2+	1+	1+	2+	2+	0	0
Trimipramine	1+	4+	0	2+	2+	0	3+
Amoxapine	2+	2+	2+	2+	3+	0	1+
Maprotiline	2+	4+	0	0	1+	0	2+
Trazodone	0	4+	0	1+	1+	1+	1+
Bupropion	0	0	2+	0	1+	1+	0
Fluoxetine	0	0	2+	0	0	3+	0
Paroxetine	0	0	2+	0	0	3+	0
Sertraline	0	0	2+	0	0	3+	0
Monoamine oxidase inhibitors	1	1+	2+	2+	0	1+	2+

[a] Numerals indicate the likelihood of side effect occurring ranging from 0 for absent or rare to 4+ for relatively common.

[b] Dry mouth, blurred vision, urinary hesitancy, constipation.

From **Depression Guideline Panel.** *Depression in primary care: detection, diagnosis, and treatment.* Quick reference guide for clinicians, No. 5. Rockville, MD: U.S. Department of Health and Human Services, Public Health Service, Agency for Health Care Policy and Research; 1993:14; AHCPR pub no 93-0553, with permission.

Table 12.5. Compounds Used for Anxiety

Medication	Trade Name	Rate of Absorption[a]	Half-Life[b]	Active Long-Acting Metabolite	Comments
Benzodiazepines					
					Metabolism of benzodiazepines is inhibited by cimetidine, disulfiram, isoniazid, and oral contraceptives. Metabolism of benzodiazepines is enhanced by rifampin.
Alprazolam	Xanax	Intermediate	Intermediate	No	Preferred in elderly patients or patients with poor hepatic functions.
Chlordiazepoxide	Librium, others	Intermediate	Intermediate	Yes	
Clonazepam	Klonopin	Long	Long	No	
Clorazepate	Tranxene, others	Short	Short	Yes	
Diazepam	Valium, others	Short	Long	Yes	Half-life increased 3 or 4 times in elderly patients.
Lorazepam	Ativan, others	Intermediate	Intermediate	No	Preferred in elderly patients or patients with poor hepatic function.
Oxazepam	Serax	Long	Intermediate	No	Preferred in elderly patients or patients with poor hepatic function.
Prazepam	Centrax	Long	Short	Yes	
Atypical agent					
Buspirone	BuSpar	—	—	—	Not effective in panic disorder, little sedation, little risk of dependence or tolerance.

[a] Long ≥2 hours; Intermediate = 1–2 hours; Short ≤1 hour.
[b] Long >20 hours; Intermediate = 6–20 hours; Short <6 hours.
From **Gilman AG, Rall TW, Nies AS, et al.** *The pharmacological basis of therapeutics,* 8th ed. New York: McGraw-Hill, 1990.
From **Stotland NL.** Psychiatric and psychosocial issues in primary care for women. In: **Seltzer VL, Pearse WH,** eds. *Women's primary health care: office practice and procedures.* New York: McGraw-Hill, 1995.

Appendix V: Benign Gynecologic Conditions

Table 13.1. Classification of Benign Conditions of the Vulva, Vagina, and Cervix

Vulva

Skin conditions
Pigmented lesions
Tumors and cysts
Ulcers
Nonneoplastic epithelial disorders

Vagina

Embryonic origin
 Mesonephric, paramesonephric, and urogenital sinus cysts
 Adenosis (related to diethylstilbestrol)
 Vaginal septa or duplications
Disorders of pelvic support
 Anterior vaginal prolapse
  Cystourethrocele
  Cystocele
 Apical vaginal prolapse
  Uterovaginal
  Vaginal vault
 Posterior vaginal prolapse
  Enterocele
  Rectocele
Other
 Condyloma
 Urethral diverticula
 Fibroepithelial polyp
 Vaginal endometriosis

Cervix

Infectious
 Condyloma
 Herpes simplex virus ulceration
 Chlamydial cervicitis
 Other cervicitis
Other
 Endocervical polyps
 Nabothian cysts
 Columnar epithelium eversion

Table 13.2. Benign Ovarian Tumors

Functional

Follicular
Corpus luteum
Theca lutein

Inflammatory

Tuboovarian abscess or complex

Neoplastic

Germ cell
Benign cystic teratoma
Other and mixed

Epithelial

Serous cystadenoma
Mucinous cystadenoma
Fibroma
Cystadenofibroma
Brenner tumor
Mixed tumor

Other

Endometrioma

Table 13.3. Causes of Bleeding and Pelvic Mass By Approximate Frequency and Age Group

Causes of bleeding by approximate frequency and age group

—	*Prepubertal*	*Adolescent*	*Reproductive*	*Perimenopausal*	*Postmenopausal*
—	Vulvovaginitis	Anovulation	Exogenous hormone use	Anovulation	Exogenous hormone use
—	Vaginal foreign body	Exogenous hormone use	Pregnancy	Fibroids	Endometrial lesions, including cancer
—	Precocious puberty	Pregnancy	Anovulation	Cervical and endometrial polyps	Atrophic vaginitis
—	Tumor	Coagulopathy	Fibroids	Thyroid dysfunction	Other tumor—vulvar, vaginal, cervical
—	—	—	Cervical and endometrial polyps	—	—
—	—	—	Thyroid dysfunction	—	—

Causes of pelvic mass by approximate frequency and age group

Infancy	*Prepubertal*	*Adolescent*	*Reproductive*	*Perimenopausal*	*Postmenopausal*
Functional cyst	Functional cyst	Functional cyst	Functional cyst	Fibroids	Ovarian tumor (malignant or benign)
Germ cell tumor	Germ cell tumor	Pregnancy	Pregnancy	Epithelial ovarian tumor	Functional cyst
—	—	Dermoid/other germ cell tumors	Uterine fibroids	Functional cyst	Bowel, malignant tumor or inflammatory
—	—	Obstructing vaginal or uterine anomalies	Epithelial ovarian tumor	—	Metastases
—	—	Epithelial ovarian tumor	—	—	—

Table 13.4. Causes of Vaginal Bleeding in Prepubertal Girls

Vulvar and external

Vulvitis with excoriation
Trauma (e.g., straddle injury)
Lichen sclerosus
Condylomas
Molluscum contagiosum
Urethral prolapse

Vaginal

Vaginitis
Vaginal foreign body
Trauma (abuse, penetration)
Vaginal tumor

Uterine

Precocious puberty

Ovarian tumor

Granulosa cell tumor
Germ cell tumor

Exogenous estrogens

Topical
Enteral

Table 13.6. Abnormal Menses—Terminology

Term	Interval	Duration	Amount
Menorrhagia	Regular	Prolonged	Excessive
Metrorrhagia	Irregular	±Prolonged	Normal
Menometrorrhagia	Irregular	Prolonged	Excessive
Hypermenorrhea	Regular	Normal	Excessive
Hypomenorrhea	Regular	Normal or less	Less
Oligomenorrhea	Infrequent or irregular	Variable	Scanty

Table 13.7. Etiology of Postmenopausal Bleeding

Factor	Approximate Percentage
Exogenous estrogens	30
Atrophic endometritis/vaginitis	30
Endometrial cancer	15
Endometrial or cervical polyps	10
Endometrial hyperplasia	5
Miscellaneous (e.g., cervical cancer, uterine sarcoma, urethral caruncle, trauma)	10

From **Hacker NF, Moore JG.** *Essentials of obstetrics and gynecology,* 3rd ed. Philadelphia: WB Saunders, 1998:635, with permission.

Table 13.8. Conditions Diagnosed as a Pelvic Mass in Women of Reproductive Age

Full urinary bladder

Urachal cyst

Sharply anteflexed or retroflexed uterus

Pregnancy (with or without concomitant leiomyomas)
    Intrauterine
    Tubal
    Abdominal

Ovarian or adnexal masses
    Functional cysts
    Inflammatory masses
      Tuboovarian complex
      Diverticular abscess
      Appendiceal abscess
    Matted bowel and omentum
    Peritoneal cyst
    Stool in sigmoid
    Neoplastic tumors
      Benign
      Malignant

Paraovarian or paratubal cysts

Intraligamentous myomas

Less common conditions that must be excluded:
    Pelvic kidney
    Carcinoma of the colon, rectum, appendix
    Carcinoma of the fallopian tube
    Retroperitoneal tumors (anterior sacral meningocele)
    Uterine sarcoma or other malignant tumors

Table 13.9. Ultrasonographic Scoring System for Adnexal Masses[a]

Clear cyst and smooth borders	1
Clear cyst with slightly irregular border; cyst with smooth walls but low-level echoes (i.e., endometrioma)	2
Cyst with low-level echoes with slightly irregular border but no nodularity (i.e., endometrioma); clear cyst in postmenopausal patient	3
Equivocal, nonspecific ultrasonographic appearance: solid ovarian enlargement or small cyst with irregular borders and internal echoes (hemorrhagic cyst or benign ovarian tumor)	4–6
Multiseptate or irregular cystic mass consistent in appearance with ovarian tumor (7, 5 less nodularity; 8–9, 5 more nodularity)	7–9
Pelvic mass as above, with ascites	10

[a] 1, benign; 10, malignant.
From **Finkler NJ, Benacerraf B, Lavin PT, et al.** Comparison of CA 125, clinical impression, and ultrasound in the preoperative evaluation of ovarian masses. *Obstet Gynecol* 1988;72:659, with permission.

Table 13.10. Subacute and Chronic Recurrent Conditions of the Vulva

Noninfectious	Infectious
Acanthosis nigricans	Cellulitis
Atopic dermatitis	Folliculitis
Behçets's disease	Furuncle/carbuncle
Contact dermatitis	Insect bites (e.g., chiggers, fleas)
Crohn's disease	Necrotizing fasciitis
Diabetic vulvitis[a]	Pubic lice
Hidradenitis suppurativa[a]	Scabies
Hyperplastic dystrophy	Tinea
Lichen sclerosus	
Mixed dystrophy	
Paget's disease	
Pseudo folliculitis	
Razor bumps	
Psoriasis	
Seborrheic dermatitis	
Vulvar intraepithelial neoplasia	

[a] Etiology unknown, often secondarily infected.

Table 13.11. Types of Vulvar Tumors

1. **Cystic Lesions**	3. **Anatomic**
Bartholin duct cyst	Hernia
Cyst in the canal of Nuck (hydrocele)	Urethral diverticulum
Epithelial inclusion cyst	Varicosities
Skene duct cyst	
	4. **Infections**
2. **Solid Tumors**	Abscess—Bartholin, Skene, periclitoral, other
Acrochordon (skin tag)	Condyloma lata
Angiokeratoma	Molluscum contagiosum
Bartholin gland adenoma	Pyogenic granuloma
Cherry angioma	
Fibroma	5. **Ectopic**
Hemangioma	Endometriosis
Hidradenoma	Ectopic breast tissue
Lipoma	
Granular cell myoblastoma	
Neurofibroma	
Papillomatosis	

Appendix VI: Pelvic Pain

Table 14.2. Nerves Carrying Painful Impulses from the Pelvic Organs

Organ	*Spinal Segments*	*Nerves*
Perineum, vulva, lower vagina	S2–S4	Pudendal, inguinal, genitofemoral, posterofemoral cutaneous
Upper vagina, cervix, lower uterine segment, posterior urethra, bladder trigone, uterosacral and cardinal ligaments, rectosigmoid, lower ureters	S2–S4	Sacral afferents traveling through the pelvic plexus
Uterine fundus, proximal fallopian tubes, broad ligaments, upper bladder, cecum appendix, terminal large bowel	T11–T12, L1	Thoracolumbar splanchnic nerves through uterine and hypogastric plexes
Outer two thirds of fallopian tubes, upper ureter	T9–T10	Thoracolumbar splanchnic nerves through mesenteric plexus
Ovaries	T9–T10	Thoracolumbar splanchnic nerves traveling with ovarian vessels through renal and aortic plexus and celiac and mesenteric ganglia

Table 14.3. Peripheral Causes of Chronic Pelvic Pain

Gynecologic

Noncyclic

1. Adhesions
2. Endometriosis
3. Salpingo-oophoritis
   a. Acute
   b. Subacute
4. Ovarian remnant syndrome
5. Pelvic congestion syndrome (varicosities)
6. Ovarian neoplasms
7. Pelvic relaxation

Cyclic

1. Primary dysmenorrhea
2. Secondary dysmenorrhea
   a. Imperforate hymen
   b. Transverse vaginal septum
   c. Cervical stenosis
   d. Uterine anomalies (congenital malformation, bicornuate uterus, blind uterine horn)
   e. Intrauterine synechiae (Asherman's syndrome)
   f. Endometrial polyps
   g. Uterine leiomyoma
   h. Adenomyosis
   i. Pelvic congestion syndrome (varicosities)
   j. Endometriosis
3. Atypical cyclic
   a. Endometriosis
   b. Adenomyosis
   c. Ovarian remnant syndrome
   d. Chronic functional cyst formation

Gastrointestinal

1. Irritable bowel syndrome
2. Ulcerative colitis
3. Granulomatous colitis (Crohn's disease)
4. Carcinoma
5. Infectious diarrhea
6. Recurrent partial small bowel obstruction
7. Diverticulitis
8. Hernia
9. Abdominal angina
10. Recurrent appendiceal colic

Genitourinary

1. Recurrent or relapsing cystourethritis
2. Urethral syndrome
3. Interstitial cystitis
4. Ureteral diverticuli or polyps
5. Carcinoma of the bladder
6. Ureteral obstruction
7. Pelvic kidney

Neurologic

1. Nerve entrapment syndrome
2. Neuroma

Table 14.3. — *continued*

Musculoskeletal

Low back pain syndrome

1. Congenital anomalies
2. Scoliosis and kyphosis
3. Spondylolysis
4. Spondylolisthesis
5. Spinal injuries
6. Inflammation
7. Tumors
8. Osteoporosis
9. Degenerative changes
10. Coccydynia

Myofascial Syndrome

Systemic

1. Acute intermittent porphyria
2. Abdominal migraine
3. Systemic lupus erythematosus
4. Lymphoma
5. Neurofibromatosis

Appendix VII: Chemotherapy

Table 32.4. Combination Chemotherapy for Advanced Epithelial Ovarian Cancer: Recommended Regimens

Drugs	Dose	Administration (hr)	Interval	No. of Treatments
Standard regimens				
Paclitaxel	175 mg/m^2	24	Every 3 weeks	Six cycles
Carboplatin	AUC = 5–6			
Paclitaxel	135 mg/m^2	3	Every 3 weeks	Six cycles
Cisplatin	75 mg/m^2			
Alternative drugs[a]				
(Can be given with *platinum*)				
Cyclophosphamide	600–750 mg/m^2	—	Every 3 weeks	—
Topotecan	1.0–1.25 mg/m^2	—	Daily × 5 days every 3 weeks	—
Gemcitabine	800–1000 mg/m^2	—	Every 3 weeks	—

AUC, area under the curve dose by Calvert formula (181).
[a]Drugs that can be substituted for *paclitaxel* if hypersensitivity to that drug occurs.
From **Berek JS, Hacker NF,** eds. *Practical gynecologic oncology,* 3rd ed. Philadelphia: Lippincott Williams & Wilkins, 2000:493, with permission.

Table 32.6. Combination Chemotherapy for Germ Cell Tumors of the Ovary

Regimen and Drugs	Dose and Schedule[a]
BEP	
Bleomycin	15 units/m^2/week × 5; then on day 1 of course 4
Etoposide	100 mg/m^2/day × 5 days every 3 weeks
Cisplatin	20 mg/m^2/day × 5 days, or 100 mg/m^2/day × 1 day every 3 weeks
VBP	
Vinblastine	0.15 mg/kg days 1 and 2 every 3 weeks
Bleomycin	15 units/m^2/week × 5; then on day 1 of course 4
Cisplatin	100 mg/m^2 on day 1 every 3 weeks
VAC	
Vincristine	1–1.5 mg/m^2 on day 1 every 4 weeks
Actinomycin D	0.5 mg/day × 5 days every 4 weeks
Cyclophosphamide	150 mg/m^2/day × 5 days every 4 weeks

[a]All doses given intravenously.

Table 32.7. POMB-ACE Chemotherapy For Germ Cell Tumors of the Ovary

POMB

Day 1	*Vincristine* 1 mg/m^2 IV; *methotrexate* 300 mg/m^2 as a 12-hr infusion
Day 2	*Bleomycin* 15 mg as a 24-hr infusion: *folinic acid* rescue started at 24 hrs after the start of *methotrexate* in a dose of 15 mg every 12 hrs for 4 doses
Day 3	*Bleomycin* infusion 15 mg by 24-hr infusion
Day 4	*Cisplatin* 120 mg/m^2 as a 12-hr infusion, given with hydration and 3 g magnesium sulfate supplementation

ACE

Days 1–5	*Etoposide* (VP16-213) 100 mg/m^2, days 1–5
Days 3, 4, 5	*Actinomycin D* 0.5 mg IV, days 3, 4, and 5
Day 5	*Cyclophosphamide* 500 mg/m^2 IV, day 5

OMB

Day 1	*Vincristine* 1 mg/m^2 IV; *methotrexate* 300 mg/m^2 as a 12-hr infusion
Day 2	*Bleomycin* 15 mg by 24-hr infusion; *folinic acid* rescue started at 24 hrs after start of *methotrexate* in a dose of 15 mg every 12 hrs for 4 doses
Day 3	*Bleomycin* 15 mg by 24-hr infusion

IV, intravenous; hCG, human chorionic gonadotropin; AFP, α-fetoprotein; PLAP, placental alkaline phosphatase; LDH, lactate dehydrogenase.

The sequence of treatment schedules is two courses of POMB followed by ACE. POMB is then alternated with ACE until patients are in biochemical remission as measured by hCG and AFP, PLAP, and LDH. The usual number of courses of POMB is three to five. Following biochemical remission, patients alternate ACE with OMB until remission has been maintained for approximately 12 weeks. The interval between courses of treatment is kept to the minimum (usually 9 to 11 days). If delays are caused by myelosuppression after courses of ACE, the first 2 days of etoposide are omitted from subsequent courses of ACE.

From **Newlands ES, Southall PJ, Paradinas FJ, et al.** Management of ovarian germ cell tumours. In: **Williams CJ, Kaikorian JG, Green MR, et al.,** eds. *Textbook of uncommon cancer.* New York: John Wiley and Sons, 1988:47, with permission.

Appendix VIII: Staging of Cancer

Table 30.5. FIGO Definition for Grading of Endometrial Carcinoma

Histopathologic degree of differentiation:
G1: >5% nonsquamous or nonmorular growth pattern
G2: 6%–50% nonsquamous or nonmorular growth pattern
G3: >50% nonsquamous or nonmorular growth pattern

Notes on pathologic grading:
Notable nuclear atypia, inappropriate for the architectural grade, raises a grade 1 (G1) or grade 2 (G2) tumor by one grade.
In serous adenocarcinoma, clear cell adenocarcinoma, and squamous cell carcinoma, nuclear grading takes precedence.
Adenocarcinomas with squamous differentiation are graded according to the nuclear grade of the glandular component.

FIGO, International Federation of Gynecology and Obstetrics.

Table 30.7. FIGO Surgical Staging for Endometrial Carcinoma (1988)

Stage	*Finding*
Ia G123	No myometrial invasion
Ib G123	< $^1/_2$ Myometrial invasion
Ic G123	> $^1/_2$ Myometrial invasion
IIa G123	Extension to endocervical glands
IIb G123	Cervical stromal invasion
IIIa G123	Positive uterine serosa, adnexa, and/or peritoneal cytology
IIIb G123	Vaginal metastasis
IIIc G123	Metastasis to pelvic and/or paraaortic lymph nodes
IVa G123	Tumor invasion of bladder and/or bowel mucosa
IVb	Distant metastasis including intraabdominal and/or inguinal lymph nodes

FIGO, International Federation of Gynecology and Obstetrics.

Table 31.1. FIGO Staging of Carcinoma of the Cervix Uteri

Preinvasive Carcinoma

Stage 0 Carcinoma *in situ,* intraepithelial carcinoma (cases of stage 0 should not be included in any therapeutic statistics).

Invasive Carcinoma

Stage I[a] **Carcinoma strictly confined to the cervix** (extension to the corpus should be disregarded).

Stage Ia Preclinical carcinomas of the cervix, that is, those diagnosed only by microscopy.

Stage Ia1 Lesion with ≤3 mm invasion.

Stage Ia2 Lesions detected microscopically that can be measured. The upper limit of the measurement should show a depth of invasion of >3–5 mm taken from the base of the epithelium, either surface or glandular, from which it originates, and a second dimension, the horizontal spread, must not exceed 7 mm. Larger lesions should be staged as Ib.

Stage Ib Lesions invasive >5 mm.

Stage Ib1 Lesion less than or equal to 4 cm.

Stage Ib2 Lesions larger than 4 cm.

Stage II[b] **The carcinoma extends beyond the cervix but has not extended onto the wall.** The carcinoma involves the vagina, but not the lower one third.

Stage IIa No obvious parametrial involvement.

Stage IIb Obvious parametrial involvement.

Stage III[c] **The carcinoma has extended onto the pelvic wall.** On rectal examination, there is no cancer-free space between the tumor and the pelvic wall. The tumor involves the lower one third of the vagina. All cases with hydronephrosis or nonfunctioning kidney.

Stage IIIa No extension to the pelvic wall.

Stage IIIb Extension onto the pelvic wall and/or hydronephrosis or nonfunctioning kidney.

Stage IV[d] **The carcinoma has extended beyond the true pelvis or has clinically involved the mucosa of the bladder or rectum.** A bullous edema, as such, does not permit a case to be allotted to stage IV.

Stage IVa Spread to the growth to adjacent organs.

Stage IVb Spread to distant organs.

[a]The diagnosis of both stages Ia1 and Ia2 should be based on microscopic examination of removed tissue, preferably a cone, which must include the entire lesion. The depth of invasion should not be more than 5 mm taken from the base of the epithelium, either surface or glandular, from which it originates. The second dimension, the horizontal spread, must not exceed 7 mm. Vascular space involvement, either venous or lymphatic, should not alter the staging but should be specifically recorded because it may affect treatment decisions in the future. Lesions of greater size should be staged as Ib. As a rule, it is impossible to estimate clinically whether a cancer of the cervix has extended to the corpus. Extension to the corpus should therefore be disregarded.

[b]A patient with a growth fixed to the pelvic wall by a short and indurated, but not nodular, parametrium should be allotted to stage IIb. At clinical examination, it is impossible to decide whether a smooth, indurated parametrium is truly cancerous or only inflammatory. Therefore, the case should be assigned to stage III only if the parametrium is nodular to the pelvic wall or the growth itself extends to the pelvic wall.

[c]The presence of hydronephrosis or nonfunctioning kidney due to stenosis of the ureter by cancer permits a case to be allotted to stage III even if, according to other findings, it should be allotted to stage I or II.

[d]The presence of the bullous edema, as such, should not permit a case to be allotted to stage IV. Ridges and furrows into the bladder wall should be interpreted as signs of submucous involvement of the bladder if they remain fixed to the growth at palpation (i.e., examination from the vagina or the rectum during cystoscopy). A cytologic finding of malignant cells in washings from the urinary bladder requires further examination and a biopsy specimen from the wall of the bladder.

FIGO, International Federation of Gynecology and Obstetrics.

Table 31.2. Staging Procedures

Physical examination[a]	Palpate lymph nodes
	Examine vagina
	Bimanual rectovaginal examination
	(under anesthesia recommended)
Radiologic studies[a]	Intravenous pyelogram
	Barium enema
	Chest x-ray
	Skeletal x-ray
Procedures[a]	Biopsy
	Conization
	Hysteroscopy
	Colposcopy
	Endocervical curettage
	Cystoscopy
	Proctoscopy
Optional studies[b]	Computerized axial tomography
	Lymphangiography
	Ultrasonography
	Magnetic resonance imaging
	Radionucleotide scanning
	Laparoscopy

[a]Allowed by the International Federation of Gynecology and Obstetrics (FIGO).
[b]Information that is not allowed by FIGO to change the clinical stage.

Table 31.6. FIGO Staging of Vaginal Cancer

Stage 0	Carcinoma *in situ,* intraepithelia carcinoma.
Stage I	The carcinoma is limited to the vaginal wall.
Stage II	The carcinoma has involved the subvaginal tissue but has not extended to the pelvic wall.
Stage III	The carcinoma has extended to the pelvic wall.
Stage IV	The carcinoma has extended beyond the true pelvis or has involved the mucosa of the bladder or rectum.
Stage IVa	Spread of the growth to adjacent organs.
Stage IVb	Spread to distant organs.

FIGO, International Federation of Gynecology and Obstetrics.

Table 32.2. FIGO Staging for Primary Carcinoma of the Ovary

Stage I	Growth limited to the ovaries.	
	Stage Ia	Growth limited to one ovary; no ascites containing malignant cells. No tumor on the external surface; capsule intact.
	Stage Ib	Growth limited to both ovaries; no ascites containing malignant cells. No tumor on the external surfaces; capsules intact.
	Stage Ic[a]	Tumor either stage Ia or Ib but with tumor on the surface of one or both ovaries; or with capsule ruptured; or with ascites present containing malignant cells or with positive peritoneal washings.
Stage II	Growth involving one or both ovaries with pelvic extension.	
	Stage IIa	Extension and/or metastases to the uterus and/or fallopian tubes.
	Stage IIb	Extension to other pelvic tissues.
	Stage IIc[a]	Tumor either stage IIa or IIb but with tumor on the surface of one or both ovaries; or with capsule(s) ruptured; or with ascites present containing malignant cells or with positive peritoneal washings.
Stage III	Tumor involving one or both ovaries with peritoneal implants outside the pelvis and/or positive retroperitoneal or inguinal nodes. Superficial liver metastasis equals stage III. Tumor is limited to the true pelvis, but with histologically proven malignant extension to small bowel or omentum.	
	Stage IIIa	Tumor grossly limited to the true pelvis with negative nodes but with histologically confirmed microscopic seeding of abdominal peritoneal surfaces.
	Stage IIIb	Tumor of one or both ovaries with histologically confirmed implants of abdominal peritoneal surfaces, none exceeding 2 cm in diameter. Nodes negative.
	Stage IIIc	Abdominal implants >2 cm in diameter or positive retroperitoneal or inguinal nodes or both.
Stage IV	Growth involving one or both ovaries with distant metastasis. If pleural effusion is present, there must be positive cytologic test results to allot a case to stage IV. Parenchymal liver metastasis equals stage IV.	

These categories are based on findings at clinical examination or surgical exploration or both. The histologic characteristics are to be considered in the staging, as are results of cytologic testing as far as effusions are concerned. It is desirable that a biopsy be performed on suspicious areas outside the pelvis.

[a]In order to evaluate the impact on prognosis of the different criteria for allotting cases to stage Ic or IIc, it would be of value to know if rupture of the capsule was (a) spontaneous or (b) caused by the surgeon and if the source of malignant cells detected was (a) peritoneal washings or (b) ascites.

**Table 32.9. Modified FIGO Staging of Fallopian Tube Cancer
(Based on Operative Findings Before Debulking and Pathologic Findings)**

Stage 0	Carcinoma *in situ*[a] (limited to tubal mucosa).[b]
Stage I	Growth is limited to the fallopian tubes.
Stage Ia	Growth is limited to one tube with extension into the submucosa[c] and/or muscularis but not penetrating the serosal surface; no ascites.
Stage Ib	Growth is limited to both tubes with extension into the submucosa[c] and/or muscularis but not penetrating the serosal surface: no ascites.
Stage Ic	Tumor either stage Ia or Ib but with tumor extension through or onto the tubal serosa; or with ascites present containing malignant cells or with positive peritoneal washings.
Stage II	Growth involving one or both fallopian tubes with pelvic extension.
Stage IIa	Extension and/or metastasis to the uterus and/or ovaries.
Stage IIb	Extension to other pelvic tissues.
Stage IIc	Tumor either stage IIa or IIb but with tumor extension through or onto the tubal serosa; or with ascites present containing malignant cells or with positive peritoneal washings.
Stage III	Tumor involves one or both fallopian tubes with peritoneal implants outside of the pelvis and/or positive retroperitoneal or inguinal nodes. Superficial liver metastases equals stage III. Tumor appears limited to the true pelvis but with histologically proven malignant extension to the small bowel or omentum.
Stage IIIa	Tumor is grossly limited to the true pelvis with negative nodes but with histologically confirmed microscopic seeding of abdominal peritoneal surfaces.
Stage IIIb	Tumor involving one or both tubes with histologically confirmed implants of abdominal peritoneal surfaces, none exceeding 2 cm in diameter. Lymph nodes are negative.
Stage IIIc	Abdominal implants greater than 2 cm in diameter and/or positive retroperitoneal or inguinal nodes.
Stage IV	Growth involving one or both fallopian tubes with distant metastases. If pleural effusion is present, there must be positive cytology to be stage IV. Parenchymal liver metastases equals stage IV.

FIGO, International Federation of Gynecology and Obstetrics.

[a]The staging system does not distinguish between microscopic foci or replacement of tubal epithelium by malignant epithelium and grossly evident masses in the tubal lumen that do not penetrate the wall beyond the epithelium. The former have not been reported to spread beyond the tube, whereas the latter can extend beyond the tube, recur, and be fatal.

[b]The *mucosa* presumably refers to the epithelium because involvement of the lamina propria component of the mucosa requires staging of the tumor as Stage Ia.

[c]Because the fallopian tube has no *submucosa,* this designation presumably refers to the lamina propria.

From **Berek JS, Hacker NF,** eds. *Practical gynecologic oncology,* 3rd ed. Philadelphia: Lippincott Williams & Wilkins, 2000:546, with permission.

Table 33.4. Revised FIGO Surgical Staging for Vulvar Cancer (36)

FIGO Stage	TNM Classification	Clinical/Pathologic Findings
0	Tis^a	Carcinoma *in situ*, intraepithelial carcinoma
I	$T_1N_0M_0$	Tumor confined to vulva and/or perineum, $\leq$2 cm in greatest dimension, nodes are negative
Ia^b		Stromal invasion $\leq$1 mm
Ib		Stromal invasion >1 mm
II	$T_2N_0M_0$	Tumor confined to vulva and/or perineum, >2 cm in greatest dimension, nodes are negative
III	$T_3N_0M_0$ $T_{1-3}N_1M_0$	Tumor of any size with 1. Adjacent spread to lower urethra, vagina, or anus or 2. Unilateral regional lymph node metastases
IVa	$T_4N_{any}M_0$ $T_{any}N_2M_0$	Tumor of any size with 1. Adjacent spread to upper urethra, bladder mucosa, rectal mucosa, pelvic bone or 2. Bilateral regional lymph node metastases
IVb	$T_{any}N_{any}M_1$	Any distant metastases, including pelvic lymph nodes

[a]TNM Classification:

T: Primary tumor
Tx: Primary tumor cannot be assessed
T_0: No evidence of primary tumor
Tis: Carcinoma *in situ* (preinvasive carcinoma)
T_1: Tumor confined to the vulva and/or perineum, $\leq$2 cm in greatest dimension
T_2: Tumor confined to the vulva and/or perineum, >2 cm in greatest dimension
T_3: Tumor invades any of the following: lower urethra, vagina, anus
T_4: Tumor invades any of the following: bladder mucosa, rectal mucosa, upper urethra, pelvic bone

N: Regional lymph nodes
Regional lymph nodes are the femoral and inguinal nodes
Nx Regional lymph nodes cannot be assessed
N_0 No lymph node metastases
N_1 Unilateral regional lymph node metastases
N_2 Bilateral regional lymph node metastases
M Distant metastases
Mx Presence of distant metastases cannot be assessed
M_0 No distant metastases
M_1 Distant metastases (including pelvic lymph node metastases)

[b]The depth of stromal invasion is measured from the epithelial–stromal junction of the adjacent most superficial dermal papilla to the deepest point of invasion.

Table 33.6. Microstaging of Vulvar Melanoma

	Clark Level (117)	Chung Depth of Invasion (115)	Breslow Tumor Thickness (118)
I	Intraepithelial	Intraepithelial	<0.76 mm
II	Into papillary dermis	<1 mm from granular layer	0.76–1.5 mm Superficial invasion
III	Filling dermal papillae	1.1–2.0 mm from granular layer	1.51–2.25 mm Intermediate invasion
IV	Into reticular dermis	>2 mm from granular layer	2.26–3.0 mm Intermediate invasion
V	Into subcutaneous fat	Into subcutaneous fat	>3 mm Deep invasion

Table 34.2. Staging of Gestational Trophoblastic Tumors

Stage I	Disease confined to uterus
Stage Ia	Disease confined to uterus with no risk factors
Stage Ib	Disease confined to uterus with one risk factor
Stage Ic	Disease confined to uterus with two risk factors
Stage II	**Gestational trophoblastic tumor extending outside uterus but limited to genital structures (adnexa, vagina, broad ligament)**
Stage IIa	Gestational trophoblastic tumor involving genital structures without risk factors
Stage IIb	Gestational trophoblastic tumor extending outside uterus but limited to genital structures with one risk factor
Stage IIc	Gestational trophoblastic tumor extending outside uterus but limited to genital structures with two risk factors
Stage III	**Gestational trophoblastic disease extending to lungs with or without known genital tract involvement**
Stage IIIa	Gestational trophoblastic tumor extending to lungs with or without genital tract involvement and with no risk factors
Stage IIIb	Gestational trophoblastic tumor extending to lungs with or without genital tract involvement and with one risk factor
Stage IIIc	Gestational trophoblastic tumor extending to lungs with or without genital tract involvement and with two risk factors
Stage IV	**All other metastatic sites**
Stage IVa	All other metastatic sites without risk factors
Stage IVb	All other metastatic sites with one risk factor
Stage IVc	All other metastatic sites with two risk factors

Risk factors affecting staging include the following: (a) human chorionic gonadotropin > 100,000 mIU/ml and (b) duration of disease longer than 6 months from termination of antecedent pregnancy.

The following factors should be considered and noted in reporting: (a) prior chemotherapy has been given for known gestational trophoblastic tumor, (b) placental site tumors should be reported separately and (c) histologic verification of disease is not required.

Table 35.1. Official Screening Recommendations

Bilateral mammograms:
  By age 40: baseline mammogram
  Age 40–49: every 1–2 years
  Age >50: every year
  If family history of breast cancer, may consider baseline mammogram age 35, or 10 years younger than earliest family member was diagnosed, whichever is younger.

Self-examination:
  Premenopausal: 5–7 days after menstrual period monthly
  Postmenopausal: same day every month

Clinical breast examination:
  Age 20–40: exam by physician every 3 years
  Age ≥ 40: exam by physician every 2–3 years
  (May do annually if there is a positive family history)
Tumor markers (CA27–29, CA15–3): not recommended as screening tests

From American Cancer Society, Workshop on Guidelines for Breast Cancer Detection; March 7–9, 1997; Chicago, 11. National Cancer Institute Advisory Board issues on mammography screening recommendations; Bethesda, MD NIH; March 27, 1997; **Dodd GD.** Screening for breast cancer: practical considerations. *J Surg Oncol* 1995;60:1–3, with permission.

Table 35.2. Tumor–Nodes–Metastasis (TNM) System for Staging of Breast Cancer

Primary tumor (T)

TX	Primary tumor cannot be assessed
T_0	No evidence of primary tumor
Tis	Carcinoma *in situ:* intraductal carcinoma, lobular carcinoma *in situ,* or Paget's disease of the nipple with no tumor
T_1	Tumor 2 cm or less in greatest dimension
T_{1A}	0.5 cm or less in greatest dimension
T_{1B}	More than 0.5 cm but not more than 1 cm in greatest dimension
T_{1C}	More than 1 cm but not more than 2 cm in greatest dimension
T_2	Tumor more than 2 cm but not more than 5 cm in greatest dimension
T_3	Tumor more than 5 cm in greatest dimension
T_4	Tumor of any size with direct extension to chest wall or skin
T_{4A}	Extension to chest wall
T_{4B}	Edema (including *peau d'orange*) or ulceration of the skin of breast or satellite skin nodules confined to same breast
T_{4C}	Both T_{4A} and T_{4B}
T_{4D}	Inflammatory carcinoma

Lymph node (N)

NX	Regional lymph nodes cannot be assessed (e.g., previously removed)
N_0	No regional lymph node metastasis
N_1	Metastasis to movable ipsilateral axillary lymph node(s)
N_2	Metastasis to ipsilateral axillary lymph node(s) fixed to one another or to other structures
N_3	Metastasis to ipsilateral internal mammary lymph node(s)

Pathologic classification (pN)

pNX	Regional lymph nodes cannot be assessed (e.g., previously removed or removed but not for pathologic study)
pN_0	No regional lymph node metastasis
pN_1	Metastasis to movable ipsilateral axillary lymph node(s)
pN_{1A}	Only micrometastasis (none larger than 0.2 cm)
pN_{1B}	Metastasis to lymph nodes, any larger than 0.2 cm
pN_{1bi}	Metastasis in one to three lymph nodes, any more than 0.2 cm and all less than 2 cm in greatest dimension
pN_{1bii}	Metastasis to four or more lymph nodes, any more than 0.2 cm and all less than 2 cm in greatest dimension
pN_{1biii}	Extension of tumor beyond the capsule of a lymph node metastasis less than 2 cm in greatest dimension
pN_{1biv}	Metastasis to a lymph node 2 cm or more in greatest dimension
pN_2	Metastasis to ipsilateral axillary lymph nodes that are fixed to one another or to other structures
pN_3	Metastasis to ipsilateral internal mammary lymph node(s)

Distant metastasis (M)

MX	Presence of distant metastasis cannot be assessed
M_0	No distant metastasis
M_1	Distant metastasis (includes metastasis to ipsilateral supraclavicular lymph node[s]).

From **Fleming ID, Cooper JS, Henson DE, et al.,** eds. *AJCC cancer staging manual,* 5th ed. Philadelphia: JB Lippincott, 1997:171–180, with permission.

Appendix IX: Reference Values

Measure	SI	Conventional (C)	Conversion Factor (CF) C × CF = SI
Acetoacetate, plasma	<100 μmol/l	<1.0 mg/dl	97.95
Adrenal steroids, plasma			
Aldosterone, supine, saline suppression	<220 pmol/l	<8 ng/dl	27.74
Cortisol			
8:00 AM	220–660 nmol/l	8–24 μg/dl	27.59
4:00 PM	50–410 nmol/l	2–15 μg/dl	27.59
Overnight dexamethasone suppression	<140 nmol/l	<5 μg/dl	27.59
Dehydroepiandrosterone (DHEA)	0.6–70 nmol/l	0.2–20 μg/l	3.467
Dehydroepiandrosterone sulfate (DHEAS)	5.4–9.2 μmol/l	820–3380 ng/ml	0.002714
11-Deoxycortisol (compound S)	<60 nmol/l	<2 μg/dl	28.86
17α-Hydroxyprogesterone, women	1–13 nmol/l	0.3–4.2 μg/l	3.026
Adrenal steroids, urinary excretion			
Aldosterone	15–70 nmol/d	5–26 μg/d	2.774
Cortisol, free	30–300 nmol/d	10–100 μg/d	2.759
17-Hydroxycorticosteroids	5.5–28 μmol/d	2–10 mg/d	2.759
17-Ketosteroids, women	14–52 μmol/d	4–15 mg/d	3.467
Ammonia (as NH_3), venous whole blood	6–45 μmol/l	10–80 μg/dl	0.5872
Angiotensin II, plasma, 8 AM	10–30 ng/l	10–30 pg/ml	1.0
Arginine vasopressin (AVP), plasma, random fluid intake	2.3–7.4 pmol/l	2.5–8 ng/l	0.92
Bicarbonate, serum	18–23 mmol/l	18–23 meq/l	1.0
Calciferols (see vitamin D)			
Calcitonin, serum	<50 ng/l	<50 pg/ml	1.0
Calcium			
Ionized serum	1–1.5 mmol/l	4–4.6 mg/dl	0.2495
Total serum	2.2–2.6 mmol/l	9–10.5 mg/dl	0.2495
β-Carotene, serum	0.9–4.6 μmol/l	50–250 μg/dl	0.01863
Catecholamines, plasma			
Epinephrine, basal supine	170–520 pmol/l	30–95 pg/ml	5.458
Norepinephrine, basal supine	0.3–2.8 nmol/l	15–475 pg/ml	0.005911
Catecholamines, urinary			
Epinephrine	<275 nmol/d	<50 μg/d	5.458
Normetanephrine	0–11 μmol/d	0–2.0 mg/d	5.458
Total catecholamines (as norepinephrine)	<675 nmol/d	<120 μg/d	5.911
Vanillylmandelic acid (VMA)	<35 μmol/d	<68 mg/d	5.046
Chloride, serum	98–106 mmol/l	98–106 meq/l	1.0
Cholesterol, plasma			
Total cholesterol			
Desirable	<5.20 mmol/l	<200 mg/dl	0.02586
Borderline high	5.2–6.18 mmol/l	200–239 mg/dl	0.02586
High	≥6.21 mmol/l	≥240 mg/dl	0.02586
High-density lipoprotein (HDL) cholesterol			
Desirable	≥1.29 mmol/l	≥50 mg/dl	0.02586
Borderline high	0.9–1.27 mmol/l	36–49 mg/dl	0.02586
High	≤0.91 mmol/l	≤35 mg/dl	0.02586
Low-density lipoprotein (LDL) cholesterol			
Desirable	<3.36 mmol/l	<130 mg/dl	0.02586
Borderline high	3.39–4.11 mmol/l	131–159 mg/dl	0.02586
High	≥4.14 mmol/l	≥160 mg/dl	0.02586
Corticotropin (ACTH), plasma	4–22 pmol/l	20–100 pg/ml	0.2202
C peptide, plasma	0.5–2 μg/l	0.5–2 ng/ml	1.0
Creatinine, serum	<133 μmol/l	<1.5 mg/dl	88.40
Fatty acids, nonesterified or free (FFA), plasma	<0.7 mmol/l	<18 mg/dl	0.03906
Gastrin, serum	<120 ng/l	<120 pg/ml	1.0
Glucagon, plasma	50–100 ng/l	50–100 pg/ml	1.0
Glucose, plasma			
Overnight fast, normal	4.2–6.4 mmol/l	75–115 mg/dl	0.05551
Overnight fast, diabetes mellitus	7.8 mmol/l	>140 mg/dl	0.05551
72-hour fast, normal women	>2.2 mmol/l	>40 mg/dl	0.05551
Glucose tolerance test, 2-hour postprandial plasma glucose			
Normal	<7.8 mmol/l	<140 mg/dl	0.05551

Measure	SI	Conventional (C)	Conversion Factor (CF) C × CF = SI
Imparied glucose tolerance	7.8–11.1 mmol/l	140–200 mg/dl	0.05551
Diabetes mellitus	>11.1 mmol/l	>200 mg/dl	0.05551
Gonadal steroids, plasma			
Androstenedione, women	3.5–7.0 nmol/l	1–2 ng/ml	3.492
Estradiol, women			
Basal	70–220 pmol/l	20–60 pg/ml	3.671
Ovulatory surge	>740 pmol/l	>200 pg/ml	3.671
Dihydrotestosterone, women	0.17–1.0 nmol/l	0.05–3 ng/ml	3.467
Progesterone, women			
Luteal phase	6–64 nmol/l	2–20 ng/ml	3.180
Follicular phase	<6 nmol/l	<2 ng/ml	3.180
Testosterone			
Women	<3.5 nmol/l	<1 ng/ml	3.467
Prepubertal boys and girls	0.2–0.7 nmol/l	0.05–0.2 ng/ml	3.467
Gonadotropins, plasma			
Women, basal			
Follicle-stimulating hormone	5–20 IU/l	5–20 mIU/ml	1.0
Luteinizing hormone	5–25 IU/l	5–25 mIU/ml	1.0
Women, ovulatory peak			
Follicle-stimulating hormone	12–30 IU/l	12–30 mIU/ml	1.0
Luteinizing hormone	25–100 IU/l	25–100 mIU/ml	1.0
Prepubertal boys and girls			
Follicle-stimulating hormone	<5 IU/l	<5 mIU/ml	1.0
Luteinizing hormone	<5 IU/l	<5 mIU/ml	1.0
Growth hormone, plasma			
After 100 g glucose orally	<5 μg/l	<5 ng/ml	1.0
After insulin-induced hypoglycemia	>9 μg/l	>9 ng/ml	1.0
Human chorionic gonadotropin, beta subunit, plasma; nonpregnant women	<3 IU/l	<3 mIU/ml	1.0
β-Hydroxybutyrate, plasma	<300 nmol/l	<3.0 mg/dl	96.05
Insulin, plasma			
Fasting	35–145 pmol/l	5–20 μU/ml	7.175
During hypoglycemia (plasma glucose <2.8 nmol/l [<50 mg/dl])	<35 pmol/l	<5 μU/ml	7.175
Insulin-like growth factor I (IGF I, somatomedin-C), women	0.45–2.2 kU/l	0.45–2.2 U/ml	1.0
Lactate, plasma	0.56–2.2 mmol/l	5–20 mg/dl	0.111
Magnesium, serum	0.8–1.20 mmol/l	1.8–3.0 mg/dl	0.4114
Osmolality, plasma	285–295 mmol/kg	285–295 mosm/kg	1.0
Oxytocin, plasma			
Random	1–4 pmol/l	1.25–5 ng/l	0.80
Ovulatory peak in women	408 pmol/l	5–10 ng/l	0.80
Parathyroid hormone, serum (intact PTH using immunoradiometric assay [IRMA])	10–65 ng/l	10–65 pg/ml	1.0
Phosphorus, inorganic, serum	1–1.5 mmol/l	3.0–4.5 mg/dl	0.3229
Potassium, serum	3.5–5.0 mmol/l	3.5–5.0 meq/l	1.0
Prolactin, serum	2–15 μg/l	2–15 ng/ml	1.0
Pyruvate, blood	39–102 μmol/l	0.3–0.9 mg/dl	0.01129
Renin activity, plasma, normal-sodium diet			
Supine	3.2 ± 1 μgl/h	3.2 ± 1.1 ng/ml/h	1.0
Standing	9.3 ± 4.3 μgl/h	9.3 ± 4.3 ng/ml/h	1.0
Sodium, serum	136–145 mmol/l	136–145 meq/l	1.0
Thyroid function tests			
Radioactive iodine uptake, 24 hours	0.05–0.30	5–30%	—
Reverse triiodothyronine (rT$_3$), serum	0.15–0.61 nmol/l	10–4 ng/dl	0.01536
Thyrotropin (TSH), highly sensitive assay, serum	0.6–4.6 mU/l	0.6–4.6 μU/ml	1.0
Thyroxine (T$_4$), serum	51–42 nmol/l	4–11 μg/dl	12.87
Thyroxine-binding globulin, serum (as thyroxine)	150–360 nmol/l	12–28 μg/ml	12.87
Triiodothyronine (T$_3$), serum	1.2–3.4 nmol/l	75–220 ng/dl	0.01536
Triiodothyronine resin uptake, serum	0.25–0.35	25–35%	—
Triglycerides, plasma (as Triolein)	<1.80 mmol/l	<160 mg/dl	0.01129
Uric acid, serum	120–420 μmol/l	2–7 mg/dl	59.48
Vitamin D (as vitamin D$_3$, cholecalciferol), plasma			
1,25-Dihydroxycholecalciferol (1,25(OH)$_2$D)	36–144 pmol/l	15–60 pg/ml	2.400
25-Hydroxycholecalciferol (25-OHD)	20–100 nmol/l	8–40 ng/ml	2.496

Modified with permission from **Wilson JD, Foster DW,** *Williams Textbook of Endocrinology,* 8th ed. Philadelphia: WB Saunders, 1991.